The Politics
of Breastfeeding

The Politics
of Breastfeeding

Gabrielle Palmer

Pandora
An Imprint of HarperCollins*Publishers*

Pandora Press
A Division of HarperCollins*Publishers*
77–85 Fulham Palace Road,
Hammersmith, London W6 8JB

Published by Pandora Press 1988
Reprinted 1990, 1991
This edition published 1993

A catalogue record for this book
is available from the British Library

ISBN 0 86358 220 6

Phototypeset by Harper Phototypesetters Limited,
Northampton, England
Printed and bound by Woolnough Bookbinding Ltd,
Irthlingborough, Northamptonshire, England

For Nat and Fran

Contents

Illustrations

Foreword

This is an important book. Writing in a vivid, highly accessible way, Gabrielle Palmer examines in depth the political aspects of breast and bottle-feeding and explores the social pressures exerted on women globally to feed their babies artificially. Gabrielle Palmer has herself breastfed and brings to this book historical skills and her knowledge of the Third World and of nutrition.

The result is a cross-cultural study of breastfeeding and a pithy analysis of industrialised society, where women working in a men's world are expected to behave like men, and where fertility and responsibility for nurturing babies is a nuisance and an impediment to employment.

Women have been led to believe that breastfeeding is merely a matter of personal inclination. When a patient in an antenatal clinic is asked early in pregnancy by the midwife or nurse who takes her 'history': 'Do you want to breast or bottle-feed?' it is easy to assume that it is merely a question of personal preference, and that one choice is just as good as the other. If a woman who hopes to breastfeed replies, as she often does: 'I'd like to *try* to breastfeed,' both nurse and mother may take it for granted that it is a matter of maternal willpower and stamina, or tacitly accept that, in the end, it is as much in the hands of providence as whether the baby turns out to be a boy or a girl. In fact breastfeeding is as subject to commercial, economic and political pressures as the production of wheat or the arms race.

This book is for all those who are interested in the role of women as mothers and in the relations between men and women in a society which undervalues motherhood.   *Sheila Kitzinger*

Acknowledgements

This book expresses my own perceptions and does not necessarily reflect the views of the organisations and individuals whom I acknowledge here. Firstly, I thank the International Baby Food Action Network workers around the world who have provided so much help and information. I also thank the members of the Department of Human Nutrition at the London School of Hygiene and Tropical Medicine.

I thank Irene Elia, Julie Kavanagh, Candida Lacey and Patti Rundall who contributed so much through their discussions, suggestions and enthusiasm to the making of this book. More importantly, they were the ones who said, 'You can do it,' when I wanted to give up and like a breastfeeding woman I needed this support more than anything else.

Amongst all the writers whose research I have used, I have drawn most substantially on the work of Rima Apple, Andy Chetley and Valerie Fildes; I thank them for this and for the extra information they have given me. I also thank the following for their help and advice: Ann Ashworth, Ian Bray, Wendy Cartwright, Barbara Dinham, Marianne Eve, Chloe Fisher, Robert Hamilton, Jo Hanlon, Doug Johnson, Sheila Kitzinger, Margaret Kyenkya, Maureen Minchin, Rachel O'Leary, Andrew Prentice, Ann Prentice, Mark Ritchie, John Rivers, Jean Rowe, James Woodburn, Lisa Woodburn; also Helen Armstrong, Elizabeth Hormann, Ann Link, Andrew Radford, Felicity Savage, Betty Sterken, and all the other friends who have made such useful suggestions. The librarians at Cambridge University Library, the Cambridge Medical Library, the Fawcett Library, and the London School of Hygiene and Tropical Medicine Library have been most helpful. I also thank all the women I met and worked with in Mozambique who taught me more than anything I have ever found in books.

Most of all I thank Frances, Nat and John Palmer for their support and affection.

Preface to the Second Edition

I wish I were not writing this preface. There should be no need for this book to be in print. In a world beset by overwhelming problems, here is a resolvable issue. Seven years ago when writing the first edition, more than three thousand babies were dying every day from infections caused by bottle-feeding. This is still happening.

In the first edition I wrote about the pressures on women, on health workers and on governments. I wrote about the collusion between the baby milk and bottle companies and the medical and nutritional establishments. Both have promoted products which have contributed to the suffering, illness and death of millions of babies and sometimes their mothers too. This is still happening.

An update has been necessary because some things have changed. There has been a flowering of scientific evidence showing breastfeeding to be an even more amazing process than was ever realised before and that women's bodies are so resilient and adaptable that we can marvel at this power. It has been even easier than in the first edition to defend the case for breastfeeding. What infuriates me is that I still have to do it.

Knowledge is nothing if it is not spread around and, as the poor continue to get poorer and the rich get richer, the entrenched ignorance of the medical establishment is being kept in place. This new edition shows how the baby milk companies are as stubborn as ever, but that their power is being challenged by those who dared not do so before. It has been good to document the initiatives taken by those in high places and to note that ordinary women and men are questioning the sophisticated misinformation. The companies may not have changed their directions; they spend even more resources manipulating the media, governments and international bodies and their skills must not be underestimated, but the strength to resist them grows.

I wrote the first edition with a sense of despair because so many people greeted this subject with mockery and disbelief. Now to my amazement, I hear my own words from other mouths and read my own phrases on other pages and I feel some hope. I have been bowled over by the resilience and talents of those who have provided me with information for both editions. They are now educating the powerful, making it harder for the international policy makers to ignore the plain sense of the facts.

The unnecessary suffering of babies, the threat to long-term health and the destruction of women's confidence in their own bodies continues to be a major issue of this century. This book was not written for breastfeeding mothers, it was written for everyone, man or woman, parent or childless, old or young, because this issue concerns all of us. I have added and adapted some facts, it is updated, but the main theme remains unchanged. I hope I will never write another preface and the sooner this book is out of date, the happier I will be.

· 1 ·

Why Breastfeeding is Political

THE BASIC ISSUES: WHAT IS GOING ON

If a multinational company developed a product that was a nutritionally balanced and delicious food, a wonder drug that both prevented and treated disease, cost almost nothing to produce and could be delivered in quantities controlled by the consumers' needs, the very announcement of their find would send their shares rocketing to the top of the stock market. The scientists who developed the product would win prizes and the wealth and influence of everyone involved would increase dramatically. Women have been producing such a miraculous substance, breastmilk, since the beginning of human existence, yet they form the half of the world's people who are the least wealthy and the least powerful.

As a subject of research, breastfeeding and breastmilk have attracted increasing attention during the last twenty years, yet as more academic careers wax on the theory of human milk, fewer babies receive the product. As propaganda about the benefits of breastfeeding increases, so too do the worldwide sales of artificial milks and feeding bottles. This may surprise those who live among groups where the 'fashion' for breastfeeding has spread among women with access to information and their babies. However, worldwide more and more babies get less and less time at their mothers' breasts.

Why, after more than a million years of survival, are human beings abandoning one of the principal evolutionary characteristics by which we identify ourselves as mammals? Are women being freed from a timewasting biological tyranny to lead nobler, more fulfilling and more equal lives? In this book I examine the political reasons for a situation which is having a profound effect on our society from the macroeconomic level of a squandered natural resource to the individual misery of a sick child or a confused, unhappy woman. Why is it that whether you were breastfed yourself or whether you breastfeed your own child depends so much on your social and economic class position in your own society? How is it that in some societies, 100 per cent of poor, marginally nourished women can all breastfeed successfully, while in others, groups of privileged, well-nourished women cannot? Why is the right to breastfeed fought for so vehemently by some women and rejected so forcefully by others according to their class, education and society? And why, if women participate in the modern economic structures which are claimed to be for the benefit of us all, must the unique breastfeeding relationship be curtailed and restricted? For many women, what could be a simple compromise becomes an agonising decision.

Politics does not only refer to economic and territorial power structures, it also means sexual politics. The fact of women's separate biological capacities has been used as a pretext for excluding women from the centres of power, yet as women's reproductive functions come to be controlled both by themselves and others, there is no significant change in absolute male control. Tokenism is rife but in all the major organisations, whether they are governments, transnational companies or international bodies of experts, the men are still in charge. Often the very men who discover the excellence of breastfeeding and recommend it wholeheartedly will forbid their secretaries to bring their babies to work, do nothing to establish facilities in the workplace and little to advocate the financial benefits and flexible schedules which are essential for those mothers who must or choose to remain in the wage-earning world.

Any woman who is working in a paid job must certainly not flaunt any signs of fertility. If her breasts are functioning she must discreetly withdraw to feed her baby or express her milk, because to suckle a baby in daily public life is too disturbing a sight for the men in charge. After work those same men may well pay to watch a woman in a strip club expose her breasts for the sexual stimulation of strangers. Men may pay more in a restaurant to have their food served by bare breasted women. Though every part of a woman's body has been a focus of eroticism, our era is the first in recorded history where the breast has become a mass fetish for male sexual stimulation, while at the same time its primary function has diminished on a vast scale. Perhaps the only parallel is the phenomenon of foot binding in China, when the primary use of a part of the body was sacrificed to serve the cult of a sexual fetishism which symbolised female helplessness. In our century, women have been presented with an illusion of liberation through the bottle-feeding of babies, only to find their breasts appropriated by men. This is expressed both privately, with many men forbidding their sexual partners to breastfeed, and publicly, through pornography and the mass marketing of products and information. There is a fundamental racism in attitudes to public breastfeeding. Intrusive cameras turn the zoom lens on hungry women who, during some disaster, are keeping their babies alive with this precious fluid. As long as she is black and devastated the audience is happy to watch, but in the filming of a 1987 TV consumer programme on a baby food issue some of the film had to be reshot because the baby wanted to suckle his well-dressed, white mother and the producer considered that this would be too controversial for the viewers. [1]*

It is not a coincidence that the decline of breastfeeding accelerated as the predominantly male medical profession took over the management of childbirth and infant feeding. Nor was it chance that led to the expansion of the baby milk industry during the late nineteenth and early twentieth centuries when mechanisation of the dairy industries had resulted in large whey surpluses. When a manufacturer has a waste product his first business instinct is to search for a way of marketing that product, and the development of baby milk has been a marketing success story, not least in the skill with which the competing product has been destroyed. Women are not paid for producing or delivering breastmilk, nor for caring for we humans in this special way. Those who market the substitute product and the equipment benefit economically from keeping breastfeeding in check. There

---

*A welcome change: On a 1993 British TV programme ('Forty Minutes' BBC2, 23.3.1993) about Dr. Dee Dawson's treatment of anorexia nervosa, she suckled her toddler from time to time throughout the film.

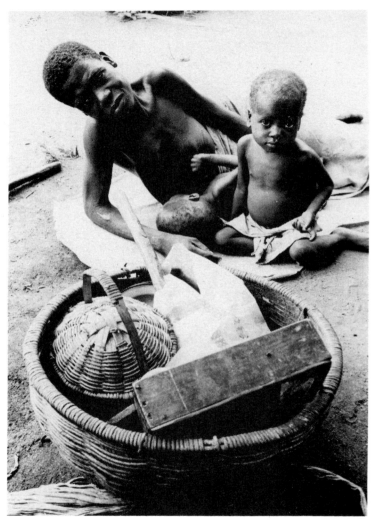

1a Mozambican refugee with all her possessions (*Photo*: Alexander Joe, 1984; courtesy of Oxfam).

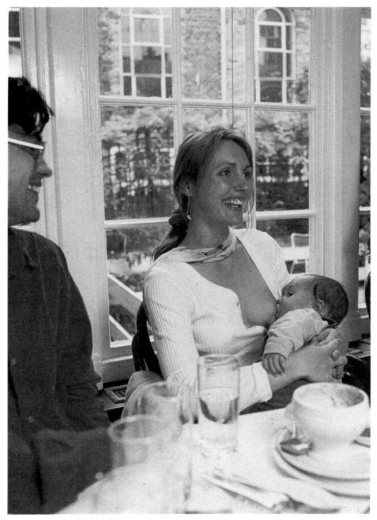

1b A woman breastfeeding in an English café. (*Photo*: Paul Smith)
Which image is more familiar on television and in newspapers?

is no equivalent vested interest group to protect breastfeeding and it is destroyed for the same reasons that forests are destroyed – for immediate profit.

In the modern world, status and often self-esteem come from a person's role in the structures of wealth creation. If a woman joins the industrial economy she must be seen to be like a man and it is taken for granted that she must adapt to the 'norm', not that social and economic organisation must adapt to all human beings. Women must prove that they are 'as good as' men, but men do not have to show that they are as good as women. To gain recognition, striving women must show that they can be as 'tough' and competitive as men. Imagine a world where men had to show that they possessed certain supposedly 'female' qualities such as sensitivity and altruism before they were allowed to enter the spheres of power and influence.

Women, whatever their class, still take the major responsibility for the care of babies. Women with children who cannot or who do not want to opt out of the wage economy are expected to delegate the tasks of baby care to another so they can function in a male world, and in the majority of cases another woman takes on the task and inevitably is underpaid. The few men who engage in childcare are a tiny minority that is not increasing because they will avoid working for such paltry economic reward, or for such low status in the complex pecking order of the modern world. In the struggle for economic and sexual justice a baby's needs are often neglected and, during this crucial phase of physical and emotional development, many are damaged for ever.

WHO PROFITS?

An estimated US $7 billion worth of baby milk is sold each year, which is around US$19 million or 380,000 tins a day. The potential market, if every baby were bottle-fed for 6 months only, is estimated to be US$38 billion.[2] Doctors and nutritionists are often investors and beneficiaries of the industry. A doctor who invents a new artificial baby milk may get a royalty on each batch sold. Many doctors might support breastfeeding in theory and try to in practice, but their careers rarely blossom as a result. Our current economic system does not encourage the promotion of products or systems which do not make an immediate financial profit. As with so many of the biological solutions to the ecological devastation of the planet, the money makers would not benefit immediately if we adopted them, though in the long term the world and all society would be wealthier.

Doctors and manufacturers are not and have not all been evil individuals consciously planning to appropriate the power of women, though certainly male-dominated, cultural attitudes to women may have distorted their judgment. Many doctors have been faced with the problem of failing lactation or with women not wanting to feed their babies, and because of their own ignorance they believed they were finding the way to solve an urgent problem. Industrial society has become geared to technological solutions and an indifference to the costs of primary extraction and it is often harder to discover why a problem occurs in the first place than to work out a stopgap way of alleviating that problem. Now that knowledge about breastfeeding has been rediscovered, there is less excuse for the medical and commercial purveyors of substitute milks to continue their practices, but so many of them are caught up in the whirlwind of career progress and profit seeking that they cannot stop to review the damage they do. There has been a curious doublethink among those scientists and manufacturers whose own interests lie in the production of breastmilk substitutes. On the one hand there is eagerness to claim that artificially fed babies are just as healthy as breastfed ones and that the choice of feeding method is an equal one; on the other there is an obsessive desire to imitate human milk, and it is used as the 'gold standard' to sell the commercial product. There is still so much to find out about breastmilk and breastfeeding and the more research is done the more fascinating the process seems. Much of the financing of research into breastmilk has come from the baby food industry. There is probably no other manufacturing industry which gains so much free access to the rival product. Drug companies are obsessive about patenting, but all over the world women unwittingly give their unique nutrient and medical product away to the very people who want to replace it. If society were reorganised so that the true infant milk manufacturers . . . women . . . earned the economic rewards they deserve for their production, the baby food industry would dwindle overnight, and a large amount of the poverty that causes infant disease and death would disappear.

Much as they would like us to think otherwise, the baby milk companies are not philanthropic organisations but commercial enterprises which must compete to survive. It is in their interests that women find it hard to breastfeed. Classical economic theory tells us that the invisible hand of the market leads only to the manufacture of products that people need. If this is so, then why do milk companies invest millions in newer and increasingly devious methods of promotion all over the world? These methods are necessary because they can only sell their product by impeding the production of the rival one. For example, companies can sabotage breastfeeding through donating architectural services. The US-based company Abbot-Ross provided free advice to hospitals for planning and layout: 'The purpose here is to impose a design that literally builds bottle-feeding into the facility by physically separating mother and infant to make bottle-feeding more convenient than breastfeeding for the hospital staff . . .. A single investment in such architectural services can create new sales opportunities for the entire life span of the building.'[3] A company can thus gain prestige as a benefactor and create customers, all through a single strategy. These marketing activities are an excellent investment because all humans have something in common; whether they are poor or rich they want their children to live. If a woman's breastmilk has been jeopardised and she sees artificial milk as the only means of her child's survival, she will sacrifice everything to buy it. The milk may use over 30 per cent of the household income and impoverish the rest of the family. The more that feeding bottles and artificial milk become acceptable and 'normal' in any society, the more stable is the manufacturers' income. Breastmilk substitutes can be useful, life-saving products, just as artificial insulin can save the lives of diabetics, but no honest doctor would ever advocate the use of insulin unless it were strictly necessary. The infant feeding

By the turn of this century, almost half of humanity will live in urban centres; the world of the 21st century will be a largely urban world. Over only 65 years, the developing world's urban population has increased tenfold, from around 100 million in 1920 to 1 billion today. In 1940, one person in a hundred lived in a city of 1 million or more inhabitants; by 1980, one in 10 lived in such a city. Between 1985 and the year 2000, Third World cities could grow by another three-quarters of a billion people. This suggests that the developing world must, over the next few years, increase by 65 per cent its capacity to produce and manage its urban infrastructure, services and shelter merely to maintain today's often extremely inadequate conditions.

*Few city governments in the developing world have the power, resources, and trained personnel to provide their rapidly growing populations with the land, services and facilities needed for an adequate human life: clean water, sanitation, schools and transport. The result is mushrooming illegal settlements with primitive facilities, increased overcrowding and rampant disease linked to an unhealthy environment. Many cities in industrial countries also face problems: deteriorating infrastructure, environmental degradation, inner-city decay and neighbourhood collapse. But with the means and resources to tackle this decline, the issue for most industrial countries is ultimately one of political and social choice. Developing countries are not in the same situation. They have a major urban crisis on their hands. (*Our Common Future*, Report of the World Commission on Environment and Development, Oxford University Press, 1987.)*

issue is frequently misrepresented as one of the individual choice between two parallel methods, the breast or the bottle, but the products are not equal and the true cost to society and the individual is seldom measured or mentioned. Women must have the right to choose how they use their bodies and women cannot in fact be 'made' to breastfeed (see page 49), but that does not mean that information should be censored. Informed choice is everyone's right and in most of the world the choice between breast and bottle is a choice between infant health and sickness, or even life and death.

The medical profession strives to maintain a 'neutrality' which belies the integration of commercial interests with medical issues. The health workers who promote breastfeeding are working against the interests of the companies, who provide not only the substitute milks but also the research grants, the health information costs, the gifts and the conferences which are felt to be so important for progress. When the industry donates expensive medical equipment this is not without a cost, for the medical workers are then under an obligation to their benefactors. In spite of an International Code of Marketing these same companies still flout basic ethical practices wherever they can get away with it, including pushing baby milk products into those communities where to bottle-feed is to play Russian roulette with an infant's life. Even those medical experts who question the superiority of breastfeeding over artificial feeding for the privileged baby concede that breastfeeding is essential in the Third World, yet the struggle of the Third World to 'catch up' with the rich nations involves a disastrous progress towards urbanisation which is linked, for many different reasons, with a decline in breastfeeding.

THE WIDENING GAP BETWEEN RICH AND POOR

The population growth which is part of rapid urbanisation is linked to a decline in breastfeeding. The conditions which make artificial feeding so lethal are part of a system which is destructive to breastfeeding. The division between the First and the Third World is an artificial one. There are many different grades of quality of life between and within different countries. A baby in the slums of Washington DC or Liverpool who is bottle-fed may be at as great a risk of illness as a baby in rural India who at least has her mother's milk. The cost of the medical services which save the life of the baby in the North are paid for by the economic exploitation of the South.

Among their many disregarded abilities, women have a unique power in breastfeeding, to maintain health, life and finite resources, yet understandably many might resist this suggestion because it is associated with the oppression of women by limiting them to their 'traditional' roles. When the visibly powerful of the world conspicuously deny the practice and influence of this activity, and women who do it are deliberately kept apart from the mainstream of admired positions, it is no wonder that confusion reigns. In a shrinking world where the consumption of finite resources and environmental degradation are reaching a crisis, here is an unacknowledged resource. Until the power structures are changed so that women are recognised and rewarded, gain full access to the means of economic independence and take a real part in decision making, another natural product will be undervalued and discarded. Just as people have come to realise that forests are not simply a source of firewood or obstacles to the 'development' of land, so economic planners must learn that human beings are part of the ecosystem and that something as unnoticed as breastfeeding contributes to a saner management of the earth's resources.

In writing this book I have discovered how ignorance and common misunderstandings have affected the way our bodies and minds work. I cannot unravel everything but what I hope to do is to encourage the reader to question all those authorities: the scientists, the doctors, the manufacturers of products and the politicians who try to convince us that everything is managed for the best. I also want to urge women who have achieved some small measure of power and influence, especially those who may have decided not to have children in order to do this, to recognise the enormous contribution that millions of women make to human prosperity and welfare through the particular process of breastfeeding. Feminist writers have already commented on what would happen if men menstruated.[4] Actually over the course of history women have produced far more milk than menstrual blood, yet it is still usually considered as an incidental phenomenon.

All over the world, in various research institutions, experiments are being carried out in an attempt to use genetic manipulation so that cows can produce 'human' milk. What is the motive for this expensive research when there is potentially more than enough human milk in humans? Will the next expensive project be to get a pig to produce human sperm so that men will be liberated from the messy task of fathering their own children?[5]

· 2 ·

The Right to Call Ourselves Mammals: The Importance of Biology

BIOLOGY AND POLITICS

I have to start with biology. For a long time I resisted this because I believed that biologists were saying that political ideas could never change our biological destiny; that the forces of natural selection, of competition and of the primal drives for survival made any attempt at the reorganisation of society a meaningless exercise. I now believe that the understanding of nature, of both the planet and our human nature and the links between the two, is vital if we are to have any hope of resolving the problems of people. Just as architects have to understand the qualities of their materials if they are to construct a sound and safe building, nature cannot be disregarded if a system of survival, justice and dignity is to be established.

Just as the 'Social Darwinists' misused Darwinian theories in the nineteenth century to endorse the economic and social structures of that time, so biological bigotry is still misused to justify the exploitation of some groups by others. The exploitation of females is a fact of human society yet it is not the norm amongst other animal groups. Many women are justifiably suspicious of any argument which glorifies motherhood, because it has frequently been used to restrict women and exclude them from positions of power. However it is those very mothering qualities which have led to traits such as intelligence, dexterity, endurance and love which are valued, and they are traits of men as well as of women. In the struggle for power, or simply survival, in the modern world, many women who have children find that they must restrict mothering if they are to achieve any measure of equality with men, and denying lactation is part of this. Yet lactation is the very core of our identity; the process evolved even before gestation and each mammal has evolved, over the millennia, a milk unique to its requirements, its behaviour and its environment. It is such a spectacular survival strategy that we call ourselves, after the mammary gland, mammals . . . animals that suckle their young.

THE VULNERABLE HUMAN BABY

Humans, like most mammals, reproduce by what biologists call the K-strategy, as opposed to the r-strategy. An example of the r-strategy is the oyster which produces millions of eggs to be fertilised in the sea and does no parenting, K-strategists produce far fewer offspring, but nurture them. If an r-strategist parent dies, the species still survives; indeed some mothers, for example mayflies, die as soon as they have laid their eggs. Humans are of course K-strategists and their young are the most vulnerable and slowest-growing of all mammals. the human baby, supposedly because of its large brain, is considered by some to be born 'prematurely', and therefore called 'the exterogestate foetus'.[1] Breastfeeding provides an intermediate environment of nurturing and security which makes the transference from womb to outside world safer and less harsh, and a mother's breast gives warmth, food, protection against disease and a learning exercise in interactions.

HUMAN GENDER RELATIONS

Before explaining how lactation works I want to explore the biological explanation of human gender relations. When people say 'its natural' for males to dominate females they ignore the behaviour of the majority of species (which are not mammals) where there are as many 'unmotherly' females as there are 'motherly' males. Amongst mammals most, but by no means all, females do the bulk of the mothering; however this does not always make them vulnerable or oppressed and in fact many females are stronger than males. Until recently, the biological observers who could write down their ideas and gain public acclaim were usually men and, however intelligent, they could not help but be biased. Arisotle assumed the queen bee was male because she was 'king' of the hive. Modern male observers of social animals have described harems as groups of females 'owned' or dominated by one male, but in fact they can also be described as females who form a band to protect those who are pregnant and lactating and who choose to allow one or two males near the band. There are many examples of non-human primates (monkeys and apes) where the female is in charge (such as the siamangs of Asia) or where the sexes are equal and share childcare.

Whenever this subject is discussed someone will say that nevertheless in most human societies males do dominate the females. Even when women do all the work or are extremely strong, men usually have the ultimate political or religious authority. Why? One possible explanation is as follows. One of the most useful survival strategies of human evolution is that humans can pack away larger fat stores in proportion to their body size than any other land mammal, even the pig, and females store more fat than males. Of course the slimming industry employs an army of researchers to look for ways of combating this characteristic, but it is probably one of the reasons why humans have been so successful in evolutionary terms; they can store food in the form of body fat during the good times and use it to survive during the hard times. This is especially useful for females who can support a growing foetus and, after the birth, produce milk to feed it without the need for a dramatic increase in food intake. This does not mean that a reduced food supply is good for a pregnant or lactating woman, but compared with many other mammals, a normal, adequate intake does not need a dramatic change for reproduction. This is a quite different physiological strategy from that of some other mammals, such as the laboratory rat, an animal whose life and times have influenced a lot of decisions about human bodies.

If you have a big skeleton, you need more muscle to carry it around and more food just to maintain that big body. Girls reach puberty, which accompanies the final phase of skeletal growth, earlier than boys, so that any surplus food eaten towards the end of this phase gets laid down as fat. Fat does not mean obesity; even slim women have proportionally more body fat than men. The fine tuning of natural selection has resulted in a compromise in women's size; to be bigger may mean easier childbirth, but to be too big means that a seasonal food shortage may carry more risk of weakness and death, especially under stress of reproduction, than if you are smaller. Modern women in rich societies can afford to be big because they are protected from such food shortages. A smaller body needs less food for basic energy and maintenance needs, so it can put any extra food available in the fat store and this can be drawn on for reproduction and lactation. Adolescent males eating the same amount as adolescent females can just get bigger.

So, human males may have grown bigger because they did not evolve the strategy of fat storage to as great an extent as the females, because it did not make any difference to their reproductive capacity. On the principle of 'power corrupts and absolute power corrupts absolutely', the larger males only had to hit out in fear to find that the recipient of the blow fell to the ground and they learned the effectiveness of physical violence for dominance and survival, which led to its further use. Endocrinologists point to the link between the male hormone testosterone and aggression, and this certainly exists, but not all males are aggressive and some females can be. Moreover any observation of primates will reveal that the groups where the males dominate are those with the greatest difference of size between the sexes. When the sexes are almost the same size, such as with siamangs and lemurs, there is equality or female dominance.

Extrapolating from 'natural' animal behaviour to our distorted human society can be misleading, but I believe there are some links. It is interesting that in Hawaii where there is a record of extremely tall women, there has been an unusual degree of sexual and political parity with men. It is physical violence or the threat of it which still brings dominance in the modern world. Language reflects the link between size and control, as in the 'superpowers', 'Mr Big', and 'a weighty matter', and research shows that the taller are more 'successful', that is dominant. Political might may be expressed through 'sophisticated' weapon systems rather than by a swipe round the ear, but it is still the fear of being crushed and destroyed that allows certain individuals and groups to be dominated by others. Once dominance is achieved it is hard to take it away. The big male gorilla may be content to let the small female eat bananas if he has a good supply, but if he has taken them all and she tries to snatch one away, woe betide her. The smaller animal soon has to learn other strategies of survival, which may actually require greater intelligence. In short, I believe that human males are still in charge because they have been able to use physical coercion, or its implicit threat, both privately and publicly, and this has developed into a range of psychological, cultural and economic methods of control. Because of this dominance, most human societies end up being organised by and for men and any exclusively female abilities are usually disregarded in the allocation of prestige and reward. The fact that a woman in power has to be like a man, in that she must hide particularly female qualities like lactation or pregnancy, is a measure of continuing male dominance. It is hard to imagine Margaret Thatcher or even Hillary Clinton with a baby at the breast while making a key political speech, yet it would be perfectly possible. This concept is often met with ridicule, yet I remember an economist and former freedom fighter in Mozambique bringing her new baby with her when she was a speaker at a meeting. She gave a powerful speech while holding her baby as though this were the most natural thing in the world, which of course it was. [2]

THE EFFICIENT FEMALE

Research indicates other useful survival strategies, besides the storage of fat and the slowness of growth. Though this is still uncertain and may depend on the amount of food available to the individual, there is some evidence that female metabolic rate is lowered during the first two-thirds of pregnancy and though it rises again during the last third, there may be a net saving of energy for the whole pregnancy. This does not mean that women should be underfed while they are pregnant, but that in comparison with most other mammals reproduction can continue successfully without women having to devote their time to eating hugely increased quantities of food. There is also an idea that lactation may involve some nutrient-sparing mechanisms, which means that women, again unlike many other mammals, can reproduce enough milk for their baby's needs without requiring a lot more food. We have populated this planet because our females can reproduce and feed their young with the help of two marvellous strategies: storing any excess food in the form of body fat as a supply of energy for the hard times, and adjusting the body's ways of using up the food supply when we are supporting a new life. Women are like a very economical car that not only has a spare fuel tank, but probably also uses up less petrol per mile when it carries an extra passenger.[3]

JUST LIKE A COW?

When young mammals die it may be because of predators, congenital weakness which might stop them getting at milk (as with the runt who gets pushed out by the siblings) or a deterioration in the habitat which reduces the weaning food supply, but it is almost unknown for a mammal in her normal environment to produce live young and not be able to suckle them. So why in twentieth-century society is human 'lactation failure' so common? Biologically it is one of nature's star turns, but culturally it has become another human mess. All other mammals suckle their young; monkeys and bats do it, so do the killer whale and the tiger. One exception is the modern dairy cow who has her calf removed a few days after the birth so that humans can take the milk, and although there is plenty for both calf and humans, modern agricultural organisation does not allow for such compromises. If the calf were left with its mother and received all the milk that was available, it would become seriously ill and the cow would develop inflammation of the udder (mastitis) because of the small calf's inability to strip out the over-abundant milk. In the development of dairying over the centuries, selective breeding has emphasised placidity, excess milk production and response to intensive feeding with high milk output, but these qualities are irrelevant to the survival of the young, which is the primary purpose of lactation. The human is not at all like a cow, yet join any discussion about breastfeeding and someone will make a comparison between humans and dairy cows: 'You've got to be placid to breastfeed'; 'I felt just like a cow'; 'you must keep eating a lot to keep your milk up, you know what happens to a badly fed cow'. To say that a woman must be like a cow in order to breastfeed is like saying everyone must do a course in muscle building in order to carry the newspaper. Tigers are not placid, yet they suckle their cubs; bats are mammals, but no one suggests that women must hang upside down in caves to be successful breastfeeders. In modern society the knowledge of dairy cows has exceeded that of human lactation and has had a misleading influence on the understanding of human mothers and babies.

THE USE OF NON-HUMAN MILK

The human species has only engaged in agriculture and pasturage for 12,000 to 15,000 years, which is a mere 1 per cent of our time on earth, so for 99 per cent of our existence humans survived without any milk other than breastmilk. Many societies have never used animal milk and indeed the majority of people in the world lack the stomach enzyme, lactose, which is necessary to digest milk fully. Only Europeans and other cattle-rearing groups have the biologically unusual characteristic of producing this digestive enzyme once they are past infancy. Many Asians and Africans suffer from pain, wind and diarrhoea if they are forced to drink milk, and some Chinese regard drinking animal milk as disgusting as the idea of drinking a glass of saliva. Until the invention of refrigeration (which is still only available to a tiny minority), milk could be a dangerous food because it is such an ideal breeding ground for bacteria. In the past, except in very cool climates most milk had to be converted into butter, cheese and yoghurt for it to be used safely. Fresh non-human milk can be useful for those communities who live in an environment suitable for stock rearing, but it is not essential for a nutritious diet and for many people it is an inappropriate food. Millions now mistakenly believe that cows' milk is essential for the health of infants and small children.

· 3 ·

Everything You Wanted To Know About Breastfeeding But Forgot To Ask

A BORN TALENT

If they are not prevented from doing so, the majority of babies have the power to stimulate the manufacture of their own food supply and to keep its production going in the quantities they need. A baby has to work for her breastmilk by asking for it, by crying when she is hungry and then suckling properly to maintain the production of milk. The influence of western medical practice has distorted this, but when it is allowed to happen, the relationship between a baby and her mother's breast is quite different from that with a bottle because it is more dynamic. A baby is actively involved in the milk manufacture, because it is the baby's suckling that keeps the whole process going. This is why the English word 'suckle' is so appropriate; it means the action of both the mother and the baby who are co-workers.

Many people still think that lactation only occurs after the birth of an infant. Certain species, for example elephants and foxes, are known to lactate and suckle young without ever having given birth. In fact most women, whether they have had children or not, can stimulate lactation and sometimes sexual partners who enjoy suckling are surprised to find the breasts producing milk.[1] There are many reports of both childless women, and mothers who stopped breastfeeding years previously, who have produced milk, simply by allowing a baby to suckle their breasts. In many traditional societies, foster mothers, often grandmothers, feed the babies of the dead, ill or absent mothers and in western society adopting mothers have used various methods to establish lactation. Some have used mechanical devices (breast pumps or the specially designed 'Lact-aid' which carries artificial baby milk through a tube into the baby's mouth while she suckles her mother's breast), but one woman I met shared the feeding with her sister, so that the baby learned to feed on a fully functioning breast and gradually stimulated his adopted mother's breast to produce his full supply.

The production of milk works on the supply and demand principle. The more often and the more vigorously the baby sucks, the more milk is made. A healthy, hungry baby is the best milk producer in the world; she produces exactly the amount she needs by suckling whenever she wants. Of course if she cannot get near the breast, because custom forbids this, then she will not be able to order her milk supply. Moreover, if she is exhausted from crying when she gets there she might not suck so well. Most people know what it is like to be hungry, yet too tired or upset to eat, but it is often forgotten that babies are people too. In the same way that most adults hate to be forced to eat when they are full, if someone has given the baby a bottle of artificial milk or even glucose water, she will not be hungry enough to stimulate the production of milk by breastfeeding.

THE GOD OF ROUTINE

Since 'medical science' began to supervise breastfeeding it has been the custom to restrict it. When babies are only fed at regular intervals and their time at the breast curtailed, then sufficient milk cannot be stimulated in most women. This is why the prevalence of 'insufficient milk syndrome' follows in the wake of medical services.

One source of the idea of feeding babies at fixed intervals was the influential eighteenth-century doctor William Cadogan. His 'Essay upon nursing and the management of children from their birth to three years of age'[2] was widely read. Among his reasonable ideas was his disapproval of tight swaddling clothes; many babies in those days were trussed up like well-packaged parcels and could barely move, let alone kick or play. He also condemned pre-lacteal feeds, often exotic mixtures of butter, wine or breadcrumbs, which their richer parents gave to their newborns. Cadogan observed that peasant women who could not afford anything but heir own milk and could not buy swaddling clothes had healthier babies than the wealthy. He advocated maternal breastfeeding and persuaded wealthy women, who usually sent their babies to a wet nurse, to feed their own children. Cadogan was an observant man who used infant mortality rates to back up his arguments, who improved the care of foundlings and saved many infant lives.

The environment of eighteenth-century London was apallingly unhygienic. Bacteria had not yet been discovered and no one really understood how disease spread. Cadogan noticed the frequent illnesses of infants and, observing that they were constantly fed with either breastmilk, cows' milk or 'paps' and gruels, he perceived a cause and effect. His reasoning was sound, for food was very likely to be contaminated and a source of infection. Though he valued breastmilk, he did not distinguish between this and other foods when he became concerned about 'overfeeding' which he believed was the cause of diarrhoea. He therefore advocated only four feeds at regular intervals in twenty-four hours and forbade night feeding. He did not however suggest limiting the length of a feed. Cadogan claimed that, as a father himself, he had practiced all his principles with success. The reader envisages a household with baby after baby thriving on the perfect routine, but if you sneak a look at Cadogan's biography[3] it appears he had just one daughter. Perhaps she happened to be one of those special babies who stick to routines and never wake at night and perhaps her mother belonged to that minority of women who do have an adequate milk supply even when they feed infrequently. It is these rare women who have inadvertently kept the gospel of routine alive, proving the point that restricted, routine breastfeeding can be achieved. Actually, I suspect that while Cadogan was attending to his wealthy clients his wife or wet nurse was sneaking in the extra feed whenever his daughter cried and not telling him. Cadogan did not think highly of women and his wife is never mentioned. He begins his essay with his relief that at last 'men of sense rather than foolish unlearned women' were taking over the supervision of infant care. This taking over of the management of infant feeding by men was significant. An illiterate, 'unlearned' mother will know about the supply and demand principle, she will feel her milk increasing after a day when the baby has been extra hungry and suckling a lot. No male doctor has experienced this.

Most of the ordinary country women whose babies Cadogan had admired carried on as they always had, without clocks or learning, but over the course of the nineteenth century ideas about regularity and routine developed to the point of tyranny and they persist to this day. The source of this religion is complex and wide-rooted. The blossoming of scientific knowledge was in part derived through disciplined exactitude and rigorous observational techniques. Mechanisation and the need for controlled production methods in the growth of industrial capitalism precipitated the need for timing, measurement, clocks and consistency. The new ideas were applied to humans, and indeed the realisation that pulse rates, blood pressure and respiration had consistent measurements and rhythms endorsed these perceptions of scientific thought. The problems arose when humans were supposed to fit in with arbitrary ideas of what the physical rhythms should be. It was when true scientific observations weakened that most problems occurred. I come from a generation where the god of routine still ruled; teatime, night prayers, bowel movements and baby's crying were all supposed to coincide with the striking of the clock and woe betide the naughty child who experienced hunger pangs, gut cramps or mysticism at the wrong time. The lucky babies were those whose own personal body rhythms happened to coincide with Greenwich mean time, but for those renegade beings who did not fit in, there was a lot of miserable adjustment for both mothers and babies.

The idea of the dangers of overfeeding persisted well into the twentieth century and any woman with access to orthodox health information would have been advised to limit feeding time. (I was accused of 'overfeeding' my second baby in 1972 because she doubled her birth weight in two months; as I had only recently been informed that my first child was undersized, I began to doubt the possibility of producing anything that met the quality control standards of the paediatric conveyor belt). The result of this certainly did avoid any 'danger' of overfeeding, for the physiological result was that many women who fed only at prescribed intervals did not stimulate sufficient milk, their babies cried, did not grow rapidly and the mothers correctly diagnosed that they did not have enough milk. To this day 'insufficient milk' is the commonest reason that women give for abandoning breastfeeding and the problem manifests itself in societies where free access to the breast becomes medically and socially deplored. Ironically, an idea that evolved from a fear of a non-existent problem – there has never been a scrap of good evidence showing the ill effects of too much breastfeeding – led to the establishment of a real problem. Separating the mother and baby so that the baby could not take the breast when he asked for it reduced the chances of establishing a cohesion between the baby's and mother's physical rhythms. The baby busily sucking at one breast would be wrenched off on to the other at the stroke of the clock. By the twentieth century, 'complementary' bottle-feeds would be given to 'top up' the baby, so he would lose his appetite for the breast and hence reduce the milk supply. Underfeeding was dreaded, but no less than overfeeding, so that test weighing of the baby before and after a feed meant that few mothers were producing the exact quantities of milk that were deemed to be 'correct'.

THE DAMAGE OF MEDICAL SUPERVISION

The disastrous advice to restrict the time the baby spends at the breast is still found in the text books and is practised in many maternity wards. The justification for this is that suckling causes sore nipples. In fact there is no evidence to indicate that duration has any effect on nipple damage; rather it is bad positioning and frequent washing of the nipples that causes this problem. Breastmilk changes in nutrient proportions as the baby suckles, and if he is taken off the breast before he is finished, he may not receive the high energy hind milk. Because mothers are told to change breasts after a set time, some babies take in quantities of lower energy fore milk and, though full, are not truly satisfied. It is like having a meal with two soups and no main course. Babies are skilled at knowing when they have fulfiled their needs, but arbitrary medical rules have sabotaged this pattern.

The nineteenth century discovery of the germ theory of disease was a breakthrough for society, but the resulting overzealous concern with hygiene proved disastrous for breasfeeding. Washing the nipples before and after feeds destroys the protective secretions, exacerbating the possibility of sore nipples and increasing the risk of infection. By the twentieth century, textbooks advised scrubbing the nipples with surgical spirit during pregnancy to 'harden them' and massaging with lanolin after the birth to 'soften them'. Some mothers and babies escaped or even survived these persecutions, but not surprisingly more and more found bottle-feeding a blessed relief and the suppliers and makers of foods and feeding equipment were eager to provide them with the goods.

Today, in spite of supposed 'demand feeding' being in fashion, it is still rare in industrialised society. Michael Latham, Professor of Nutrition at Cornell University, described real 'demand' feeding when he said, 'Asking a woman in rural Africa how often she breastfeeds is like asking someone with an itchy rash how often they scratch.'[4] Most rural African women cannot afford clocks or watches and so rarely have insufficient milk.

THE ESTABLISHMENT OF BREASTFEEDING AFTER BIRTH

Lactation depends on a group of reflexes which trigger the secretion of certain hormones. Prolactin is the key hormone for initiating and maintaining the milk output and it is this hormone that is stimulated by suckling in non-puerperal lactation. Though we do not see it as such, in a way lactation is the 'normal' state of the body because we need a special hormone (prolactin release-inhibiting hormone) to stop us lactating. It is this inhibiting factor that is removed as soon as the placenta is delivered after the birth which allows the prolactin to be released into a mother's bloodstream. The breast then starts to produce the early milk, called colostrum. This is a thick yellowish fluid which is lower in fat and lactose than mature milk and high in anti-infective properties and certain nutrients such as zinc. Many women are already secreting a fluid called pre-colostrum during their pregnancy (also some women continue to breastfeed a child through a pregnancy and then may feed both for some time; commonly called 'tandem' breastfeeding). Many cultures, both traditional and modern, erroneously consider colostrum to be bad or irrelevant and either express and discard it or wait for a day or two before letting the baby near the breast. This deprives the baby of a useful supercharge of appropriate nutrients and antibodies and in western society lessens the likelihood of successful breastfeeding. Interestingly, in societies where ability to breastfeed is taken for granted, mothers seem to withstand this early disruption with few lactation problems. If breastfeeding does not take place prolactin output will decrease and eventually the milk will disappear. The experience of this varies from woman to woman. Some will feel that their breasts are distended and full within a day of the birth, and even if they do not breastfeed may produce milk for weeks afterwards. Others never feel the sensation of full breasts and these have often been the women who believed, or were told, that their milk 'never came in'. In fact, the maintenance of prolactin depends on the baby's suckling and if this does not happen, the mother's body gets the message that the baby has died and shuts down the mechanisms of secretion. Giving most normal full-term babies anything other than the fluid from their mothers' breasts is a waste of effort and a risk. Glucose and water will diminish the new baby's appetite and thirst which are essential to make her suckle strongly and stimulate the breastmilk flow. Artificial milk has an even worse effect, for it satiates the baby even more and can also prime the baby's body for future allergic reactions, as well as establishing an inappropriate acid/alkali balance in the gut which discourages the establishment of beneficial gut flora. Significantly, during the eighteenth century, when William Cadogan advocated early, exclusive suckling, there was a dramatic fall in the infant mortality rate, due particularly to greater survival in the first month of life, which cannot be explained by other factors. Despite contempary knowledge (and a UNICEF campaign) that they are unnecessary, uneconomic and interfere with the establishment of successful lactation, pre-lacteal feeds are still used in many maternity wards all over the world.[5]

What does happen to some women after giving birth is that their breasts rapidly become overfull and engorged and without a baby to milk them, they can feel uncomfortable and painful. This can in some cases lead to the development of mastitis or a breast abscess. It can also lead to later lactation problems because the breast tissue can become damaged from this early, exaggerated distension. Conversely, for the women who do not have an immediate copious supply, the lack of stimulus can mean delay or difficulty in establishing a supply of milk, because the main worker, the baby, is not doing his part. The role of the baby in all aspects of breastfeeding has been underestimated and one scientist has described this part aptly 'the baby in the driving seat'. Full-term normal babies are not nearly as helpless at birth as has been thought and they can organise their own meals to suit themselves and their mother's bodies, if only other people will let them do it. Nevertheless it is worth adding, because I may be guilty of the crimes I criticise and be demoralising mothers of premature or low birth weight babies, that it is possible to produce milk without the baby's stimulus for the first few weeks if you get the right information and support. I have known mothers who did this for many weeks and their babies were tube or spoonfed until they were allowed to suckle at the breast, whereupon normal breastfeeding was established.[6]

POSITIONING AND THE SUCKLING REFLEX

Full-term, healthy babies are born with a suckling reflex, usually misleadingly called the sucking reflex. In industrialised societies more people have seen a baby sucking a bottle or a dummy than suckling a breast, so many are unaware of the true nature of this reflex. When a baby takes her mother's breast in her mouth, the nipple touching the roof of her mouth stimulates her to perform a milking action. The actual tip of the nipple, depending on the relative size and shape of the baby's mouth and the mother's nipples, goes quite far to the back of the mouth. The baby takes a good bit of the breast itself, particularly the underside of the areola, into her mouth too and the waves of pressure and the upward action of her tongue and lower jaw strip the milk from the milk pools behind the nipple while at the same time sending a message to the mother's brain to produce more of the breastfeeding hormones.

Some people believe that incorrect positioning is one of the most serious causes of breasfeeding failure. The influence of artificial feeding practices means that a mother may be given the new baby to hold sideways, as though her breast were a bottle, and her nipple is damaged as a result. In western society sore nipples are seen as an inevitable part of breastfeeding and women are expected to bear the pain. It is an awful experience and it is understandable that so many women give up breastfeeding as a result, yet really sore nipples need never happen. A persistent myth is that fair-skinned women are bound to suffer nipple damage, but this is because the injury from bad positioning might hurt their sensitive skins more than darker-skinned women. As midwife Chlöe Fisher has pointed out, if fair-skinned women cannot breastfeed how did blond or red-headed groups evolve? Chlöe has helped an albino woman to feed and she had no pain or soreness at all. Many of my own generation were solemnly informed by their mothers that they were born with 'one skin missing' and had to be wrapped in silk and bathed in olive oil, an idea which springs from the cult of white racial superiority. This 'princess and the pea' complex fitted in nicely with lactation failure, which was more common among the ignorant white ruling classes and made them feel superior through their 'delicacy', as well as explaining why black peasant women were so competent at breastfeeding. Because we do not see breastfeeding happening as an everyday event no one learns how to do it and unless a helper is at hand who really knows what is right, a mother and baby can become habituated to 'nipple sucking' rather than 'breastfeeding'. This damages the nipples and closes down the milk production because the breast is never properly 'stripped'.

Breastfeeding is not an instinct and it has to be learned. Non-human primates, such as chimpanzees, have to learn about both sex and suckling by observation when they are young and if deprived of this have problems with both activities when they reach maturity. Humans are the same and if they do not get a chance to learn, unless they are very lucky, it might be hard for them to get either function right without information and help. This is why expecting breastfeeding to happen, by telling women to do it, is such a ridiculous goal. It is rather like expecting good performances from choir boys who have always been forbidden to listen to music.

THE LET-DOWN REFLEX

There is another hormone, oxytocin, which plays an equally important part in breastfeeding as it controls the let-down reflex which facilitates the flow of milk. As the biologist Roger Short describes, 'Thus oxytocin serves today's meal and prolactin prepares tomorrow's'.[7] Like prolactin, the secretion of oxytocin from the brain is stimulated through the nerves in the nipple area. Oxytocin is also involved in sexual arousal and orgasm (milk may spurt from the breasts during orgasm) and in the contraction of the uterus during childbirth. All these processes can be affected by stress, which will cause another hormone, adrenalin, to inhibit the circulation of oxytocin. Most women, especially when they are experienced breastfeeders, are well aware of the let-down reflex as the tingling sensation of milk pouring from within the breast to the milk pools behind the nipples. Many mothers feel their milk coming down when they hear their baby's cry or even just think about their baby. In some societies, if a woman believes she has a curse or spell on her that is drying up her milk, it is the let-down function that is inhibited by her emotional state. If she believes her milk will go, it may. Conversely, women who have lost their milk can have it restored through their faith in a spell or a ceremony. It is disruption of the let-down reflex that causes some women to experience sudden cessation of their milk flow if they are shocked or upset. A friend told me how her milk seemed to vanish when she went to see Stanley Kramer's 1959 film *On the Beach*, because she was so disturbed by it. Fortunately for her and her baby she knew that frequent suckling would quickly restore the supply, and it did.

THE BELEAGUERED WOMAN

Consider a western woman having her first baby in hospital. She may never have seen a child suckling; her main perception of her own breasts may be as sexual objects. Maybe for her own personal sense of power or perhaps as a significant part of the social definition of her attractiveness, she may have come to value them herself in this way. A lot of women's employment is still linked to their looks. Moreover most mothers are dependent on a male sexual partner to stay out of poverty. If a woman gains social esteem and economic security through her skill in 'keeping her man' and she knows that her body's shape is part of that skill, then she has a lot to lose if she damages that nubile beauty. It is a fact of life that men do abandon women whose youthful bodies have changed and that abandoned women are poorer. The cosmetics and fashion industries thrive on women's felt need to maintain a certain prescribed ideal of physical attractiveness and they stimulate insecurities with the advertising images of impossible standards of 'beauty'. Because stereotyped ideals of breast shape and size are endorsed by commerce and the use of 'soft-porn' in the media to capture attention, many women are self-conscious about their breasts even in private relationships and crave reassurance about their acceptability. Using breasts for feeding a baby may be emotionally confusing if society and your own experience has emphasised their sexual and aesthetic functions. Some women are shy of handling their own breasts. A new baby suckling with a powerful animal reflex can be disturbing to a woman who has never seen this happen and has not been prepared for it. The unfamiliarity of the hospital ward, the busyness of the staff, the presence of strangers, the ubiquitous bottles and the promotion of artificial milks in advisory booklets, on cot cards and in gift packs can all profoundly inhibit a woman. This inhibition is not just a 'feeling' but actually affects the secretion of oxytocin and impedes the flow of milk. People often discuss why so many women do not breastfeed or give up quickly. I feel it is firm evidence of the determination of women that some actually succeed amidst such destructive supervision and in such an inappropriate environment.

Imagine a young man embarking upon his first attempt at sexual penetration. Ask him to set about the project in a special sex centre where there are 'experts' he has never met before, ready to supervise and tell him how it ought to be done. Presume that his partner is as inexperienced as himself and that he is asked if he is going to '*try* and achieve an erection'. When he starts, a

---

'After I gave birth, I couldn't imagine milk coming out of my breasts any more than I could imagine milk coming out of my elbow or my feet, so I didn't think it was going to. I think that's why a lot of breastfeeding fails: you don't believe that milk will come out of you so you just unconsciously stop it.'

The difficulty of this imaginative leap is compounded by the documented (in interviews and sociological and anthropological studies) ambivalence and discomfort of American men towards breastfeeding women, men who have grown up with the cultural value that the breast is a sexual object belonging to them, not their interloping infants. Men may indeed feel enthusiastic about the idea of breastfeeding, but good intentions, alas, do not eradicate largely unconscious mixed emotions which may remain inaccessible to the man but are picked up by, and are confusing to, a woman in her attempt to be supported in nursing. To deny her experience or suggest that her husband is unusual is to add unnecessary stress. (From 'Dancing in the dark' 1. 'Romanticized motherhood and the breastfeeding venture' by Linda Blachman in *Birth and Family Journal*, vol. 8, no. 4, Winter 1981.)

busy 'expert', who may never have personally experienced sexual relations, starts telling him how to do it and inspects his body with a critical expression, prodding him and his partner in an insensitive manner. By the bed is an artificial penis, put there, as the young man is told, 'just in case you can't manage it; many young men can't make it; it is not their fault, nature often fails'. Everyone knows how vulnerable the male penis is to psychological stress and how sensitive sexual partners must be in order to nurture the psyche, as well as the body, of the male, yet such sensitivity has been conspicuously absent from the milieu of hospitalised parturient women. There are thousands of horror stories of medical staff snapping at women, brusquely pushing the baby on to the breast, dragging her off and distributing the feeding bottles whose very presence is saying, 'You won't do it, you can't do it.' It is no wonder that, the world over, a decline in breastfeeding is linked with an increase in hospital births.

The let-down reflex may continue to be damaged outside hospital, by embarrassment at feeding amongst people who disapprove, by lack of faith of the woman herself in her ability to feed and by the stress of near-imprisonment in the home and exclusion from normal life when she lives in a society where breastfeeding is forbidden or ostracised in public. If all this psychological damage occurs as well as the baby being badly positioned and suckling restricted to certain times, breastfeeding is bound to fail, and these circumstances have been the normal experience of most women in most industrialised countries.

It has been a common assumption that breastfeeding has returned to the western nations, but the fact is that whereas many more women are attempting to breastfeed (approximately two-thirds of mothers in the UK) than twenty years ago, only about a third of these are still breastfeeding at three months.[8] A study from France showed that of the 75 per cent of women who wanted to breastfeed, only 41 per cent left hospital doing so and the description of ward practices revealed a profound ignorance of the facts of feeding. The baby food companies can maintain good profit margins while individual women hear what a wonderful thing breastfeeding is without getting the support they need to do it. The choice to bottle-feed is often a rational one, when social feedback informs women that breastfeeding is an unhappy experience. A lot of mothers advise their daughters against breastfeeding because they want to protect them from the sense of failure that they themselves endured.[9]

TRADITIONAL SOCIETIES AND WESTERN MEDICAL INFLUENCES

The situation is different in most traditional societies where strong breastfeeding support systems ensure that all babies and mothers have a period of rest and lactation establishment. Techniques are learned unconsciously at an early age through observing breastfeeding as an everyday activity. In peasant society, women's sexual attractiveness is not necessarily linked with a pre-fertile body shape and the capacity for economic production is a priority. Consequently breastfeeding does not conflict with her social image. Indeed in Papua New Guinea there is a dreaded curse that a witch may put on an enemy to make her breasts stay pert and upright like a young girl's forever.

Where women normally engage in extremely hard physical labour, the post-natal period is often one of complete rest with all normal duties performed by other women, who also give emotional support and practical breastfeeding knowledge. Newly delivered mothers are often treated like princesses and they welcome this respite from their hard-working lives. With urbanisation and increased hospital delivery, this support system is disrupted; lactation failure spreads and becomes socially accepted which in turn demoralises more women. Hospitals can be exhausting places where clattering trolleys, early waking for medical procedures, night lighting and other people's noise can mean disruption of normal sleep patterns. Staff are often overworked and stressed and their mood communicates itself to a new mother. Breastfeeding help is rarely a priority. Doctors have said to me, 'Oh I leave all that to the nurses and midwives,' as though it were a trivial concern. Nurses might be reprimanded if they are late with form filling, but not admonished if they fail to sit down with a mother to help her breastfeed. No one takes the responsibility. Western priorities spread to the developing world. When I visited a paediatric ward in Costa Rica, an enthusiastic young doctor expounded about the hospital's commitment to breastfeeding. As we peered at various babies in incubators, a sad young woman was sitting nearby, bottle-feeding her three-day-old baby, I asked the doctor why; he did not know and asked the woman. 'I have no milk,' she said in Spanish. The doctor translated the words without a flicker of reaction and we sped on to gaze at another technological marvel. It was more important for him to impress us than it was to help this woman. I am ashamed to admit that I was too intimidated by protocol to sit down and help her. Many women have no milk at three days, which is why their babies must suckle frequently so as to stimulate the supply, and this doctor's acceptance of the woman's own diagnosis confirmed her lack of confidence in her own body. Like most doctors he was probably untrained in the techniques of breastfeeding support. Health workers' experience of breastfeeding failure is often greater than their experience of success. They all know the mantra that breast is best, which is as useful as knowing that potatoes are edible without ever learning how to cook them. In fact in Brazil it was shown that the *more* breastfeeding instruction women received, the *less* likely they were to breastfeed because bad information does more harm than none at all. Health workers who really know how to explain, encourage and help position the baby on the breast save hours of future work as well as the health and lives of babies. If a mother and baby are helped at the start they are far less likely to have problems later, but hospital maternity staff do not have to deal with these, whereas a community health worker who both delivered the baby and was responsible for its health and welfare later on would have a greater interest in breastfeeding. When relatives or neighbours used to deliver babies they had an emotional interest in establishing successful lactation.

The new dissemination of breastfeeding knowledge has come from women themselves, and every doctor or midwife who is interested in the subject will acknowledge that they learned more from their own babies or from other mothers and breastfeeding

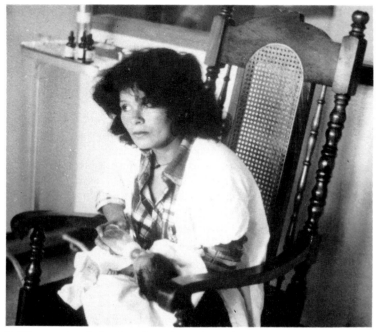

2 Woman bottle-feeding her three-day-old baby in a Costa Rican paediatric ward (*Photo:* Gabrielle Palmer 1987)

support groups than from medical training.

Faith in the process is conspicuously lacking in many health workers and this mistrust communicates itself to mothers. I recently discussed breastfeeding by childless women of adopted babies with a paediatric nutritionist. He confidently stated that this procedure was impossible because the breast had to be 'primed with the post-natal hormone influx and that this would be difficult to manage pharmacologically'. One infertile woman who has breastfed her adopted baby lives in the town where this doctor works, but because the facts do not fit in with his understanding of the way women's bodies work he could not accept them. Health workers often need more breastfeeding support than mothers. Derrick Jelliffe and Patrice Jelliffe illustrated this need with a story from a relactation unit in Uganda. There, mothers were well-fed and rested, and suckled their babies frequently in order to restimulate lactation after they had misguidedly abandoned it for bottle-feeding. They were also given a small dose of chlorpromazine, a tranquillising drug which has the side-effect of inducing lactation.* The Jelliffes' experience had taught them that relactation could happen without pharmacological assistance, but the main purpose of the drug was to inspire confidence in the health workers who could not believe that relactation could happen without western medical aids, and their drug-induced faith communicated itself to the mothers, thus aiding the process. We have to have placebos for doctors and nurses administered via the patient![10]

Faith alone does not make breastfeeding easy in a society ignorant of ordinary techniques, but in those parts of the world where breastfeeding is still a normal procedure, the fact that every woman knows rather than hopes she can breastfeed has a potent effect on her success.

THE SUSPICIOUS FEMALE FLUID

Why the medical profession, who must be credited with the discovery of the understanding of so many physiological processes, should have got this one so wrong is still a mystery. There have been lone doctors crying with the voice of sanity amidst all the nonsense, but they were rarely heard. I suspect that the dominant nineteenth-century attitude to women influenced the misunderstanding. It has to be said that the few women doctors were no better than their male counterparts in this respect. Perhaps because they were trying so hard to be treated as equals they had to show themselves to be 'as good as men' and therefore felt compelled to disregard traditional female knowledge.

---

* This was carried out many years ago. It is now advised that chlorpromazine should not be given to breastfeeding mothers.

The profound mistrust of breastfeeding is very complex, but a primitive male fear of the polluting quality of women must come into the argument. Separation of mothers and babies is so persistent a practice that in 1991 UNICEF had to launch a global 'Baby Friendly Hospital Initiative' to try and combat this and other harmful interventions. There is not a single scientific study to show that separated babies have fewer infections than those left with their mothers, indeed the contrary has been shown.[11] Why should a nurse, midwife or doctor be less of a carrier of disease than the mother who has been protecting the baby in her body for months? Rituals such as washing the nipples or wiping them with various potions before the baby is allowed to suckle strips them of their protective lubrication and increases the risk of soreness and of thrush and other infections. The breast is viewed as a carrier of disease yet, inconsistently, health workers who may be bringing infections from the environment outside the maternity ward are not compelled to scrub up every time they handle a normal baby.

Many cultures have beliefs in the power and pollution of female fluids. Zulu tradition claims that manhood may be lost if breastmilk falls on a man's skin and in Mozambique a friend assured me that women deliberately killed men by having intercourse when they were bleeding from their vaginas. Some European Christian churches have cleansing ceremonies which coincide with the cessation of the lochia, the bleeding after childbirth, and one Christian priest told me that he believed it was an irrational horror of menstruation that was behind the resistance to female ordination.

Newly delivered women are both bleeding from their vaginas and secreting from their breasts and the germ theory of disease has been used to endorse these ancient primitive fears. I would have dismissed these theories as obscure nonsense if I had not been confronted with the attitudes of so many male doctors whose expressions betray their revulsion of women. Many men twitch at the mere mention of menstrual blood and a joke nurses used to play on new young male doctors was to put expressed breastmilk in their coffee and tell them afterwards and see their disgust. In Mozambique, though the mortality rates were high it

---

Rabbis bar women

Rabbis in the northern Israel town Migdal Ha'emek have caused outrage by barring women from attending funerals in what they say is a move to ward off the evil eye and halt a series of local deaths. (*Financial Times*, 4 April 1987)

---

took the late President Machel's personal intervention to persuade male Portuguese doctors that mothers should stay with their babies in the paediatric wards. The excuse for keeping them out was 'hygiene', yet of course mortality rates plummeted when mothers were allowed to stay to breastfeed and care for their babies.

A theory that women with sexual 'hang-ups' were less likely to breastfeed came from Masters and Johnson's research in the 1960s.[12] It seemed nonsense to me when the millions of women in societies that practice genital mutilation or deny the concept of female sexuality breastfeed easily. More obvious is the fact that breastfeeding is discouraged by male sexual 'hang-ups', both within personal relationships and through the medical profession. During the nineteenth century women were socially and economically distanced from men and female stereotypes were forged into the ruling male psyche. In England, women were called 'the fair sex' and were, according to class, viewed as either ethereal, spiritually superior creatures or coarse, inferior beings. An ambiguity towards their bodies was reflected in the elaborate and restrictive clothing of the times.

Many doctors' statements about breastfeeding reveal an attitude to the breast which expresses fear as well as doubt. Dr Koplick, a leading paediatrician of his time, wrote about breastfeeding in 1903, 'The thumb may be used to exert pressure on the breast, thus aiding the flow of milk. In this way the infant is prevented from drawing the nipple too far into the mouth.'[13] The implication is that the fearful nipple could do harm if it went 'too far', when in fact this advice is a recipe for nipple damage and inadequate milk production. A widespread recommendation

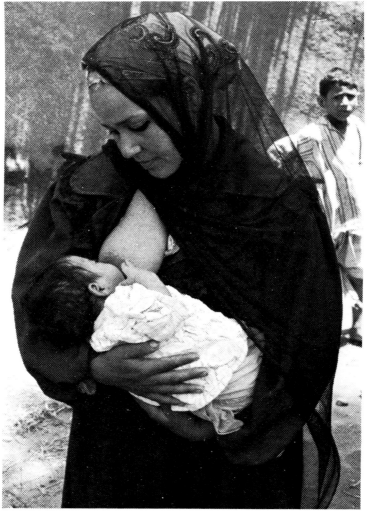

3 Egyptian woman breastfeeding her baby in the street (*Photo:* I. Lippman; courtesy of UNICEF)

which persists to this day is the advice to hold the nipple and breast between the fingers in case the baby cannot breathe.(There is not a single case of a baby being suffocated by the breast, but it is a recurring adult male fantasy: in the 1986 James Bond film *The Living Daylights* a man is killed by being crushed to death between a woman's breasts.) Influenced by Dr Koplick's and other similar ideas, thousands of women have fearfully breastfed in this way, sincerely believing that their baby could choke if they did not 'control' the procedure. The idea that the means of sustaining your baby's life could actually kill her through suffocation must have made many mothers terrified. Male fears of women's bodies were used to depict the breast as an instrument of death rather than nurturance. No wonder the bottle seemed safer. This attitude to the 'danger' of breastfeeding is enshrined in medical practice. Research from the United States with healthy pre-term babies showed, through a set of physiological indicators, that babies were far less stressed by the act of breastfeeding than by bottle-feeding, yet the rule in many hospitals is that a pre-term baby must not be allowed to breastfeed until it can take a bottle. [14]

THE MISTAKES SANCTIFIED IN PRINT

Medical traditions that destroy breastfeeding are sanctified by recommendations in textbooks and training schools. Rituals such as separation of mother and child, limited suckling time and the giving of other fluids have no justification for the majority of babies' welfare and are usually harmful. They have become sacred rites which pay more respect to the whims of long-dead doctors than to the needs of the mother and child.

I am spoilt for choice when I delve into my collection of pamphlets given through the Health Service to British mothers. The booklet I pick at random, *The Baby Book,* available free to all British mothers, says, 'Place your finger on the breast below his nose so that he can breathe freely.' It also states that the mother should put 'most' of the areola into his mouth. As some women have areolas that may spread about twenty centimetres back from the nipple, you need a baby with a mouth like a carp to achieve such a miracle. After several references to sore nipples the confident statement is made that 'overproduction' of milk is unlikely but that 'underfeeding is possible because, through no fault of your own [hinting that it could be], you may not be producing enough milk.' There follows advice to feed more frequently [a tiny gem of accuracy] or to use a pump, with no explanation as to why this is preferable to a suckling baby. Then,

> There is never anything wrong with the richness of the milk but you may not be making enough. There are two golden rules to make sure you are not underfeeding at the breast. You must make sure the weight gain is satisfactory – an average of ½lb a week for the first three months [this is misleading because babies grow in spurts]; secondly, make sure your baby is contented. Persistent crying usually means hunger *even if the weight gain is average* [my italics] because some babies need to grow faster.

Having carefully impressed on the mother the quite imaginary risks of the inadequacy of breastfeeding in the early months, on the facing page is a full-page advertisement saying,

> *Q.* My baby's always hungry. Is there a baby milk which can keep him contented?
> *A.* Yes, Ostermilk.

This is just one of hundreds of examples of misinformation that have been distributed through health care systems. This booklet was edited by the Professor of Obstetrics and Gynaecology at a leading London teaching hospital, yet it is so larded with advertisements that it conveys the message that actually producing and caring for a child is secondary to the purchase of a wide range of products. These booklets are financed by the baby product industry which exploits medical prestige in order to promote sales. I assume that the medical editors do not conspire directly with the copywriters, but the language used in both infant feeding advice and baby milk adverts is similar. The former implies that hunger and discontent are likely with breastfeeding and the latter informs us that the problem is resolvable with bottle- feeding. Both are a potent method of discouragement. In the same text the discussion of persistent crying in bottle-fed babies is categorically seen as not to do with the milk: 'If the baby seems to be crying a great deal, don't keep changing the milk from one brand to another. Take him to your doctor or clinic for advice. The chances are that the milk has nothing to do with it.'[15] Interestingly 'insufficient milk syndrome' happens to bottle-feeding mothers too. British research shows that 44 per cent of bottle-feeding mothers do change to a different milk during the early weeks, some more than once, principally because they perceive that the baby is still hungry and unsatisfied.[16]

The fact that all the hard-working, sometimes underfed mothers in the African village of Keneba can produce enough milk to maintain good growth in the first three months of their babies' lives is in part due to the fact that they were not exposed to *The Baby Book* and its nonsensical text and advertisements.[17] Tragically such information is being disseminated in developing countries, not only in company pamphlets, but also in medical textbooks. Here is an example from a Nigerian textbook, *Nutrition*.

> 5 per cent glucose water is recommended for the first 48 hours after birth, to prevent hypoglycaemia which may lead to permanent brain damage [how come the whole human race avoided permanent brain damage before the invention of glucose water?]. This is given irrespective of whether breastfeeding has been established or not. Before each breastfeed, mothers must make sure that their hands are clean. The nipples must be washed and dried before and after each feed . . . . The nipple and the areola are then held between two fingers and introduced into the baby's mouth. Care should be taken to see that the baby does not suck too quickly [how do you do this?] and that his nose is not covered by the breast. On the first day, the baby should be allowed to suck for 2 minutes at each breast, and the next day for 3 minutes, etc. etc. This timing is necessary to ensure that the nipples are not subjected to too

much friction [how can suckling be equated with friction?], which can make them sore and painful. Susceptible mothers can develop mastitis and sometimes breast abscesses result from sores acquired in this way.[18]

The tragedy is that the midwife-author, who is a nurse tutor, could probably have learned far more from her own mother and other women in her community than from her western medical training which destroyed all the useful information she may have acquired as a child.

THE VANISHING KNOWLEDGE

The people who know about breastfeeding are not the medical authorities of prestigious institutions but ordinary women who have been fortunate enough to escape one of the ravages of 'development'. In the less assaulted societies, the idea of being unable to breastfeed does not exist. When Leslie Conton[19] asked Usino women in Papua New Guinea about knowledge of breastfeeding they were amazed: 'Why does she ask us all this? All women know how to breastfeed!' and they laughed at the thought that she might not know how to feed an infant. As Conton points out, most adult skills were learned by observation and practice, rather than verbal instruction, so the idea of formulating verbal descriptions of the breastfeeding process was strange. Even if the nineteenth-century doctors had discussed techniques with ordinary women, the women might not have been good at verbally describing actions they had never analysed. Another point that Conton makes is that much of our knowledge on infant feeding comes from cultures undergoing rapid development where a crisis already exists, so that most groups we are in contact with are already being damaged by this contact. It is therefore vital to grasp the vanishing knowledge from those rare societies which are still relatively undamaged by industrialisation. When I trained as a breastfeeding counsellor, I was taught that one could avert milk leaking by holding the heel of the hand to the breast for at least one minute, and I solemnly absorbed and disseminated this 'new fact'. In Africa I noticed women unconsciously performing this action just as I might obliviously scratch my ear. In Papua New Guinea there are very few breastfeeding problems because women's knowledge has not been taken away from them, and it is one of the few countries that managed to pre-empt the tragic effects of bottle-feeding by restricting it by law at a stage of development when traditional skill was still thriving. Many infant lives have been saved as a result (see page 262).

BREASTMILK

Breastmilk contains all the nutrients necessary for infant growth and health, and these are so well absorbed that some babies excrete very little waste matter. The low proportions of some nutrients are as important as the abundance of others, because a baby's immature kidneys lack the capacity to filter out all the excess waste that a diet too high in, for example, certain proteins and minerals would produce. It is because cows' milk is 'too rich' in these nutrients that it has to be diluted and 'modified' when used for human babies. Breastmilk comes with its own regulating substances which not only raise the bioavailability of some nutrients when this is useful, but lower them when it is dangerous. For example, the breastmilk enzyme lipase makes fat available to the infant even before it has reached its own digestive processes, whereas the protein lactoferrin binds with iron to prevent too much being utilised because excess iron can encourage the growth of harmful bacteria in the gut. There are only two nutrients, vitamins D and K, whose adequacy in breastmilk is in rare cases questioned. Vitamin D is actually a hormone that is activated by the action of sunlight on the skin and enables calcium to be used for bone formation and maintenance. Deficiency causes rickets, the disease in which the bones soften, causing deformities such as bandy legs. The only rich food source of vitamin D is fish liver oil and in modern industrialised countries, most vitamin D is derived from artificially enriched foods. Dietary sources are potentially dangerous and over-enriched baby foods have caused serious illness in infants. Exposure to sunlight (or artificial ultra violet light) for thirty minutes a week, or two hours if the baby is clothed but bare-headed, maintains enough vitamin D, and this is stored in the body to last through the sunless times. Rickets is rare in sunny countries unless the baby is permanently kept covered and indoors. In the past it was primarily a disease of the industrialised cities of northern Europe, where indoor factory work, bad housing and polluted air deprived people of sunlight. There have been a few modern cases of vitamin D deficiency in some full-term, breastfed babies because their mothers were deficient, often because they stayed indoors constantly or wore over-enveloping clothing. A mother's deficiency is avoidable and its existence is therefore a sorry reflection of her ante-natal care, as ultra violet light treatment could solve the problem. If margarine can be treated, why not the few vulnerable pregnant and lactating women? For children born in the winter in the far north of the world, there may be the need for some supplementation, though in the past it seems that any slight deficiency effects healed rapidly in breastfed babies. [20]

Vitamin K is needed for blood clotting and very rarely a baby may develop haemorrhagic disease (bleeding) due to deficiency. This vitamin is made by bacteria in the gut and the baby can usually rely on stores in his liver until his own personal germ farm has got going. Before the use of enemas prior to childbirth, a woman reflexedly emptied her bowels as she pushed her baby out and inevitably he would have ingested a few useful micrograms of faeces and his gut could be quickly contaminated with the vitamin K producing bacteria. With modern obstetric practices the effect of this beneficial contamination may be prevented and routine vitamin K injections are given in many maternity hospitals (a practice which as with any injection carries some risk). Until recently it was confidently stated in medical literature that vitamin K was low in breastmilk. Recent research has revealed that there are significant levels of vitamin K in the colostrum and early milk and that the highest proportion is in the fat rich hind milk. Obviously if colostrum is denied to the baby and restricted time at the breast prevents him getting the hind milk, there could be a risk of deficiency. This is an example of arbitrary medical custom adversely affecting not only the quantity, but the quality of the breastmilk the baby receives.[21a]

There have been occasional cases of infantile beriberi (thiamin [vitamin B1] deficiency) in the babies of extremely deprived women who subsist on an inadequate diet of overpolished rice, but due to improvements in rice processing this is now rare. The world over, even undernourished women can maintain the quality of their milk and they have to be very malnourished indeed not to be able to support the growth of their infants. I quote these rare problems because they show how resilient is the nutrient quality of breastmilk for the great majority of women. Over the years breastmilk has been criticised for being too rich, too weak, too little or too much and doubt about the success of the function is widespread. The western image of traditional breastfeeding is of a hungry mother in a famine rather than of the millions of ordinary women who breastfeed extremely successfully. Reporters often refer to babies suckling on empty breasts when they have no evidence to prove this fact. A withered breast reflects a mother's weight loss, not her state of lactation. Of course hungry mothers do not have over-abundant milk, but their babies are often wasted because they have contracted an infection and are too weak to suckle, and are only alive because of the breast milk that they have managed to take in.

The more research is carried out, the more beautifully adapted for its purpose breastmilk is found to be. It has been subjected to a burden of proof which logically should have lain with artificial milk, but this doubt has acted as a 'null hypothesis' and proved its excellence.

ARTIFICIAL BABY MILK

In contrast to breastmilk, artificial milk has been a hit and miss affair relying on long-term experimentation on babies to discover what works. Its composition is as much influenced by nutritional fashions as by facts, as the tragic Syntex story in Chapter 8 illustrates. Nowadays more deference is paid to breastmilk in the design of artificial milks, simply because there is more knowledge, but it is still an entirely different substance, containing no living cells and not adapting to each baby's changing needs. Reluctantly, I compare breastmilk with cows' milk because the latter is commonly the basis of breastmilk substitutes not because it is the most appropriate substance – chimpanzee's or horse's milk might be better – but because it is the most available. Cows are not like humans and there are many risks in feeding such a dissimilar animal's milk to human infants. One example is the link between juvenile diabetes and early feeding of cows' milk based formulas.

Because of both nutritional fashion and economic expediency, baby milk manufacturers replace most or all of the butterfat in the cows' milk. Coconut oil is used because it is cheap as is beef tallow, a waste product from the meat industry. So is groundnut oil which can trigger allergy and may contain traces of cancer-causing aflatoxins. Agro-chemicals are used in most large scale oil crop production and the refining processes may remove vital nutrients. Vegetable oils cannot replace breastmilk fats which help the brain and nervous system to develop, so marine oils are coming into favour, though there may be a risk of environmental pollutants. Soya beans are used for artificial baby milks, not because different foods were analysed to find the best for babies, but because the soya industry sought profitable outlets. Soya can be as allergenic as cows' milk. Breastmilk has better quality control than any artificial milk, which may change because of an ingredient's price rise, a new cattle treatment or the quality control inspector being off work with flu. The long journey from nutritionists' theories to the babies' stomachs means the possibility of error is endless. Farm, factory, laboratory, packaging, transport, storage and kitchen are all managed by human beings who have only a lifetime to learn their tasks. Nature has had several million years. [21b]

When in the 1860s, the German chemist Justus von Liebig, invented 'the perfect substitute for mother's milk' from wheat and pea flour (see page 192), he matched it to the substances he knew how to analyse. The situation is the same today; we can only describe what is known and there is still so much to learn. By modern standards no artificial milk until the 1970s was appropriate for babies and there is still concern about many ingredients. The list of production errors is scandalously long (see Appendix 1) and these are only the recorded cases.

THE ANTI-INFECTIVE PROPERTIES OF BREASTMILK

Breastmilk is more than a food, its secretion is part of a process which affects the mother and the baby both immunologically and hormonally. Exclusively breastfed babies are less likely to get infections, especially gastroenteritis, respiratory tract and middle ear infections. This is not just due to the hygienic methods of delivery, but because breastmilk contains unique anti-infective properties. These work in a variety of ways, some acting as specific attackers of particular pathogens while others are non-specific antibodies. For example, there are macrophages, cells which gobble up invading bacteria, while others, for example some immunoglobulins, work in a preventive way by coating the baby's gut with a protective 'paint' that stops pathogens getting through. Breastmilk attacks viruses and even contains a unique factor, not found in cows' milk or human blood, which prevents the Human Immunodeficiency Virus (HIV) from attaching itself to the cell (see page 77). Scientists have discovered a beautifully economical function of the immunoproteins; they can function to attack disease, and also be digested as nutrient protein. It is as though your antibiotics were also a food supplement.[22]

A baby's immune system is not fully developed at birth. She is reliant on the antibodies she acquired in the uterus, transferred from her mother across the placenta. The protective factors in breastmilk provide an intermediate immunology system while the baby's own immune system is developing. Pathogens such as the polio virus are destroyed by the antibodies in breastmilk. A baby is challenged by many diseases and her own antibodies develop to protect her as the placental ones gradually disappear. During this crossover phase, breastmilk makes the challenge less of a risk. If she is immunised against the common infections with synthetic vaccines, breastfeeding enhances their effectiveness.

The difficult conditions in which most of the world's babies live makes this protection essential for health and life, but even in the pampering environment of wealthy society, it reduces the chance of illness. Of course breastfed babies can get ill, but the breast is like a very efficient pharmacist; it produces specific medicines to order as the message gets through that they are needed, so any disease is diagnosed by the mother's body even before anyone else has noticed it. A baby and a mother are a couple who share the same environment and are likely to be challenged by the same germs. So a mother who ingests bacteria or viruses that could cause diarrhoea will start manufacturing her own antibodies and these will be transferred to the breast which is on the immunological network. The antibodies in the milk are also believed to protect the breast itself from disease as well as the baby. Comparative research shows that women in poor environments have more antibodies in their milk, and though this has not been conclusively proven it points to the idea that the more infection there is a around, the more the breast is working to combat it. Breastmilk has been found to destroy or reduce a wide range of organisms, including cholera, the parasite giardia and fungal infections. This is one of the reasons why in poor, unhealthy environments not every baby dies. Miraculously the majority live, thanks to this efficient system of supply and demand of nutrients and disease protection.[23]

OTHER PROPERTIES

Breastfed babies are less likely to develop diabetes, childhood cancer or suffer sudden death (SIDS). Breastfeeding makes immunisation more effective and it may prevent long term bowel disease, certain autoimmune conditions and coronary heart disease. In allergic families, the breastfed baby will gain protection against eczema and wheeziness. All the fascinating properties of breastmilk cannot be described here. They include growth factors which help the tissue of the baby's body develop and hormones which trigger the ideal digestive responses to nutrients. A breastfed baby's intestine will have a different acid/alkali balance from that of the artificially fed infant and this will affect the gut flora. Also, breastmilk changes according to the needs of the infant. The milk of mothers of premature babies is different from that of other mothers and such constituents as the fat are in forms that are particularly appropriate for each phase of the baby's life. More digestible fats are in greater proportion when the baby's digestive system is still immature and others which are a basis for brain tissue and central nervous system development are at high levels at an early stage when the baby's brain is growing rapidly.[24]

Until recently, health workers worried about breastfed babies' growth because it did not conform to the 'standards' which had been established by measuring mainly bottle-fed babies. Breastfed babies were deemed to 'fall off' the charts, but what was ignored was the fact that babies breastfed on demand actually grew faster in the first three months and that this fall-off was to be expected. Nutritionists then had to acknowledge the problem of obesity in some artificially fed babies and also the existence of smaller but perfectly healthy breastfed babies. Sometimes babies do stop gaining weight and this always used to be blamed on insufficient milk in the mother; it was assumed that the weight loss preceded an infection. What is now considered is the idea that the first sign of illness is often loss of appetite, and a baby who feels unwell will not suckle the milk and as a result loses weight. In poor regions breastfed babies usually grow well in the early months and it is only at the crossover time, usually after six months when they need extra weaning foods and suitable food is scarce or contaminated, that there is an increased risk of malnutrition or illness. Researchers are now questioning the validity of weight charts that have been used the world over and which have prompted a lot of early, unnecessary and dangerous supplementation.[25]

PREMATURE AND LOW BIRTH WEIGHT BABIES

There are important differences between these babies, as to exactly why they are small and how early they are born. Among some of the known causes of growth retardation and prematurity is the effect of the mother's long-term health and nutrition, and the stress she has had to endure during her life. This is why poorer mothers are most likely to have smaller and more vulnerable babies. Industrialised countries with greater extremes of social deprivation such as the United States, have a greater proportion of low birth weight babies than in more equal societies such as Scandinavia.

Extremely premature or tiny babies may not be able to suckle and swallow but almost all mothers can express milk for them. Very early babies need supplementary nutrients and in most Scandinavian hospitals these are derived from donated breastmilk. During the 1980s, research, mostly funded by the baby milk industry, was published that claimed 'better growth' in babies who had been fed on 'special' pre-term formulas. The studies did not address the issue of inadequate support and information for the mothers. As research continued crucial differences came to light; some evidence indicated that bone density was better in the breastmilk fed babies and there were high rates among the artificially fed babies of necrotising enterocolitis (NEC), a condition where part of the gut lining 'dies'. NEC is almost unknown in countries where breastmilk is the normal food of low birth weight babies, but elsewhere hundreds of babies died who might have lived if they had received their mother's or even donated breastmilk.

A mother's own milk is always the best but donated breastmilk, is still better than artificial milk as long as it is properly collected and pooled so as to maintain the right balance of nutrients. Awareness of HIV has led to routine pasteurisation of all donated milk and testing of all breastmilk donors. Regrettably many milk banks have closed down, often on the pretext of fears of HIV infection. The reality is that companies give free milk to hospitals (a violation of the WHO/UNICEF Code) and doctors and hospital managers who feel more loyalty to companies than to breastfeeding avoid the tedious logistics and costs of breastmilk collection.

Of course health workers in this field care about saving the lives of these vulnerable infants, but there is a horrible irony that while a lot of money is spent on technology and doctors gain prestige from its use, other babies suffer and die the world over because their basic needs are not met. In Columbia, one doctor has found that many low birth weight babies who were able to suckle could be kept constantly between their mother's breasts. The humidity and temperature matched sophisticated incubators and they received enough of the right milk for their needs. [26] Technology can be a blessing, but it is sometimes used because of its intrinsic fascination to researchers rather than for broad social progress. Its use sometimes obliterates simpler and more appropriate solutions and occasionally babies have been kept in special care baby units unnecessarily. Meanwhile healthy, full-term babies still die from tetanus because the knowledge to prevent it does not get disseminated. There is financial profit to be made from sophisticated technology, but no money is made when a traditional midwife sterilises her razor blade to cut the umbilical cord.

WEANING FOODS*

The majority of babies probably need no supplementation until six months and the WHO/UNICEF guidelines, which recommend four to six months as the age of supplementation, are designed to cover the needs of all babies, including the minority who might need early supplementation. Most foods are nutritionally inferior to breastmilk, lessen the baby's appetite for the breast and therefore reduce milk supply. Brazilian research showed that supplementation with infant formula, cows' milk, water, juice and 'teas' increased the risk of infection and death, but that solid foods (at the right time) lowered it. There is often a crucial period at around three months when the baby does seem hungrier and many mothers interpret this as a sign of inadequate lactation. In response they may introduce other foods and thus diminish their supply, proving their inadequacy to themselves. Letting the child suckle more frequently or for longer during this

* The term 'to wean' means to accustom to foods and liquids other than breastmilk, but I do not use it to mean the complete cessation of breastfeeding. For this I use the word 'sevrage'.

phase would maximise the output and defer the risks of weaning foods. These can be a source of infection, intolerant and allergic reactions, and they disrupt the benefits of breastfeeding; for example both pears and cows' milk reduce iron absorption.

Timing of the introduction of other foods varies greatly from culture to culture and may be given as early as the first week, as with rice in parts of Asia, or not until the child walks as in some groups in Africa. Babies also vary a great deal and do not conform to standards. There is a child in Australia who was growing well on exclusive breastfeeding at fifteen months. Though this living advertisement for breastmilk delights me, I would love to know how they stopped him from grabbing the food off the family table. Babies at about six months start reaching out and putting things in their mouths, which indicates that this might be an appropriate time to try other foods. Also, the average age of eruption of the first tooth is around six months, though it can be as late as thirteen or fourteen months. This is another indicator of a 'natural' time for eating solid food. Our nearest relatives, chimpanzees, depend on breastmilk for about three years and then for another two to three years on a combination of breastmilk and other foods, until their mother finally denies the infant her breast. It is interesting that it is the mother who initiates the process of complete 'sevrage' and the infant often resists it with displays of temper. The primate mother deals with this with great sensitivity and tenderness.[27]

Some babies suffer rare digestive disorders where breastmilk is the only food they can absorb, even after one year. When there were difficulties with supplies of donated milk at a leading children's hospital, it was suggested to a nutritionist that the mother of one of these children could relactate. The nutritionist said that it was simply too 'way out' a suggestion to put to the mother. It seems incredible that in a world where people walk about with other people's organs surgically grafted, carry complex plastic heart pacemakers in their bodies and send cameras down into stomachs, the simple process of triggering a natural function is viewed with alarm, even if it can save a life. How did such an irrational taboo evolve?

ENVIRONMENTAL POLLUTION

The pollutants that most threaten our health and lives are chlorine-based compounds (organochlorines) such as PCBs, and their by-products such as dioxins. Their production and use in PVC plastic, electrical equipment, pesticides, the paper industry, timber treatments and many other products have proliferated since the 1940s, and the damage outweighs any benefits. They are highly toxic and some are carcinogenic. Through waste incineration, seepage and contamination, they enter the air, water and soil, get into the food chain and are stored in our body fat. These pollutants have been found in breastmilk and in some areas, particularly Germany, mothers have been scared away from breastfeeding. This advice is unsound for the benefits of breastfeeding still outweigh the risks of artificial feeding, which is itself not free of pollution. In one study breastfeeding even appeared to counteract the neurological effects of contaminants before birth. Damage can happen in the uterus or through the father's sperm. Dioxins may cause male infertility but if a damaged sperm does fertilise an ovum this may lead to miscarriage, birth defects or childhood cancers. Evidence from Vietnam where 'Agent Orange', an organochlorine defoliant, was used as a weapon, shows an association between heavily-sprayed areas and birth defects. However, breastfeeding, normal for all babies in Vietnam, has not been shown to do harm. Indeed Vietnam's progress in child health, despite its poverty, has been attributed to good social support for breastfeeding mothers.

Despite the reassuring evidence that breastmilk has not yet been polluted so as to destroy all its amazing powers, there is no room for complacency. Mothers can try to minimise individual risk by avoiding polluted food, such as fish from contaminated areas, and not 'crash diet' which may release contaminants stored in the body fat into the bloodstream. The most important action is to do everything possible to halt the production and careless disposal of these deadly poisons, otherwise our grandchildren may never have the chance to bear healthy babies. If breastmilk becomes too contaminated to use, then it is likely that our chances of having healthy children, or even being able to reproduce at all, will be in jeopardy. The irony is that hospital incinerators are among the worst polluters and doubtless some of the disposable medical supplies they burn are used to treat illnesses triggered by lack of breastfeeding. Artificial feeding does not guarantee a pollutant-free diet. One US study revealed 78 per cent of milk samples from 1200 cows to be contaminated. No company could monitor its milk continuously for every possible contaminant. Dioxins are found in the cream of cows' milk and although some manufacturers replace this with vegetable oils, there is no guarantee that these were produced without pesticides or in uncontaminated soil.

Water is also a risk. In the USA, two Abbott-Ross formulas were found to contain carcinogenic chemicals, traced to a polluted well (see Appendix 1). 'Blue-baby' syndrome, when deoxygenated blood circulates, is a risk for artificially-fed babies if nitrate levels (from fertilisers) in water are too high, but water engineers are most worried about organochlorine residues. In the UK, bore holes have been closed because of permanent contamination, but as the cases were settled out of court this information was never publicly documented. It is often forgotten that you only find a substance if you have a specific test for it and it would be impossible to search for every pollutant, especially those present in minute (but dangerous) quantities. One chemical engineer tried out a new test on his own tap water and discovered a dangerous chemical (tetrachloroethylene) in it. One man's incidental curiosity revealed that a whole town had been drinking dangerously-contaminated water for years. Sex changes in fish supposedly due to oestrogen hormones (from contraceptive pills) in drinking water have caused alarm. Because most dairy cows are pregnant, cows' milk contains oestrogens; soya products contain plant oestrogens, so there is little chance of avoidance. Bottled waters (whose packaging and distribution cause pollution) are too high in minerals and salt to be safe for babies and they also contain microorganisms which can increase in the bottle, especially plastic ones. A proven danger is lead poisoning which affects mental development. 'Soft' water (ie low in calcium salts) absorbs lead from pipes. Twenty per cent of homes in the USA have water with high lead levels and in one magazine article about lead-damaged babies, the issue of why the babies were not breastfed was not even addressed. Another hazard is aluminium which is associated with brain damage and is easily absorbed in babies' bodies. Milk from cows grazing in areas with acid rain damage has high levels as do soya beans which avidly take up aluminium from the soil. Cows' milk based formulas can contain 10 to 20 times more aluminium and soya formulas a hundred times as much as breastmilk. It is also in some water. Premature babies have suffered permanent kidney and brain damage from aluminium in their feeds.

Radioactive contamination is also a matter of concern. Following the Chernobyl accident (1986), information from Italy and Austria showed that breastmilk contained one-three-hundredth the amount of radioactive iodine and caesium found in cows' milk. Sweden had comparable results in the most affected areas, except for one woman who had eaten an unusually large amount of local fish and reindeer meat. Strontium 90, resulting from the nuclear testing which we have been exposed to for decades, was not a risk in breastmilk and was ten times lower than in cows' milk. Radiation levels in breastmilk were much lower than in the woman's own body. Radioactively contaminated milk was exported from Europe to poor countries in the South. After Chernobyl, Poland appealed for artificial baby milks because of fear of contamination of both cows' and human milk. Months later consignments of Polish baby milks turned up in Bangladesh. There were reports from Egypt, Nepal, Ghana, India, Mexico, the Philippines and Sri Lanka of imported milks containing unacceptably high levels of radioactive contamination. Brazil returned large quantities of contaminated milk to its manufacturers in Ireland and the Gambia was subsequently flooded with mysteriously underpriced milks. Thailand banned the sale of several European branded baby milks which were radioactively contaminated whereupon an EC official warned that European aid would be cut off if they did not lower their stringent safety standards.

HIV INFECTION

Like syphilis in the sixteenth century, the human immuno-deficiency virus (HIV) has frightened the world. Many forget that new diseases have been evolving since life began and only in our age have we had the knowledge and technology to witness the arrival of a new organism. Despite these skills, our attitudes to HIV are still primitive, and fear, irrationality and bigotry abound as society tries to come to terms with the malign powers of nature and the limits of medicine. The role of breastfeeding in transmission of HIV is difficult to understand, but we can interpret a little from the way other viruses which are found in breastmilk behave, such as cytomegalovirus (CMV). Most of us have been exposed to CMV, it may be in our breastmilk and do no harm, but sometimes it does. The timing of infection and the amount of virus in the body seem to be the key factors. Up to a third of babies born to mothers with HIV become infected but it is hard to know whether transmission happens during pregnancy, delivery or breastfeeding. Babies are born with their mothers' antibodies so you cannot be sure whether they have their own HIV infection until around 18 months. There is a difference in risk between women infected after the birth and those who have an established HIV infection at delivery. Mothers with AIDS (the illnesses that HIV positive people develop when their immune systems fail) are at higher risk of infecting their babies. It is rarely possible to know when a woman contracted HIV, but whether it was before or during the pregnancy may be important in relation to breastfeeding.

Women who received HIV-contaminated blood transfusions at delivery or who contracted HIV, probably from a sexual partner, after the birth, seem to be at greater risk of infecting their babies through breastfeeding, perhaps because there is more virus in your body when you first contract HIV. In Rwanda, researchers observed 212 mothers, supposedly all HIV negative at their babies' births; sixteen mothers and nine babies later became HIV positive and breastfeeding seemed to have been the route of transmission. Seven babies did stay healthy and who can tell why? Perhaps their mothers had less of the virus in their body. One possible explanation is that some babies who are recorded as breastfed may get water or other liquid. Perhaps these or the infections they might carry could interfere with breastmilk's anti-infective factors, such as immunoglobulin A (IgA) which stops harmful microorganisms crossing through the gut wall.

Some evidence about women infected before delivery comes from the European Collaborative Study, which collates HIV data and found that 31 per cent of babies breastfed by their HIV positive mothers eventually developed their own HIV infection, whereas only 14 per cent of bottle-fed babies did so. These percentages must be regarded cautiously as there were over 700 bottle-fed babies and only 36 breastfed. The HIV positive mothers in Europe were discouraged from breastfeeding so those few who did must have been unusual women to defy the doctors. Perhaps they had been HIV positive for longer and were closer to developing AIDS when again there are higher levels of virus in the body. Regrettably their infection levels were never measured. Also it is likely that these babies received pre-lacteal fluids.

In contrast to semen, or blood in needles – where a few drops transmit HIV – breastmilk is a body fluid delivered in substantial amounts yet most breastfed babies of HIV positive mothers remain infection free. An explanation may lie in the fact that breastmilk, irrespective of the mother's HIV status, contains a unique substance which can prevent the virus from attaching itself to receptor cells. This is a hopeful sign but nevertheless the evidence of the risk of HIV transmission through breastfeeding means that infant feeding decisions must be considered carefully by mothers who know they are HIV positive. In May 1992, WHO and UNICEF issued a statement in which they advised that in 'settings' where infectious diseases are a major cause of baby deaths then breastfeeding must be promoted and supported, but in 'settings' where it is possible to use an alternative method, then HIV positive mothers should not breastfeed. The safest alternative to breastfeeding is donated, pasteurised breastmilk, given in a clean cup if bottle sterilisation is difficult. Breastmilk banks now test their donors for HIV and also pasteurise the milk. Unlike blood transfusion there has been no case of contaminated breastmilk.

The best way to protect babies is to protect women. Women's lack of power influences HIV transmission for few are able to make choices about sexual protection, to control their partners' sexual behaviours or persuade them to use condoms. Women also have less access than men to information because of lack of education, freedom and mobility. Some women become sex workers to survive and feed their children when there are few other ways of earning a living. The structures of economic oppression and inequality are making HIV and AIDS spread more rapidly. [30]

PSYCHOLOGICAL AND EMOTIONAL ASPECTS

It is breastfeeding rather than breastmilk that is the powerful emotional factor for the interaction between mother and child. When Brazilian law demanded facilities for breastfeeding at work, some factory employers organised for mothers to express and pool their milk for the crèches rather than allow them time off to suckle. This is sabotaging an important function of breastfeeding, the close skin-to-skin contact and the pleasure and love for both mother and baby. Expressing milk can take as long as suckling, but it is done outside the employer's time, so the pursuit of profit will not be interrupted. In fact breastfeeding can coincide with the mother's breaks, and the International Labour Organisation laid down that every woman has the right to two nursing breaks a day without loss of pay. A job that does not allow such time is in any case over-exhausting for a worker. Expressed milk is a useful back-up when it is impossible for mother and baby to be together, but all too often it is social prejudice and lack of organisational imagination, rather than logistics, which keeps them apart. It was 'discovered' in this century that babies in orphanages who received all their supposed nutritional requirements did not grow because they were not cuddled. Everyone needs to be stroked and touched and these actions actually influence hormone release, including digestive hormones such as gastrin and insulin. [31] Lonely people visit the hairdresser or the doctor more than necessary because it is their way of getting the touching they need. Pets are kept for stroking, cuddling and close physical contact with another live creature, and people buy 'cuddly' toys rather than hard ones for babies because of the tactile sensation. Women who have bottle-fed foster children after breastfeeding their own expose their breast so that the baby has the skin contact which they intuitively know is important for happy feeding. With bottle-feeding, the milk goes down rather quickly and not with the stop-start rhythm of breastfeeding, and the baby feels full before his oral and touching needs are satisfied. That is why a baby often needs a dummy or a thumb to make up for this lack, and it is remarkable how absent thumb or object sucking is in societies where prolonged breastfeeding is universal. It has become socially acceptable for a baby to suck anything, be it bottle, dummy, soft toy, blanket or the nearest adult finger, when the ideal object, a breast, is denied. Because babies are often less secure in the presence of strangers this is when they need the breast most, yet in industrialised society this is the time mothers are most discouraged from giving it. An empty breast can provide comfort and in some cultures men may offer their nipple to comfort a crying baby whose mother is absent. Breastfeeding is an inadequate word because it is not merely putting food in a stomach, it is also our first experience of love and it works both ways. Brazil has noted a reduction in the numbers of abandoned babies since breastfeeding rates have increased. Of course bottle-feeding mothers love their babies and in western society breastfeeding has been so damaged that it could actually spoil a mother/child relationship because of the tension that unhappy feeding could induce, but a bit of glass or plastic and rubber does not convey to the baby the primal contact that a soft, warm body can. Nor can bottle-feeding convey the warm sensual feelings that many women experience through suckling a baby.

BONDING

The concept of bonding was launched into paediatric consciousness in the 1970s with the work of Klaus and Kemmel. Observation of animals revealed the fact that infants were rejected

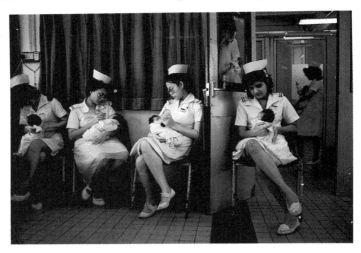

4a Nurses bottle-feeding newborns in a Singapore maternity ward (*Photo:* Raghu Rai)

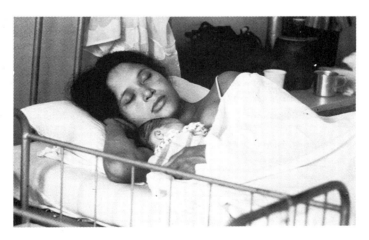

4b Woman sleeping with her newborn baby in a hospital bed (*Photo:* courtesy of UNICEF)
Who is bonding with whom?

if the mother could not nuzzle them within a certain time. Researchers who separated primate mothers and infants experimentally observed that the loss of contact was devastating and the effects could last through generations. Skin to skin contact after the birth affects the hormone levels and behaviour of both mother and baby. One observational film vividly illustrates the power of spontaneous mother/baby interaction. As the birth attendant gently places the baby on his mother's abdomen, he gradually crawls towards her breast, smelling, nuzzling, mouthing and exploring with little hands. At first the mother just holds her baby tenderly, but after about half an hour, oxytocin is coursing through her body, prompting her instinct to stroke and talk to her baby, who too makes little communicative noises, and as this happens, the mother's nipples slowly change shape. Eventually after around two hours of 'talking' and touching between mother and baby, the baby gapes his little mouth and suckles his mother's breast with consummate skill. It is a measure of the universal perversion of these natural talents that in 1991 UNICEF had to launch its global 'Baby Friendly Hospital Initiative', in an attempt to halt the 'normal' practice of babies being snatched away and bottle-fed, leaving mothers bereft and confused.

As hospitals routinely separated mothers and babies this made it much harder for women to feel comfortable with their newborns and therefore more inhibited about breastfeeding. For many ordinary people in the world to whom the idea of not cuddling babies as early and as often as possible is unthinkable, this revelation of research was a case of reinventing the wheel. The maternity ward supervision of bonding has been subject to ridicule because typically in some hospitals it has been made into a uniform, time-measured ritual. This is surely better than the cold callousness of the 'nursery' full of bawling newborns where there has been immeasurable and unnecessary suffering. However, every mother reacts differently, some take longer than others to fall in love with their babies and others never do. If an infant or mother is seriously ill, bonding may have to be deferred, but fortunately there seems to be human scope for emotional healing and love can survive many setbacks.

If you compare the breastfeeding couple with the relationship which seems to preoccupy twentieth-century western culture the most, the romantic attraction, 'bonding' is presumed to occur with the first kiss or meaningful physical contact. It is taken for granted that couples need to cuddle and that this strengthens the emotional bond, yet mothers are supposed to love their babies while at the same time unrestricted physical contact is discouraged. A baby's crying is biologically designed to motivate us to stop it. A breast is the best pacifier, yet in western society it is viewed merely as a conveyor of 'feeds'. Actual physical cruelty to babies is often triggered by an infant's ceaseless crying and many parents have felt an impulse to hurt their own child when they cannot stop this noise. I have not yet come across a case of this level of cruelty to small infants who are unrestrictedly breastfed, probably because the mother can always shut up the child by giving the breast. There are breastfed babies who continue to cry, but this is a much greater problem in western society. Among many possible causes are not only the loss of skills in holding and positioning babies, but also maternal dietary factors, with the baby possibly reacting to factors in the milk to which she may have been sensitised in the uterus. The German word for breastfeeding, *stillen*, means to quieten and soothe rather than to give food. This function is just as important as conveying nutrients to a stomach.

My own culture views physical contact with alarm. Many English feel unable to express their feelings physically. Touching strengthens the bonds of friendship and it is sad when custom inhibits actions such as stroking and holding hands which can diffuse aggression and misunderstanding. Jane Goodall has shown in her work with chimpanzees how effective these actions can be, enabling them to transcend their fear of one another. Television programmes reflect our social values when they show heterosexual contact and aggressive conflict as everyday images, but rarely showing non-sexual physical contact (except violence), such as suckling. A breastfeeding mother is being caressed and loved by her baby so it may be easier to love him or her, especially as babies are more contented when close to a human body. A tragic fact of life is that both physical and sexual abuse of small children is widespread and though not exclusively their crime, men are the principle abusers. Infants who spend their early life close to a mother's body are better protected than those left alone in cots and prams. Modern western society appears to be terribly confused about the borderline between physical closeness and genitally focused sexuality. Breastfeeding is on the borderline of these feelings and if our taboos are in turmoil, this may explain some of the rejection of breastfeeding.

BRAINS AND BREASTFEEDING

There is evidence that breastfeeding improves learning ability attributed by some scientists to the unique pattern of fats which build the brain tissue. Others attributed this to the notion that the 'type' of woman who breastfeeds (as usual ignoring societies where all women breastfeed) is more likely to stimulate her child. A significant advantage in intelligence quotient (IQ) was discovered in children born pre-term and who had breastmilk (through a feeding tube), and it was dose-related, the more breastmilk the higher the IQ. The researchers speculated that special fats, hormones and growth factors only found in human milk might be at work but they stressed that their results must not be extrapolated to full term babies. More serious are the long-term effects of inappropriate substitutes, for example both high protein and low chloride formulas (see page 240) are linked with later learning problems. [33]

BOTTLE-FEEDING AND BOTTLED-FEELINGS

I know that stating these facts can be painful or even enraging to some women who have not breastfed their children, but the continued denial of the superiority of breastfeeding and breastmilk, supposedly to spare women's feelings, is a patronising deception. The whine about 'not making mothers feel guilty' is such a cop-out. If someone told me I had been driving my car incorrectly or dangerously for years, of course I would be upset, but I do not think I should be denied that information just to spare my feelings. No woman need feel guilty for 'failing' to breastfeed. She has the right to feel angry for being denied support and information when she needed it. I did not bring up my first baby in the way I now believe is best. I tried to suckle him to a routine. I let him cry, I weaned him too early. He has survived physically and I hope emotionally. Luckily tough human babies can survive a lot of mistakes, but the more vulnerable ones cannot and it would be better not to have to put so many babies to the test.

One argument put forward in favour of bottle-feeding has been the fact that the father can feed the baby. Advertisers use this to sell their products. One such advertisement is in a US medical journal. [34] However I have not heard of large numbers of US doctor/fathers taking a career break to bottle-feed their children. It is ironic that only as breastfeeding has been becoming more common in the industrialised countries have fathers suddenly expressed interest in taking over this aspect of childcare. The reality is that few fathers actually do take the whole responsibility of infant care and most bottle-feeding is still done by mothers. I often wonder whose emotional needs we are discussing when this subject arises. A lot of honest men admit that they are jealous of breastfeeding babies and mothers; it is something that men cannot do and it can make them feel excluded. Actually there is some evidence that men can lactate, so maybe there is hope for them yet! Babies need other care besides feeding. Bottoms and noses have to be wiped, nappies changed; bathing, cuddling and massage are all important, and there are many months of weaning foods before they can feed themselves entirely. Lots of fathers and babies have warm, close relationships without the symbolic bottle- binding them together. New parents often forget that babies have a habit of hanging about the house for twenty years, so there is plenty of scope for paternal bliss. If fathers did everything for children except breastfeed they would be the main childcarers.

If breastfeeding is so wonderful, how is it that so many have survived artificial feeding? Firstly we have to remember that adaptation is part of evolution and the fact that humans are omnivores is a tremendous advantage. A survivor is just that and

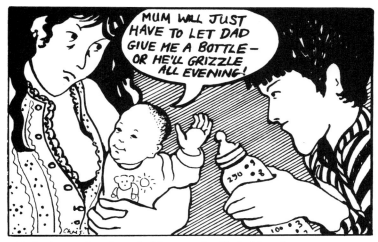

5 Father's emotional needs (Cartoon by Chris Mann)

many animals get by in less than ideal conditions. Survival involves a wide range of factors and food, though a priority, is only one. Genetics, living conditions, birth weight, birth spacing and a host of known and unknown factors all play a part. It is the increasing control of these factors, as well as the quality of the management of substitute feeding, that have contributed to the fall in infant mortality in the industrialised world. An exclusively breastfed child can die, just as an artificially fed child can thrive, because of the range of risk factors, but this does not mean the risk is equal. There is an account of a seventeenth-century man who, having been orphaned at two weeks old, was reared on beer and lived to be 70.[35] He was clearly rather special as are those babies today who survive without breastmilk; they do only because they live in the protectively organised environment of industrialised society.

What has happened in the industrialised world is that, while taking the risk of removing the ideal food and feeding method, there has been a progression in the elimination of many other immediate risk factors. It is important to remember that it is still only a minority of the world's population that can afford to take this risk and among this minority it is the better off who survive with no problems at all. There is a tremendous back-up system for those babies, not just clean water and dry housing but also of immunisation, health surveillance and speedy treatment in the case of illness. The poor bottle-fed child in Liverpool may develop severe diarrhoea, but health visitor surveillance, transport and medical services means there is the opportunity for speedy diagnosis and treatment. The poor rural breastfed baby in Africa might get malaria, but it can be more than a day's walk to the nearest clinic, and if it is planting or harvest time a mother cannot take a day or two off to get the baby there because the whole community's food supply for the year might be jeopardised by her absence. Without telephones, ambulances or decent roads there is no safety net for emergencies. This is what the real world is like for most people in it, and because people who live in industrialised countries are often unclear as to why artificial feeding is so dangerous in poorer countries I believe it is important to spell the reasons out in detail.

NORMAL CONDITIONS

Safe water

About one fifth of the world's population, just over a billion people, lack access to clean water. [36] Even uncontaminated water may not be safe for a child if it comes from a container rather than a tap, for however clean you are, contamination is more likely to occur. Running water from a tap inside your own home is one of the most effective health protections. Only 1 per cent of rural people in most of the poor countries have an internal tap. In urban areas the rate varies from 10 to 50 per cent, but those who do have inside water taps will be the rich. Every home in an elite suburb of Manila may have a luxury kitchen and bathroom, but in the urban squatter slums a family will be lucky if there is a water tap in their street. In many parts of the world people have to buy their water by the bucketful and therefore have to limit the amounts. Even if the water for a bottle-feed is boiled there is another problem. How do you cool a feed quickly if there is no running cold water? Everything stays hot for a long time when temperatures are normally high, and the more slowly milk cools the more time there is for bacteria in it to multiply.

An uncontaminated environment

Almost a third of the world's population, 1.7 billion people, lack access to adequate sanitation. [37] Disposal of waste, sewage treatment and vermin extermination are taken for granted in western society. If you live in one of the squatter slums of the world's cities, the only place to excrete may be in the street, your house is a breeding ground for insects and you will share your living quarters with many more people than the average North American or European. Consequently your baby will be exposed to more infections. In warm climates refrigeration could prevent food contamination, but only a tiny minority of households can afford fridges and with unreliable fuel supplies or shortage of spare parts, even those that exist might not always function.

Fuel

Even in wealthy regions where water is supposed to be safe, it is still necessary to boil water for a baby's feed as well as sterilise the bottle, teat and utensils in either boiling water, steam or a costly sterilising fluid. In Jakarta it costs US$30 million a year to boil water for home use. Whether it is wood, kerosene, charcoal or bottled gas, fuel is a major drain on the household budget. In Maputo families may spend half their income on fuel. It takes 200 grams of wood to boil a litre of water and it is women who gather wood, using up their scarce time and energy. A baby needs at least five feeds a day, yet poor people light the fire twice a day at the most so boiling water and utensils for every feed is impossible.

Money

Money is needed for fuel and in many places water, but the baby milk is often the most expensive food item ever purchased. In

Nigeria, it costs 264 per cent of the minimum urban wage to buy SMA infant formula. In one year the same money could purchase 158 kilos of fish, 137 of cow peas and 305 of cassava. Other children and mothers often go hungry in order to buy artificial milk. In Uganda baby milk would cost 900 per cent of a hospital cleaner's wages which means you would need 9 adults working full time to buy milk for one baby. Sometimes mothers who cannot find the cash to buy the next tin, 'stretch' the milk by overdiluting it. The feeding bottles and teats cost money too and as they become scratched and worn are even harder to clean.

Literacy

Even experienced health workers make errors in measuring out milk powder. You certainly need to be able to read the instructions on the label. Continued resistance to female education means that female illiteracy is higher than male, yet it is usually women who do the bottle-feeding. In twenty six countries over 75 per cent of women are illiterate. Many bottle-fed babies are fed by servants who often dare not admit they have problems understanding label instructions.

Medical care

In much of the world access to medical care is scarce and the services overstretched. In a relatively sophisticated country like Argentina only 21 per cent of rural people can get to health services and in Benin it is only 18 per cent of the entire population.[40] Even if parents can get to a clinic or hospital, children die because the queues are too long and there are not enough health workers to treat everyone quickly. You need transport to take your child to the health centre and you may have to pay. An episode of diarrhoea may need only oral rehydration therapy (ORT) (see box page 91), but if your child has a respiratory infection the doctor may prescribe antibiotics which are expensive. Women are usually employed in the informal sector where time off work means no pay. A mother may decide she cannot risk missing work, so she may buy one of the inappropriate drugs which are distributed and sold unethically. When a child gets diarrhoea, the gut can stay damaged for some time after the episode has ended and this affects the absorption of nutrients, so the child can become severely malnourished within a very short time. Conversely, if a child is undernourished by being fed diluted milk, the resulting malnutrition can lower resistance to infection and the child is more likely to succumb to attacks of gastroenteritis. This vicious cycle of infection and malnutrition has killed millions of children.

I wonder how many baby milk manufacturers have themselves bottle-fed babies in conditions of extreme poverty? In Mozambique I worked in an orphanage where we bottle-fed the babies. Our conditions were much better than in most homes. We had a clean, flat surface where we could prepare the bottles. We had an indoor tap which usually functioned, though it could take more than an hour to fill the kettle when water pressure was low. We usually had running water, though supply sometimes stopped for a day or so when something broke down at the pumping station or when the multinationals' sugar estates were being irrigated over the border in Swaziland. We washed our hands thoroughly, with soap when it was available. The place was cleaned daily, but that did not stop the mosquitos and flies coming in. We relied on bottled gas for fuel, but if there was a hitch in the supplies we had to make wood fires and bottle sterilisation was a real chore when you had to lug a great vat of boiling water from outside. We were lucky enough to have a fridge, but of course that depended on the electricity supply working. When the fridge broke down there were no spare parts. In spite of these relatively good conditions, there was more or less endemic diarrhoea. Once, when some tiny babies were very ill, we tried foster feeding, which the women involved were more than willing to do. It took half the time of preparing the milk feeds and saved those babies' lives.

CONFOUNDING VARIABLES

Breastfeeding is still better for babies in rich countries but there is a body of medical opinion which refutes this claim with the argument of 'confounding variables', a statistical nicety, which runs thus: 'When you "adjust" for other factors in a baby's life such as the mother's education, the family's social and economic status or the number of children in the household, then there is little difference between the effects of bottle or breastfeeding.' This means, quite correctly, that ignorance, poverty and overcrowding all affect infant health just as diet does. Of course there is a simple answer to this: merely provide every mother with a good education, a decent income, a warm, roomy house and effective, safe contraception and perhaps the breast and bottle debate could fade a little. Some members of the medical profession and managers of the baby food industry, who both profess their zeal for improving child health, are inhibited about publicly advocating these important changes. At the same time this lobby claims that 'we need industry' and that the more profitable transnational companies become, the more likely it is that Utopia will be achieved for all. However, as companies expand and become more profitable, so do the number of impoverished people.

Strangely enough, the confounding variables argument is not used by the same researchers when discussing extreme poverty. No one says, 'When you "adjust" for unsafe water, open sewers, flies and cardboard houses, there is no difference between bottle and breastfeeding.' What the 'confounding variables' arguments are really saying about data in industrialised countries is that if you are poor and uneducated, your baby is more likely to get ill and that if he were breastfed he might have a bit more protection against this likelihood. The fact that many poor mothers in industrialised countries have lost the skill and confidence to breastfeed, when poor mothers in some of the poorest regions have not, is in part due to the historical effects of the commercial/medical liaison which is a major topic of this book.

Other researchers have found that even after the statistical biases have been eliminated, that is, when 'adjustment' has been made, breastfeeding still saves lives and prevents disease.[41] In an intervention study to try to reduce 'possibly preventable' deaths in Sheffield, England, the largest single factor in the saving of life was the increase in breastfeeding.[42] When I quoted this to a

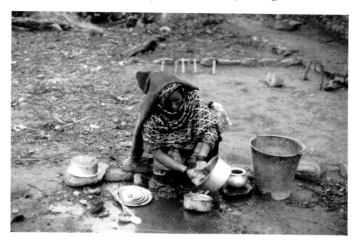

6a Normal conditions: an Asian woman cleans the cooking pots and
6b rubbish problems in urban South America (*Photo:* courtesy of
UNICEF)

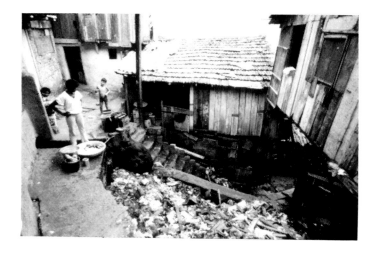

Anti-diarrhoeal drugs which immobilise the gut harm and kill babies, but are available all over the world.

Diarrhoea is dangerous because it depletes the baby's small body of water. Plain water does not rehydrate the body cells, because absorption is only facilitated by the presence and proportion of salts which are naturally present in the body's water. Doctors used to treat dehydrating babies with rehydration fluid through a drip into the veins. This is a skilled procedure which must be carried out by a trained person with a ready supply of drips and needles. By the 1970s researchers had discovered that a simple solution of boiled water, salt and sugar approximately matched the rehydration solution, that it was well absorbed when given by mouth and could be made up and administered by even an illiterate person. This meant that thousands of babies who were literally drying to death could be saved by their own mothers. This simple idea is called oral rehydration therapy; it has been found that many traditional diarrhoea remedies, such as coconut or rice water, provide a similar salt balance. Both traditional and orthodox western medical practice have often erroneously advocated stopping breastfeeding if a child has diarrhoea. The proportions of water, sodium, sugar and potassium in rehydration fluid are the same as in breastmilk. Ironically, water can carry diarrhoea-causing organisms yet is mistakenly given to breastfed babies. A study in hot, dry India found that breastfed babies given extra water took in less fluid overall than exclusively breastfed babies.
Sachdev et al *The Lancet* 1991

doctor with a vested interest in the baby food industry, he responded that it was not the actual breastmilk that had the effect, but some special quality about the 'type' of mother who wanted to breastfeed. It would be lovely if some intangible spiritual factor about women could actually save babies' lives and perhaps it does, but it is a rather unscientific claim. As Maureen Minchin points out, why should a father's occupation explain a child's illness more readily than the immense differences between a live biological fluid and a dead processed one?[43] A British study found that even after adjusting for all confounding variables, a bottle-fed child was five times more likely to suffer a significant episode of gastro-intestinal disease.[44a] Collecting feeding method data is difficult as breastfeeding is rarely defined and risky practices such as giving water go unrecorded.

The 'adjusters' argue as though bottle and breast were an equal choice. Do they imagine it is easier for a poor, uneducated mother to leap into a safe, wealthy environment than to breastfeed her baby? Social class is an important factor in infant feeding 'choice', though choice is a dubious term in societies where few people learn how to breastfeed and its practice is hidden and restricted by social and economic pressures. Moreover, the very same class who 'choose' to breastfeed in one society are the most consistent rejectors of the process in another. Educated women in Mozambique are more likely to stop breastfeeding earlier and bottle-feed than urban factory workers, yet in the UK the situation is the reverse. What the breast-feeding women in both societies had in common was access to good information and support, in Mozambique from their female friends and relatives and in the UK from the breastfeeding support groups and from books. Educated women in Mozambique were often cut off from female support structures and many had been exposed to western mores and misinformation. Social pressures compelled them to behave in a 'western' way. They were inhibited about bringing their babies to work. This was discouraged, but hospital cleaners would break the rules and just bring their babies because they felt it was more important to breastfeed their child than to conform to man-made restrictions. Less educated women in Britain have little access to the relearning sources of new information and help and their female relatives have often lost breastfeeding knowledge.

Increasing attention is being given to the effects of early nutrition on later health. Early abandonment of breastfeeding is associated with heart disease in later life. In Hong Kong where social conditions and infant survival have improved alongside breastfeeding decline, there is an alarming rise in high cholesterol levels among seven year olds.[44b] Early onset diabetes is clearly linked with absence of breastfeeding and may be triggered by cows' milk protein.[45] Even kidney transplants are significantly more successful if the patient was breastfed and even more so if a breastfed sibling donated the kidney.[46] Beef farmers know that an animal reared on its mother's milk produces better quality meat and even leather than one who is not. Even calves fed on processed cows' milk do not do as well as when suckled by the own mothers. Perhaps if you adjust for the confounding variables it will be found that it is just the calves born to well-educated, middle-class cows that do better.

WOMEN'S CAPACITY TO BREASTFEED

Women's capacity to produce milk varies widely, but their maximum potential output is rarely needed. As women can feed twins and triplets, being physiologically unable to produce enough milk for one baby is a rarity. Once again the concept of the 'good milker' comes from dairy cows. In fact a 'good milker' is a better description for the baby rather than the mother for usually if there is a problem it lies with the infant. For example, babies with cleft palates find suckling difficult because, depending on the severity of the condition, they actually lack the physical equipment needed for full milk stimulation, so unless the mother has another baby to keep the milk going she might find it hard to feed for an extended period.* However many women do succeed in expressing milk for many weeks either by hand or with a breast pump. Interaction with the baby is often forgotten. A woman who breastfed her premature baby told me how during the period when he had to be tube- and later spoonfed with her expressed milk, she always cuddled him before using a breastpump so as to stimulate her let-down reflex. Sadly she was the only mother on the ward for premature babies who continued breastfeeding, for none of the others had been helped to do this.

Experts have devoted much energy to expounding the reasons for not breastfeeding and they have made many mistakes. I used to accept that cleft-lip babies were, like those with cleft palates, impossible to breastfeed until I met a big, healthy, breastfed cleft-lipped toddler in Africa. Again I accepted the enduring medical folklore that 'successful breastfeeding is difficult with twins and virtually

*Some mothers do succeed in breastfeeding babies with cleft palates.

impossible with triplets'[47] until I met an African woman with seven-month old triplets all exclusively breastfed and, though small at birth, all the ideal weight for their age. This woman had five older children and was wryly amused by the Europeans' gasps of wonder at her capacity for something she took for granted. In 1991, two sets of quadruplets were fully breastfed by their mothers. One mother, whose babies were born at 28 weeks and in special care, was, within one week, producing a litre of milk each time she expressed. The account of the wet nurse Judith Waterford on page 160 shows that milk output can continue well into old age.

A baby may be born with a problem such as an inborn error of metabolism, a genetic 'mistake' which might mean he cannot process breastmilk. An example is galactosaemia, a condition occurring in perhaps one in 80,000 babies, whereby the absence of an enzyme in the blood means milk sugar cannot be metabolised, and neither breast nor any other milk can be taken. Before the discovery of this condition, these babies would obviously have died. This is where modern scientific knowledge is so useful, when it can actually manipulate and redirect these natural errors and protect parents from the sorrow of an infant death; in such cases the inventors of synthetic baby foods have played a useful part. Where medical science and its close companion, commerce, has been destructive is where, as in the case of infant feeding, it has tried to manipulate and redirect a very successful evolutionary strategy at the expense of health and lives of millions of babies.

IS BREASTFEEDING GOOD FOR YOU?

Humans being 'K strategists' (see page 32), it is unlikely that human reproduction would have evolved in such a way as to harm the mother. Once a woman has survived childbirth, 'nature' needs her to be able to reproduce again and there would be no evolutionary 'incentive' for lactation to be harmful. However, just as there existed in some cultures mythologies about male ejaculation 'draining' away a man's strength, so our ambivalent feelings about body fluids, together with our ruined experience of modern breastfeeding, have led to the idea that lactation is a 'drain' on the woman and is in some way harmful. In fact the opposite may be true.

Many people have looked with understandable sympathy at the overworked, underfed poor women, experiencing a lifetime's cycle of pregnancy and lactation, and have suggested that reducing the period of lactation would be of some relief. Because many western women find breastfeeding difficult they perceive it as a burden and because of ambiguous attitudes to the ties of motherhood, the baby is seen as a parasite. In fact women certainly need more food, their work burdens reduced and support in avoiding pregnancy if they choose, but lactation may have protective effects on the mother and when it is not perceived as burdensome it is not. I do not want to deny that some women do feel tired when they are breastfeeding, but I think that sometimes this tiredness is too readily attributed to the secretion of a fluid when the cause may be too much work, the stress of the experience and demands of a new baby and a lack of proper recuperation and support after what may have been a traumatic birth. When society is against what you are doing the emotional sense of isolation can be draining and many western mothers who dare not sleep with their babies often have their sleep broken excessively.

Breastfeeding and menstruation

A fully breastfeeding woman does not menstruate. There has been little detailed research into this possibly protective conservation of iron. The theoretical calculations indicate that the iron secreted into the breastmilk is equal to the iron that would have been lost in menstrual blood of the *average* woman. The quantity of iron in breastmilk is fairly consistent and extra iron in the diet does not increase the amount of iron in breastmilk. The *average* loss of iron at each menstrual period is 30 grams, which means that approximately 50 per cent of women might be protected from iron deficiency through breastfeeding by not having their usual heavy periods. There is also the factor that several diseases, for example endometrial (lining of the womb) cancer, are statistically linked to the number of menstrual periods a woman experiences in a lifetime, so that amenorrhoea may be a benefit in more than one way.[48] The contraceptive effect of lactational amenorrhoea is fully discussed in Chapter 4; it need only be said here that, worldwide, breastfeeding has prevented, and continues to prevent, more births than all other forms of birth control put together. Of course, not having periods also means no monthly pain or tension and saves money on tampons and sanitary towels or the chore of washing the cloths that many poor women use.

Bone disease

A controversial theory suggests an inverse link between osteoporosis, the brittle bone disease that is the curse of ageing women, and breastfeeding. Contrary to the popular idea that lactation drains the body of calcium, which does happen with cows, human lactation may even improve calcium metabolism and bone health. In one study, the women who had breastfed longer actually ate less protein, calcium, phosphorus and vitamin D (the nutrients thought important for bone condition), but had not developed osteoporosis. Those with less latational experience but 'better' diets had developed the disease. Prolactin (the milk-making hormone) speeds up the conversion of vitamin D to its active form which enhances calcium utilisation. Bone fractures have risen steeply in recent decades among western women, who have six times more fractures than Chinese women (whose rate equals that of Chinese men) who have less dietary calcium. Researchers speculate that inactivity, nutrition and use of prescription drugs are a cause, but forget to note that those Chinese old ladies probably breastfed for much longer than their western counterparts.[49]

Breast cancer

Breast cancer is a leading cause of death in industrialised society, but its causes are still not fully understood. As with other cancers of the reproductive system, the number of menstruations a woman experiences is significant. Protection has been attributed to early childbearing, diet and other environmental factors, but a group of women in China who customarily only breastfed from one breast were found, when they developed breast cancer, to have it only in the breast they had never used. Studies show that among both premenopausal and post-menopausal women, the risk of breast cancer decreased with increasing duration of lifetime lactation experience, although the effect was consistently stronger for pre-menopausal women. Among the many theories of breast cancer cause, one implicates a latent virus in cows' milk which when given in the form of processed baby milk during the neo-natal period may programme a female body for breast cancer in later life. [50]

NUTRITION AND THE DEMANDS OF LACTATION

The increased nutritional demands of lactation have probably been overestimated. What is clear is that no woman should be hungry or lack a nutritious diet whether she is breastfeeding or not. Women who are habitually well-nourished do not have to eat more food in order to breastfeed, though they may feel like it and should do so if they want to. Worldwide, women come last when it comes to food distribution, for two reasons. Firstly, as the poorest, their limited purchasing power means they cannot buy the food they need. Secondly, within the household women come last in the distribution system. Many cultural practices assume that a woman goes without in order to feed the family or, as in parts of India, she fasts in order to bring holiness on the household. In the industrialised societies slenderness is so prized that women will often try to 'slim' and go on an exhausting crash diet, the aim being to resume a pre-pregnancy figure as quickly as possible. Increasing poverty in the developed world is reviving the tradition of 'mum going without' to feed the family.

Women do still maintain adequate growth in their babies even when they are undernourished. During the West Darfur famine in the Sudan in 1984 and 1985, the infant mortality rate did not increase whereas the child mortality rate quadrupled. This protection for babies was attributed to exclusive breastfeeding. Moreover, the mothers' mortality rates were lower than the overall adult death rate. These facts contrast tragically with those of the 1991 plight of the Kurdish refugees whose babies died because, unlike the Sudanese women, their mothers believed they could not breastfeed. Some ill-informed aid workers supplied bottles and powdered milk, thus contributing to the death rates.

It is still controversial whether food supplements have any effect on milk output and the baby's behaviour is thought to be far more crucial. I believe that extra food may increase the supply and that when this happens the baby suckles less avidly and the amount decreases to whatever the baby was demanding before the food was given. There is no evidence to show that prolonged or repeated lactations (as opposed to too many pregnancies or overwork) ever damaged any woman. The mother of a colleague of mine brought up ten healthy children, all breastfed for two years, and she always observed the Ramadam fast. Others experience a reduction if they do not eat and drink a lot, but they usually live in western society where anxiety about breastfeeding is maintained by social messages and frequent suckling is discouraged. There are many foods which are used as milk stimulants (called galactagogues by lovers of arcane definitions) and they appear to be effective. As they have not been fully researched it is unknown whether their effects are physiological or psychological. If they work they are useful, and women's own personal reports have convinced me of their efficacy. The only time some women can relax and stop work is to feed their babies, and though this should be a right whether they are breastfeeding or not, the suggestion that women should cease breastfeeding because they are badly nourished implies an indifference to the maltreatment of women. The right to food and rest for a woman should have an equal place with the concern about the life of her child. The zeal to reduce the tragic infant mortality rates in poor communities is sometimes accompanied by a more passive acceptance of the hard lives of women, as though it is beyond the scope of a health worker to change this situation. The problem is that reduced infant mortality rate statistics are a very clear indicator of a health worker's successful input whereas the statement that mothers felt less tired has not yet become scientifically respectable. Most women are justifiably proud of suckling their children; the fact that a baby can quickly double its birth weight just from a mother's breast is a satisfying experience. Producing a new life gives pride to many women, however much discrimination they suffer as a result, preserving that new life with their own milk confirms that pride. Taking away this gift can be damaging to women as well as babies. [51]

Population, Fertility and Sex

ARE DEAD BABIES USEFUL?

When I started to write this book, a friend asked how breastfeeding would possibly have anything to do with politics. In answer I described the circumstances of a woman in a South American slum who was forbidden to take her baby to work and left it to be bottle-fed by an older child while she earned the pittance to feed the whole family. In the slum where they lived artificial feeding was clearly unsafe and the baby died. My friend responded, 'But isn't it a good thing if those babies die as there are far too many of them anyway?' As residents of Britain, both she and I live in one of the most densely populated areas of the world, which contributes more pollution to the seas and air of Europe than any other country and where in England alone well over 400,000 people are homeless.[1] Yet if I had suggested we should leave her daughter to die of pneumonia as a contribution to the UK overcrowding problems she would have understandably broken off our friendship.

I quote this story because I think my friend's reaction is not unusual and it encompasses a series of popular ideas about the causes of world poverty. She, like so many people, believes that there is a problem of overpopulation in the poorer countries of the world and that increasing the infant mortality rate will resolve this. Linked with this belief is the assumption that somehow the poor are the cause of their own poverty because they reproduce themselves excessively. Overpopulation is perceived to be a problem partly because of the intense competition for resources, yet the poor utilise far fewer of these than the rich. It has been calculated that the average North American uses in one day what a poor person in India might use in a year. The 16 million babies born each year in the rich world will have four times as great an impact on earth's resources as the 109 million born in the poor world. There is much publicity about tiny groups of the poorest people in the Sahel or Nepal using up sparce firewood that they collect with their own energy input, but scant mention of the 26 million tons of water, 21,000 gallons of gasoline, 10,150 pounds of meat, and 9,000 pounds of wheat, all produced at a very high energy input, that the average US citizen or western European uses up in a lifetime.[2] Furthermore, whereas every poor person is struggling simply to stay alive, every rich person is energetically contributing to a system of economic 'growth' which depends on increasing consumption and production which poisons the environment and will eventually exhaust the finite resources of the earth. The poor are only usually damaging their environment because the alternative is death; we, however, do it because we live in a system which must stimulate desires rather than merely satisfy needs in order to perpetuate itself. Rather than redistribute resources we engage in a system which is designed to stimulate and fulfil greed and we damp down the consciousness of injustice within the industrialised nations by making the gain or deprivation of non-essential consumer goods the primary motive of many people's lives. We, and also some of the elite of the developing countries, do this on the backs of the world's poorest people. Instead of acknowledging that it is their labour, their raw materials and their contribution to the debt repayment structure which provide us with our daily bread, we convince ourselves that they are dependent, incompetent and too numerous. The very dependency and supposed incompetence of the poor is essential for our own survival, however, for if no one borrowed money, how could 'our' money 'grow' and the financial system function? If no one were diagnosed as incompetent, to whom would the experts sell their expertise? If the birth rates were not so high, to whom would we peddle our contraceptives? The population explosion may be a problem for poor countries, but only because the population explosions of the industrialised countries were linked to the establishment of a system which required the continued extraction of resources from those countries at a deliberately maintained low and unfair price.

Until the nineteenth century in England, and probably in other parts of Europe, it was the rich who produced the very large families and not the mass of the people, who controlled their fertility quite consistently through late marriage, breastfeeding, and traditional birth limitation methods. These include *coitus interruptus*, abstinence and also the use of such 'mechanical' methods as vaginal sponges, herbal potions and induced abortion, which was morally condoned by religious authority if it occurred before the 'quickening' of the foetus which was believed to be the moment the soul entered the body.

Because most researchers with influence in high places have been men and most of this knowledge has lain with women, there has been an information gap and an arrogant assumption that until recent times people were passively fertile. A Ugandan friend told me how her grandmother had been sexually active all her life and yet only wanted and had one child: 'I wish I knew how she managed this', my friend recounted. Most 'primitive' tribes have always planned their reproduction far more carefully than, until recently, industrialised society has. Moreover, polygamous groups are often more sexually restrained than many individuals in allegedly monogamous societies.

Wealthy families are left out of the argument. The Kennedys in the US were known for their numerous children, yet they are not cited as contributing to the population problem. In Britain, HRH the Duke of Edinburgh cited in a TV programme the increasing population as the cause of environmental degradation in Africa.[3] As the father of four children, twice the amount recommended for population stability, resident in an oversized house in a city with horrendous housing shortages and himself a more avid consumer of natural resources than any nomad, his castigation of poor Africans has a curious irony. The 'population problem' is seen as something that happens in the Indian countryside or a Nairobi slum is cited as the cause of hunger and poverty, yet our own population explosions reshaped world economic structures to the permanent disadvantage of the now poor countries and of the environment. The idea that more dead babies will reduce world population is nonsense and in fact has the opposite effect. It has been demonstrated repeatedly that when people are certain their children have more chance of surviving, they will voluntarily reduce family size. This happened in Europe in the twentieth century when public health measures and better living standards made life less hazardous. It also happened in poor regions. The state of Kerala in India is an example of an area where improved health and education services had a significant effect on family limitation. These changes often take place within a region on a class basis, which has contributed to the idea of the poor being the principal culprits in the breeding game. The better-off have greater access to medical services, health benefits and information, so if a child gets ill they can be confident that help will be available quickly (speed of action is more often the life and death factor than the nature of treatment). Poor children often die needlessly because they reach the clinic or hospital too late. Rural people may continue to have more children because several could die and they know this. Chances of survival are crucial in decisions about family size which are made rationally, often for sound economic reasons.

What is more shocking is that I have to justify in demographic terms that babies should not die unnecessarily, implying that if it were good for the world as a whole we should accept it. My friend who did not accept it had never lost a child, but those I know who have, whatever society they come from, never lose the pain, however much joy other children give them. She, I am sure, would have been filled with compassion if my baby had died, but she calmly countenanced the death of 'their' babies. It is this ability to detach ourselves from other people's tragedies that is so dangerous. It is this 'switching off' which allowed the Nazis to deal as they did with another group they defined as a 'problem'. We are properly horrified when we hear of the deliberate slaughter of children but when the only cause of a baby's death is that his mother cannot have him near her to feed and protect, this is a kind of murder – a murder through indifference.

BREASTFEEDING AND FERTILITY

Some people see the rapid expansion of population as the most serious of the world's problems, while others believe that the attempt to control that expansion is genocide. High populations are seen both as the triggers of beneficial change and as the cause of increased poverty and degradation. Religious and political ideas about population control arouse furious debate and national and international policies can be reversed overnight, often with no consultation with those most affected by such changes. Why did a population explosion happen? There are many and complex reasons and expert demographers will continue to debate them, but I want to examine here two aspects which particulary affect women.

It has been taken for granted that in pre-industrial Europe both birth and death rates were high and that the benefits of industrialisation, such as medical knowledge and greater food supply, led to the survival of more babies thus precipitating the population explosion. As I will explain further in Chapters 5 and 6, certainly for England this is a false picture. Though overall deaths did fall, during the nineteenth century in England the infant mortality rate rose. Marriage and childbearing began earlier as the nineteenth century progressed and pregnancies were more closely spaced probably because unrestricted breastfeeding gradually declined.

Another important factor was that during the nineteenth and twentieth centuries in the industrialising countries there was a fall in the age of menarche. In the middle of the last century girls started their periods at about 16 years or older; now the average age is about 13 in most industrialised countries and in the USA it is even younger. Theories about the cause of this trend include climatic changes, the influence of artificial light and psychosexual stimulation. Early menarche is also linked to earlier increased height and body weight. The child growth expert J. M. Tanner states that the causes are probably multiple, but that 'better' nutrition is a major factor, perhaps in particular more protein and calories in infancy.[4] This idea of 'better' nutrition is a controversial claim in relation to women, for early menarche increases the likelihood of health problems such as breast and uterine cancer (see pages 96 and 97); it also increases the chances of conception way beyond most women's desired number of children. I do not know whether the development of sexual drive is linked to the onset of menstruation, but I do know that modern teenage girls have problems coping with their own sexual desire and with social pressures to appear sexy and heterosexual, and yet avoid sex and pregnancy.

Tanner's claim that nutrition in early infancy plays a part in age of menarche indicates that perhaps earlier weaning or early introduction of supplementary foods to a girl baby might play a crucial part and be a disadvantage in a woman's long-term reproductive life. If breastfeeding can alter something as subtle as kidney transplant acceptance (see page 93), why not lifetime endocrinological patterns? Certainly earlier menarche seems to go hand in hand with industrialisation and 'progress'. Changes in infant feeding habits are linked with these and it will be interesting to see whether the daughters of women who have exclusively breastfed and have not introduced weaning foods early will conform to the trend. This idea is speculative, but it ties in with the common biological feedback pattern that when messages get through that there is excess food in the habitat, then reproduction can be maximised.

Because of earlier menarche, the likelihood of teenage pregnancy increased throughout the nineteenth and twentieth centuries and this probably contributed to the rising illegitimacy rates in England during the nineteenth century. The devastating effects of this change on the lives of millions of teenage girls persecuted for their fertility have not been fully explored. To this day 'under age' mothers suffer appalling discrimination as a result of this effect of 'better' nutrition. Whether surviving children in the nineteenth century were abandoned to orphanages and 'baby farms' or absorbed into the family, this would have contributed to population increase, for these children would themselves have reached reproductive age while their mothers were still fertile. Age of childbearing and child spacing are two crucial factors in demographic patterns. It has been calculated that the population stabilising effect of the controversial Chinese one-child policy could be equally achieved by a policy of universal postponement of marriage (meaning first pregnancy) until over the age of 25 and the birth of two children per family as long as they were four years apart.[5] The pattern of well-spaced births and late marriage existed in England before the Industrial Revolution and probably in other parts of Europe too. Both late menarche and breast-feeding contributed significantly to child spacing in pre-industrial Europe and still does in the developing world, for breastfeeding prevents more births worldwide than all other forms of contraception put together.

Demography is too complex an issue to explore thoroughly in this book, but what is clear is that the west's export and promotion of artificial baby foods, together with the grosser errors in infant feeding techniques disseminated by health workers, have had a serious effect on birth spacing, which is a key factor in both demographic trends and in the well-being of individual women. This method of fertility control had been recognised since ancient times, but its importance was forgotten and ignored during the last two centuries because the changes in social organisation and in breastfeeding practices damaged its effectiveness. A seventeenth-century working Englishwoman married late and had well-spaced pregnancies. She used breastfeeding both to supplement her living and to space and limit her own childbearing. As unrestricted breastfeeding was the normal practice in those days she would have been unlikely to ovulate. Wealthy women were discouraged from feeding their own babies in order to reproduce greater numbers of the nobility. Slaves had their breastfeeding time limited so that they could breed more slaves for their owners. Yet by the twentieth century in Europe the use of lactation as a means of child spacing was not discussed or considered by doctors or advocates of birth control. The concept survived in the folklore, but usually as a warning that 'it didn't work'. The information was probably passed from woman to woman and became one of the much-despised 'old wives' tales'. My own mother (born in 1912) recounted that as a child she was shocked to see an Irish relative suckling her 2-year-old and said, 'I suspect she was doing it to try and avoid getting pregnant but you know that's an old wives' tale'. As scheduled and limited feeding times and earlier introduction of other milks and foods became commoner, more women probably found that breastfeeding 'let them down'. Unaware of the mechanisms that controlled ovulation and of the damage to breastfeeding practices, they believed their grand-mothers to be ignorant and mistaken.

KICKING THE BABY OUT OF BED

By the twentieth century breastfeeding in much of western Europe and North America was quite different behaviourally from what it had been and what it still is in the areas of the world where it has not been disrupted. As the 'men of sense' (see page 41) took over the management from women, new ideas came into vogue. First came the limiting of feeds to an ideal of not more than five times a day, the prohibition of night feeding and then a limiting of the actual feed times. Only someone who did not spend twenty-four hours a day with a baby could have thought of restricting feeding time. These ideas had arisen from the dread of overfeeding, but they actually caused the problem of under-feeding, as the baby was prevented from stimulating the amount of milk she actually needed. Consequently there was a greater requirement for supplements which in turn decreased the baby's control of the breast milk supply. The discouragement of sleeping with the baby at night, which had been the norm since the dawn of human life, spread throughout the nineteenth century. In England, the early twentieth century health visitors zealously handed out banana boxes (available via cheap colonial labour) to serve as cradles in order to try and stamp out the habit of mothers and babies sleeping together. This was to prevent overlaying, supposedly a common cause of infant death, though this is debatable. Such deaths are unreported in those countries where it is still custom for babies and mothers to sleep together. What this separation did do was increase the risk of infant hypothermia, maybe cot (crib) death and lessen the important contraceptive protection of night suckling which is crucial for the maintenance of the frequent nipple stimulation necessary to maintain anovulation. A mother sleeping with her baby in her arms might not even be awakened, but that occasional mouthing is an important contraceptive. With these reductions in suckling time and the increasing promotion and use of other infant foods, mothers were truly breastfeeding less and less. Even the use of a dummy or boiled water given by spoon can reduce the nipple stimulation needed to maintain infertility.

THE MECHANISMS OF LACTATIONAL FERTILITY CONTROL

Most women who are breastfeeding do not menstruate and for thousands of years many have known that there is a connection between the resumption of menstruation and fertility. Certain groups actually shortened the period of breastfeeding so as to increase their birth rate. There has not been a great deal of communication between ordinary women (who may be reticent about discussing their bodies' functions) and researchers who until recently had mostly been men. Consequently this 'old wives' tale' was disregarded for many years.

> The tribe I was with must have used some method of contraception, possibly an abortifacient, although I never managed to find out how they worked it. Anyway, the women had children more or less once every four years and for the first four years of the child's life its mother was never out of its sight. (Crashaw the anthropologist, speaking in *Savages*, a play by Christopher Hampton, 1974.)

The strength and amount of the baby's suckling influences the brain's output of the hormones which control a woman's fertility. As long as the baby is suckling at least six times a day, amounting to sixty-five minutes in total and preferably including some night feeding, a woman is unlikely to release a ripe egg (ovulate) from her ovary. Most women do not ovulate until after they have resumed menstruation, though about 10 per cent might do so prior to their first period. This is more likely to happen the longer the lactation lasts, so that women who breastfeed for several years are the ones who are most likely to have a pre-menstrual ovulation. So for most women, in the early months, as long as they and their babies are together and they can suckle whenever they want, infertility is maintained. The factor which dramatically decreases suckling and therefore increases the possibility of pregnancy, if the woman is heterosexually active, is the introduction of supplementary foods to the baby. This means that juices, water, artificial baby milk, gruels, dummies or even sucking a thumb or a blanket could alter the suckling behaviour and hence the contraceptive effect of breastfeeding. If suckling is frequent then duration of suckling is less important, but the western habit of 'feed' times with clock watching and boiled water in between 'feeds' would certainly have disturbed this biological mechanism. The number of unwanted pregnancies (and miscarriages) will have increased all over the world where medical advice and commercial misinformation has interfered with normal breastfeeding.

This breastfeeding infertility is thought to be due to the suppression of the release of a hormone called gonadotrophin-releasing hormone (GnRH), necessary for the secretion of luteinising hormone (LH) which is needed for the maturation of the egg (ovum). This activity happens in the hypothalmus, that part of the brain above the pituitary gland which controls thirst, hunger and sexual function and is also believed to be linked with emotional activity and sleep patterns. The precise mechanism is not understood but one theory, derived from animal studies, is that suckling might increase the opiate activity, in the hypothalmus and that this suppresses the GnRH release. Interestingly, heroin use suppresses gonadotrophin and causes an increase in prolactin levels just as in lactation. There has been a recent interest in natural opiate activity; breastfeeding does make some women feel great and perhaps this is one reason why. Because when blood serum levels of prolactin (the milk-making hormone) were measured, investigators noticed a rise that correlated with infertility, it used to be thought that this hormone was itself the inhibitor of ovulation, but now it is thought merely to accompany the process. Prolactin is also stimulated by frequency suckling, so that the levels measured in a woman's blood serum can indicate her likelihood of being fertile. The problem is that women can vary and one woman may be infertile at a certain level of serum prolactin while another is not. Because of this, it is difficult to lay down a norm which could indicate to individual women when they are infertile; there are always the exceptional mothers and babies. Alan McNeilly, who has researched this subject, told of one woman who had such a rapid let-down reflex that her baby took all the milk needed in two minutes and did not demand more than around twelve minutes' suckling time during the twenty-four hours so that it was impossible to reach the level of suckling needed to prevent ovulation. [6]

The biochemical tests used to assess prolactin and ovulatary state are designed for scientific research and for batches of a hundred samples. There are home tests on the market for non-lactating women to assess their hormone levels, but they are expensive and designed for use once a month. A lactating woman wanting to know whether she has ovulated might need to test every day. Women trying to assess their return to fertility might be forced to achieve a level of self-observation regarding frequency and duration of feeds which spoils the spontaneity of breastfeeding. One contraceptive that is being developed is a nasal spray which influences the hormone activity of the hypothalmus so as to suppress ovulation. It has been tested on breastfeeding women and allegedly has no biological activity in the baby. [7] However many women are suspicious of 'scientific' control of their bodies, both because any adverse effects can only be discovered by long-term use by large numbers of women and because it means they are dependent on the pharmacologist for their fertility control. What seems important in this issue is for all women to have access to knowledge of breastfeeding anovulation patterns and to work out their own ways of using it, if they wish, to manage their fertility in the way they finds suits them. As food supplements to the baby have such a dramatic effect on suckling frequency, it would be easy for a mother to understand that when she decides to introduce other foods, that is the time to know she is at the risk of conception, even if she has not resumed her periods. A lot has been learned about this subject through observations in different communities. The

!Kung women of the Kalahari desert have a nomadic lifestyle and a completed family size of four to five children, with an average birth interval of just over four years. The !Kung women start menstruating late (at about 15½ years) and reproducing even later (19½). The effect on fertility of breastfeeding was noticed because if a !Kung baby died the mother very soon became pregnant again. Contraception is not used, nor are their any sex taboos during lactation. A baby really does suckle on demand, about four times an hour and all through the night while her mother is sleeping, and this continues for three or four years. The baby stays close to her mother's body and helps herself at will. A woman who feeds like this is not burdened by breastfeeding, indeed it is almost unconscious behaviour. In fact, although she might feed forty-eight times in the twenty-four hours, in contrast to Scottish or US women's six to eight times, the total feeding time is the same.[7b]

As soon as breastfeeding behaviour is controlled, its contraceptive effect is lessened. The Hutterites, a religious community in North America who use no birth control methods, breastfeed to a schedule for one year and supplement early. Their average family size is just over ten children with about two years between each baby. Then there are examples from industrialised society where the custom until recently has been either not to breastfeed or to breastfeed to a schedule and usually (because of the schedule) with supplemental artificial foods. Mrs Margaret McNaught, one of Britain's 'champion mothers', had twenty-two single children in twenty-eight years, which is a mean interval of 1.3 years between each birth.[8] Mrs McNaught did not breastfeed her children, and was given stilboestrol as a lactation suppressant at birth. If she had breastfed each child for just three months the McNaught family might have been five fewer and this little family population explosion would have been reduced by almost a quarter. I do not wish to show any disrespect to the McNaught family, but their example shows how significant lactation suppression can be on one woman's fertility. The health workers persuaded women around the world to reduce their duration of breastfeeding and the companies which managed to get women to stop even earlier have had a potent effect on the world's population explosion, yet the false presentation of this situation as a problem caused by irresponsible individuals has prompted the unthinking genocidal sentiments of many people like my friend.

What appeals to me about this fascinating strategy of anovulation during lactation is that it destroys the arguments made by some religious and cultural groups that nature designed sexual activity only for procreation.

THE NUTRITIONAL ANGLE

For several years a team of researchers have been investigating the inhabitants of Keneba, a village in the Gambia in West Africa. One of their projects was to supplement lactating women's diet to see if this would increase their milk supply. The women do extremely hard agricultural work on a much lower energy diet than western women eat and are either pregnant or lactating for most of their adult lives. The supplement did not appear to make any significant difference to their milk output as measured by the baby's intake, and on the whole the researchers had to conclude that food intake did not influence milk supply. What did happen was that after taking the dietary supplement, the mothers' prolactin levels went down and some of them ovulated; the scientists were faced with the dilemma that in recommending more food for lactating women they might be harming their health by creating the risk of a too-early pregnancy. The Keneba women observed strict sexual taboos during lactation so they were not actually at risk, but the scientists were seeking general data for all women, particularly in poor countries. It would have been nice to show conclusively that you only had to feed women more food and they could produce more milk. Several other researchers had shown this could happen but there was always criticism of the study methods.

Some deduced that nutritional status itself influenced prolactin levels, but others thought that what had happened was that the supplement had in fact increased the rate at which breastmilk was made and consequently the babies had suckled less (that is for a shorter time and perhaps less avidly), thus decreasing the level of stimulation, and so the final quantity of milk was the same as before. This is borne out by the fact that when comparisons are made between well-nourished English mothers and the less-nourished Keneba women, their milk output is found to be the same. The African woman suckles more frequently and therefore has greater nipple stimulation which maintains her infertile status. This makes biological sense because in the food-abundant western environment, a woman who is capable of producing lots of milk with minimal stimulation from her baby can sustain another pregnancy and lactation with less risk to herself and her child than the mother in the precarious environment of seasonal food shortages. However this does not mean that fertility is not suppressed in well-nourished women. A study of Scottish women showed strong correlations between night feedings, frequency of feedings, the delayed introduction of supplements and ovulation. Whereas bottle-feeding mothers ovulated, on average, eleven weeks after delivery, the breastfeeders ovulated forty weeks later. In Chile, a group of 422 middle class women were informed and helped to use breastfeeding as a family planning method during the first 6 months after childbirth. The result was a 99.5 efficacy rate which is similar to other contraceptive methods.[9]

WHY DO WE DISLIKE BABIES?

I know of several breastfeeding women, all well-nourished, who have used lactation successfully as a means of birth spacing, and some stopped breastfeeding specifically because they were anxious to conceive. What is relevant is how despised still are women who actually want to feed their babies frequently and exclusively. There is terrific pressure from health workers, relatives and society as a whole for mothers to 'get back to normal'. That means not having a baby close to their body or in their bed and most definitely not giving the child totally free access to a breast. People will accept any means of shutting up a child's crying except putting a breast in its mouth. The negative feelings about this behaviour are astonishingly strong, especially for older babies. The fact that responding to a child's cries by giving her the breast was normal for 99 per cent of our existence and was a reason for survival of human beings makes current standards of normality questionable. Why do people in modern industrialised society feel so disturbed by seeing a mother and baby in close contact? Perhaps they are experiencing powerful unconscious feelings derived from their own infancy. Many adults around today would not have had the kind of cuddly babyhood experience that so many people in other societies had. With the cultural acceptance of frequent crying, the enforced physical separation from our mothers and the contact with a parent who would inevitably have been tense from having to tolerate the noise of a wailing baby, most of us would have experienced sadness very early in our lives, well before we could understand or cope with it. Babies tend to be loathed by many people, especially where rigidity in childcare has been well established for several generations. It seems likely that the presence of a baby stirs up feelings of a sad period in our own lives and we can project that onto the baby. People in western society get angry or upset when they think a baby is dominating the attention of an adult, perhaps because it unconsciously reminds them of their own inability to get their needs met as a baby. The 'loud noise at one end and no sense of responsibility at the other' definition of a baby denies the vulnerability of a new child. Similar factors may influence the rates of post-natal depression. Post-natal depression is considered by some to be hormonal in origin, yet why the hormonal state is assumed to precede the emotional state is unexplained. It is well known that fear stimulates adrenalin, not vice versa; why, then,

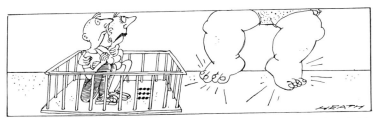

7   Our terror of babies. (Cartoon by Michael Heath, reprinted with his permission)

cannot sorrow stimulate certain hormonal states? When a woman has a baby it may trigger unconscious memories of her own birth and babyhood, which may have been very sad if she were separated at birth, left to cry and only cuddled at infrequent intervals, as was the rule for many years. Indeed one writer on post-natal depression, who experienced it herself, then goes on to say that she was left to cry as a baby and it did not do her any harm. [10]

It is so evident in those societies where babies are nurtured, never left to cry and breastfed whenever they ask, that not only are the babies far more socially pleasing in that they are more content and alert, but also that adults in those societies do not view babies with the alarm and revulsion that so many people show in my own society. Also, where babies are cherished, children usually appear better socially integrated than in some western societies. One rarely meets the whining 'brat' who so often justifies the exclusion of children from adult company. The extremes of bitchiness and horror shown by some adults' over-attention to a baby is more than cultural habit; it has some deeper emotional cause. Attention shown to a new car is tolerated far more.

Here is an account from travellers in Nepal.

> We stopped one night in a tea house in the Himalayas. The mother was cooking, but stopped to breastfeed the baby and the father took over at the stove. After the meal, when everything was cleared and put away, the parents began what was obviously a nightly ritual. The baby was lovingly massaged with oil and it was evident that both the parents and the baby thoroughly enjoyed the procedure. The baby was gurgling, the parents were smiling and sharing the task, one doing between the toes while the other concentrated on another area. Eventually the baby fell into a profound and peaceful sleep and the whole family retired contentedly to bed. [11]

Compare this with a typical British scene where the family are watching television and groan when they hear the baby wake up in its expensively equipped nursery upstairs. There might be a bit of bickering as to who should have to go and get it back to sleep. If a few minutes of jiggling does not work, or a dummy or bottle poked in its mouth, then the parents may have to resort to a dose of pharmacological tranquilliser. I am well aware that poor Nepal has high infant mortality rates and therefore babies are more precious, but it would be nice if western babies gave as much pleasure, especially to their poor, baffled parents. Babies who do not sleep twelve hours a night alone in a cot, a few weeks after birth, are seen as a 'problem'. Certainly, I know myself, it is, but as much because the baby is not conforming to a false ideal as because of the mother's tiredness. Because we have lost the art and joy of baby care, parenthood can often be a devastatingly painful experience and a lot of this ineptness may come from our own lack of mothering. Many parents who are physically violent with their infants are found to have suffered the same damage themselves as babies. Most of us did not experience this extreme, but rather a misguided neglect because a few influential, and usually male, gurus dictated childcare practices. One of the best known of these was Truby King, a New Zealand doctor whose ideas gained a foothold during the 1920s, 1930s and 1940s. He was very 'pro' breastfeeding and a stickler for rigid routines. Just like his predecessor William Cadogan, he propagated a mixture of sensible and ridiculous theories. To his credit he was effective in reducing the infant mortality rate in New Zealand and establishing infant welfare as a topic of importance. Dr King was obsessed, as were many of his colleagues, with 'resting the stomach': 'A clean-swept stomach effectively scotches microbes which might otherwise cause fermentation, indigestion, diarrhoea, etc.' Also in common with his eighteenth-century predecessor, he regretted the fact that women were the childcarers:

> Were the secretion of milk and the feeding of the baby the functions of men and not women, no man – inside or outside the medical profession – would nurse his baby more often than five times in the twenty-four hours, if he knew that the baby would do as well or better with only five feedings. Why should it be otherwise with women? [12]

Perhaps it was because many mothers were not so emotionally crippled as Dr King and his peers, able to ignore the cries of a child in need of food or physical contact. However a couple of generations of women bravely attempted to deny their own and their child's feelings, and even today many mothers who 'give in' to their babies still meet disapproval in everyday life in the western world.

These misguided and cruel ideas were able to gain a foothold because of widespread literacy, control of women by medical authority and the breakdown of traditional support systems. The focus on the mother alone to provide all nurture is a cruel and unjust burden which is linked to the economic system. A rural Thai woman remarked incredulously to Penny van Esterick, 'How can a woman give birth and raise a child without her mother's assistance?'[13] In her society babies are cherished, give a lot of joy and are never physically chastised.

On the positive side of this cyclical/cultural effect of baby care is the response of a mother who told me that she had discovered her own infantile sadness through psychotherapy, but that loving her own child and responding to his needs through breastfeeding and close physical contact helped heal her own pain. This endorses the fact that babies are born able to take an equal part in their first relationships, and if they are not distorted by outside influences the relationship between a baby and her carers can help the adults to grow as well as the child.

SEX AND BREASTFEEDING

Some societies advocate sexual abstinence during lactation. This taboo is supposedly unknown in hunter-gatherer societies, but appears among early agriculturalists. This may have evolved in food-abundant societies (many areas of the world where hunger is now normal were formerly producers of surplus foods and agricultural products, which is why they were so attractive to colonial invaders) where women found that they were becoming pregnant earlier than was desirable. This indicates that though people might have been aware of the lactational protection, they also knew that in some regions it was not always 100 per cent effective, and it was so important to space births that they would not take any risks. It would be interesting to find out whether these sexual taboos are commoner amongst groups who have traditions of early food supplementation. Sometimes the taboo is backed up with a prohibitory myth, such as belief that semen will poison the milk. When Dr David Morley first worked in Nigeria, women told him they had stopped breastfeeding because they were pregnant and he believed them, but when he kept records of dates he discovered they had their babies about fourteen months after they had announced their pregnancies. They stopped breastfeeding their babies when they felt ready to conceive another, often on the advice of the older women. It was common knowledge that complete sevrage was precarious and the fact that foreigners would often see sickly-looking 2-year-olds on the breast led Europeans, accustomed to stopping breastfeeding before the first year, to state dogmatically that breastmilk had no nutritional value after a year and that 'prolonged' breastfeeding 'caused' malnutrition. In fact the community recognised that a weak or ill child would probably only survive if his mother continued to suckle him. [14]

Abrupt sevrage is a problem in some societies because many people believe that with a new pregnancy the milk belongs to the new foetus and will poison the suckling child. Under colonial influence and with 'development' there has been a breakdown of traditional mores and authority. As monogamy is encouraged women may feel pressured to engage in frequent sexual relations with their husbands in order to deter them from having sex with other women. Some husbands believe that semen does poison milk and persuade their wives to bottle-feed so that sex can be resumed soon after the birth.

Sexual abstinence exists in both monogamous and polygamous societies, and though twentieth-century ideas emphasise the ill-effects of sexual repression, there is scant evidence that periods of celibacy or non-coital sex do much harm. Being sexually repressed is not the same as being celibate. Also, the idea of polygamy being more exploitative of women than monogamy is inaccurate. In a polygamous society, adultery or promiscuity are often as strictly proscribed as in those that profess to be monogamous. In some African societies, if a man has two wives but both are lactating, he still has to be celibate. I was told of one man whose two wives had their babies within nine days of each other five times in succession so that he had a couple of years' abstinence between each bout of lovemaking and was the subject of some good-humoured teasing in his village. He survived this ordeal without becoming neurotic. A friend in Mozambique had made his own taboos, that he must abstain from sex with anyone until his baby was three months old and then he could have sex with another woman, but not with his wife until the baby was seven months. The idea of restraint in the first period was due to the concept that after sexual intercourse the body gives off heat and this could damage the baby. There are numerous beliefs from many societies, and contrary to western prejudices it seems that often the more 'primitive' the society the more restraints there are on sexual intercourse. Women in Mozambique laughed at my attempts to generalise about people, and the phrase 'it depends on the person' put paid to my attempt to herd individuals into a cultural box. When I asked midwives what lactating women felt about enforced celibacy they said that they accepted it un-questioningly. Who knows how frustrated the women felt? Sexuality is so culturally dominated that often the individual feels what she or he is conditioned to feel and this domination leads people to give 'acceptable' answers to intrusive questions. It is hard enough for those drawn into the western cult of the priority of personal fulfilment to discover their own true desires.

THE WESTERN TABOO

Breastfeeding in industrialised society is closely bound up with perceptions of sexuality. The very reason it is frowned upon in public is that breasts are perceived exclusively as objects of sexual attention. The extremity of this attitude was brought home to me when a male friend, responding to my statement that I could not see any good reason for women not being able to leave their breasts showing, stated that after all men did not walk about with their penises hanging out. He quite unthinkingly equated breasts with genitals. Breasts are sexually stimulating, but so are legs, lips and the nape of the neck, to name a few focuses of visual eroticism. In societies where there is no shame about breastfeeding, the ordinary man is not driven into a frenzy by the sight of a female breast, but he may be embarrassed or aroused by a woman wearing shorts as Victorian men supposedly were by female ankles. Until recently women have been able to feed their babies in the most sexually repressive societies; women who dared not even show their faces could expose their breasts to feed a baby. In Victorian England, famous for its prudery, a respectable woman could feed openly in church (see page 181), yet in contemporary industrialised society where women's bodies and particularly breasts are used to sell newspapers, cars and peanuts, public breastfeeding provokes cries of protest from both men and women.

I believe the reaction comes from something more complex than the mere discomfort of unsatisfied sexual arousal. While I was discussing this issue with a successful woman journalist who works in a 'male world', she expressed concern about the embarrassment of middle-aged men when I suggested that a woman could breastfeed in the board room. These same middle-aged men survive the discomfort of erotic advertising hoardings, 'soft porn' pictures on wall calendars and the voluptuousness of classical painting. If they nip through the club areas in their lunch hours they have to resist explicit invitations to voyeuristic activities and may be propositioned by prostitutes. In spite of this harassment, which they tolerate so patiently, they survive to run vast enterprises and organise the leading structures of our society. However if one colleague breastfed a child during a business meeting the embarrassment would be too overwhelming. The poor dears must be protected from such pressure.

The feeding of a baby does provoke something far stronger than sexuality. It is a demonstration of power that is exclusively female and it is unacceptable for a woman who has claimed some of the supposedly male power to show she can have both. A male television producer recounted that a successful and assertive colleague breastfed her baby ' aggressively' during work meetings. He perceived this most tender of human activities as a threat

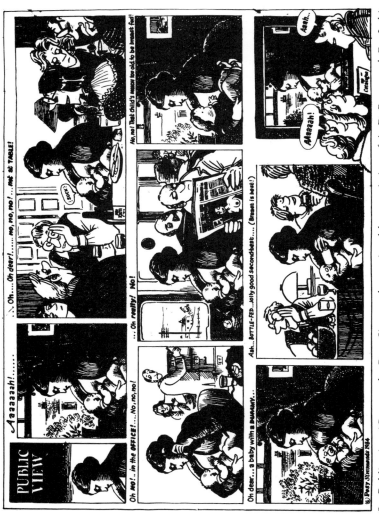

8 Public view (Cartoon by Posy Simmonds, reprinted by permission of A. D. Peters and Co. Ltd.)

because he disliked the woman. It was as though he could compete with her when she played the dirty political career games, but that by revealing other strengths which he knew he could never match she was attacking him.

The fact that such abhorrence is absent in some other societies may have another foundation. Few of us in industrialised society can remember suckling our own mothers. Many women have denied themselves the experience of reproduction because they know what a handicap it can be in the economic and career stakes. Others have children but do not breastfeed for the same reason or because it went wrong in the hopelessly unsupportive medical and social systems. When we see a suckling pair it does not summon up associations of tenderness and pleasure, but of rejection, failure and pain both in our relationships with our own mothers and with our babies if we have them. Men who are jealous of their partners' breastfeeding may have had damaged feeding relationships with their own mothers and seeing the same scene in public may be too inexplicably painful. Women who have not fed their own children, *especially if they had wanted to*, may feel terrible seeing a breastfeeding pair. My sister taught me this when she admitted how angry she felt whenever she saw a breastfeeding couple. She could not feed her first baby because, as she realised when she was helped with her second, she had never been taught to position him properly. Until she understood her own experience better she had unconsciously projected her anger at failure, and betrayal by those who should have helped her, on to other, luckier women.

LIBIDO AND BREASTFEEDING: LOSS OF INTEREST IN SEX

There are endless debates about the state of female libido during lactation, originally sparked off by Masters and Johnson's research in the 1960s claiming that breastfeeding women were more libidinous than bottle-feeders.[15] Much research is contradictory. One male doctor claims that women are desperately randy because of their 'unique hormonal state', but another informed me that breastfeeding induced 'menopausal' signs. (Why not say that the menopause induces 'lactational' signs?) Another researcher links breastfeeding with post-natal depression and loss of libido is perceived as a symptom of this.[16] These attitudes reflect a basic assumption in western society, which is that it is culturally desirable for women to be libidinous as long as the libido is directed towards their husband. Contemporary researchers record that breastfeeding mothers do not resume 'normal' sexual relations as quickly as bottle-feeding mothers. This is assumed to be a negative fact. Many husbands do not like their wives to breastfeed and this seems to be motivated by more than the state of their wives' libidos. Some men are jealous of their own children and the overt demonstration of closeness between 'their' wives and the baby is more than they can bear. In a way the modern woman is as oppressed as the 1900s woman who felt she must 'submit' to her husband to prevent him being unfaithful (see Page 186). The modern wife must do more than submit, she must be positively lustful and orgasmic and no pretence either. The response to a letter in the problem page of a popular supermarket magazine illustrates this attitude.

'Lost interest in sex'

Q: Since I had my last child three months ago I have lost interest in sex. I only make love with my husband when I have to, although when we do, I enjoy it. The trouble is I find myself using every excuse I can to get out of it. So far my husband has been very understanding and hasn't put a strain on our marriage, but I'm terrified that sooner or later he will.

A: A three-month-old baby has a lot to do with not feeling very sexy – not least because babies are very exhausting and constant fatigue is not the best recipe for sexual desire. But also, if you are breastfeeding it's quite likely that your loss of interest is caused by hormonal changes connected with the suckling. As you stop breastfeeding, your interest should return. You only need become anxious if by that stage your sex urge still hasn't returned.

Very occasionally the hormones connected with breastfeeding remain at a specially high level and need to be lowered to their usual level by drug treatment. Even if you haven't breastfed at all, these hormone levels may become too high and require the same treatment. So give yourself a bit more time before panicking, discuss it with you husband and show your appreciation of him in other ways. [17]

THE RAMPANT MALE
AND THE VARIABILITY OF DESIRE

What is remarkable about the response is the focus on the supposed needs of the husband rather than of the baby and the woman. The baby is seen as the cause of the problem and breastfeeding is an incidental obstacle to the main purpose of the woman's life which, the agony aunt assumes, is to maintain a sexual relationship with the baby's father. The letter indicates that the husband appreciates the situation more than the agony aunt, presumably because he actually loves his child and his wife. The response shows no awareness that breastfeeding could continue for two years. There is an obsession with the maintenance of libido: 'You need only become anxious . . .' The woman is exhorted to worry if her feelings do not conform to a culturally approved norm. What about all the thousands of people whose libidos are low (and who defines this?) for the greater part of their lives? Should they become anxious? The implication is that the stability of the marriage rests on the adaptation of the woman's sexual drive to the perceived needs of the man, otherwise he might seek alternative sexual fulfilment and then the relationship is threatened because coital sex above all is the bond that keeps them together. There is no allusion to the woman's sexual or affectional needs. There is no suggestion that if simple physical frustration is the problem the man can masturbate.

I am reminded of Bryan Forbes's 1974 film *The Stepford Wives*, where the women are changed into robots so as to conform to the male ideal. In real life, women are not only under pressure to make themselves appear sexually stimulating through clothes, cosmetics and body care, but must also adjust themselves biochemically if they do not match up to the required standards of behaviour, either through tranquillisers or artificial hormones. Sometimes the pro-breastfeeding lobby have cited the libido-enhancing value of breastfeeding as a sort of sales gimmick to convince the modern couple that it is literally a 'sexy' thing to do whilst those who are doubtful about breastfeeding suspect it of interfering with the 'normality' of women's lives. This 'normal' woman must be a responsive partner in a heterosexual relationship where absence of courtship-phase passion is viewed as a threat to its stability.

The main goal of the advice in most baby care books, which are invariably directed at women, and from health workers, is 'how to keep your man happy while you care for the baby', the assumption being that she is supremely responsible for the welfare of both child and adult. If forcing yourself to be libidinous is necessary then you must do it. At all costs (including depriving the baby of breastfeeding) the baby's father must continue to feel cherished and sexually served. The responsibility for both the man and the baby is assumed to lie with the woman. This is profoundly insulting to all those mature men who love their babies and, as women do, are prepared to make profound adjustments to their lives in their children's interest. It also demonstrates the urgent need for changes in the education of boys and men. What if that letter had been written by a man?

Q: Since I was made inside left for Wolverham Rangers three months ago I have lost interest in sex. I only make love with my wife when I have to – although when we do, I enjoy it. The trouble is I find myself using every excuse I can to get out of it. So far my wife has been very understanding and hasn't put any strain on our marriage, but I'm terrified that sooner or later she will.

A: A new football team has a lot to do with not feeling very sexy – not least because football is very exhausting and constant fatigue is not the best recipe for sexual desire. But also if you are training it's quite likely that your loss of interest is caused by hormonal changes connected with the physical movements. As you stop playing football, your interest should return. You only need become anxious if by that stage your sex urge still hasn't returned.

Very occasionally the hormones connected with playing football remain at a specially high level and need to be lowered to their usual level by drug treatment. Even if you haven't played football at all, these hormone levels may become too high and require the same treatment. So give yourself a bit more time before panicking, discuss it with your wife and meanwhile show your appreciation of her in other ways.

What the original letter writer could not see was that her husband was showing her he loved her and the baby by being understanding. It is taken for granted that a woman should be patient with a husband who is not very sexy when life changes lower his libido. In fact some breastfeeding women do feel much randier, but is anyone suggesting hormone treatment to keep their husbands in trim? I can think of many unhappy women confused by the conflicts between their attempts to be a loving mother and a wife. There is the unlibidinous breastfeeder who feels guilty because she actually prefers suckling her baby to having sex with her partner, and then there is the woman who stops breastfeeding 'for her marriage's sake' and feels guilty about her baby. Sexuality is so culturally conditioned that it is hard to find out what people really feel, but biologically a reduction in libido makes sense and if breastfeeding and low libido cause post-natal depression why are not all women in traditional societies in a permanent state of gloom? In spite of such hard lives many seem less miserable than women in industrialised society. The rates of severe post-natal depression are the same tiny percentage in all societies, and most of the depression suffered by new mothers in western society arises because they lose all social and economic recognition as individuals and are shut up in their homes. In societies where reproduction is admired and women are not excluded from economic activity through childbearing, most women are proud and happy to be mothers. What is a dominant ideology in many societies is the cult of the permanently rampant male who has to thrust his penis into a vagina otherwise he will experience unendurable suffering. This may sound exaggerated, but in the summer of 1987 the British junior health minister, Mrs. Edwina Currie, recommended that businessmen take their wives on foreign trips with them to protect them from the risk of HIV infected prostitutes, the idea being that men cannot possibly control their desperate biological urges and that a 'clean' wife can spread her legs at the right moment to intercept the lures of a prostitute and thus protect the poor husband from disease. Why men cannot be persuaded that, if they are desperate, masturbation can relieve their tension and cause no risk of infection is, of course, because sexuality has as much to do with expressing power and dominance as with the relief of appetite. The fact is that individual sexual drive varies greatly, that penetrative intercourse is not the only means of sexual satisfaction and that celibacy never killed anyone. The Eritrean People's Liberation Front had a mixed army that remained celibate. These were young, healthy people who had to share tents and whose common ideals made them feel emotionally close. After four years they decided to permit marriage because they did feel the need for sexual and affectionate relationships, but in common with many people throughout history, celibacy was maintained without health or sanity collapsing, as many individuals know is possible from their own experience.[18] In modern western society, commercial and cultural images provide a barrage of stimuli to maintain flagging libido in the consumer society. The primacy of sexuality in the marital relationship is endorsed by advertising and the content of many magazines, books and films. Women desperately try to compete with the images of pornography, sales of erotica soar and men demand that their wives and mistresses wear certain clothes or conform to particular commercial images of sexuality. Breasts must be firm and youthful, stomachs flat and movements frisky. Maureen Minchin describes the situation as mentally immature men going on about physically immature females'.[19]

Sex can be both fun and a profound experience, but for millions of women their sexuality is a trade-off for an illusion of economic, emotional or physical security. Many women must use their bodies to survive in a world where the woman without a man is marginalised, both economically and socially. Breastfeeding and a physically close mother-child relationship, inevitably conflicts with the current values of the ideal, heterosexual relationship. I know of a woman who had no desire for sexual intercourse for a year after childbirth, but who felt guilty and went for advice to her doctor, a man, who prescribed tranquillisers and said 'You'll just have to force yourself'. She did, so presumably the doctor can credit himself with 'saving the marriage'. I happen to believe that a baby's needs are more important than an adult man's. I am also appalled that a woman should have coitus when she feels no desire for it, yet we are still so hooked on the tradition of marriage being a sort of containment of sexuality that these solutions are still endorsed, at the expense of mother-child relationships and by the smothering of women's feelings.

From the Stone Age to Steam Engines: A Gallop Through History

PREHISTORIC WOMAN

The children's encyclopaedias of my youth were impressively illustrated with the prehistoric family scene. A woman would be sitting demurely at the entrance to a cave, surrounded by a gang of little children, while a large and muscular man, a club in one hand and a large dead animal in the other, would be striding towards them. Somehow I absorbed the idea that our male ancestors habitually dragged 'their' women about by their hair and that the staple food was woolly mammoth. The inaccuracy of these images is a distortion that endorses a contemporary set of lies. The widespread message is that all women in the past were made vulnerable by their burdensome fertility and were dependent on their men to feed and protect them. The accompanying myth is that the techniques of fertility control are a twentieth-century 'scientific' invention and that all 'primitive' women were more oppressed than their 'lucky' descendants. Fertility is seen as a female 'problem', and whether it is discouraged or enforced by the arbitrary vagaries of political, demographic and cultural decisions, it must at all times be kept in its 'traditional' place, preferably out of sight from the prestigious and power-loaded male world. In the same way breastfeeding is seen as the woman's topic, and though they are often told whether or not they should do it, it is unacknowledged as women's power but viewed as another female handicap and a pretext for discrimination. The idea that women have, in all societies and at all times, been dependent on men for food and survival because they have been handicapped by the production and nurture of children is simply not true.

Many of the deductions about our ancestors' way of life come from observations of the groups of the women and men known as hunters and gatherers, I will call them gatherer/hunters because that reflects the priority of activity. It is an oversimplification to assume too many similarities, but groups such as the Australian Aborigines, the inhabitants of the Amazonian rain forest and the !Kung of the Kalahari desert are all believed to have led a life, until very recently, that has much in common with how people have lived for the greater part of human existence. It is one of the many tragedies of the twentieth century that just as the knowledge of the value of these systems is filtering through to the narrow-visioned industrialised society, these societies are being destroyed by the relentless processes of 'development'. Whereas agricultural society is about 10,000 years old and industrial society a mere 200 to 300 years, gathering and hunting has endured for over a million years. Surviving peoples often only exist now because they occupy marginal lands that have not excited the attention of colonisers. There is a wide variety of economic systems and cultures but there are certain universal characteristics which many groups have in common.

WOMAN THE BREADWINNER

Whether a society has equal status of the sexes, as do the !Kung of the Kalahari desert, or are male-dominated as the Australian Aborigines are, women in gatherer/hunter societies usually provide the bulk of the food and are indeed the 'breadwinners'. Most men do hunt, but hunting for larger game is a precarious method of acquiring food; it entails a huge investment in risk, skill and time, not only in the hunt itself, but in the manufacture of the necessary weapons. Women are usually the ones who collect, gather and dig out all the berries and fruits, roots and tubers, leaves and shoots, as well as catch the insects and small animals that are the mainstay of survival of the whole group. They also, of course, suckle their children, often for three or four years.

They realise a much higher return in daily nutrition than the hunting men. The reasons why women do not usually hunt are complex, but it is certainly not because they lack the ability or strength. (Women's hunting skill was vividly illustrated for me in Mozambique where I saw fisherwomen wading through the sea, wielding their tridents to spear fish.) Young boys are trained to use smaller weapons, so size is not the issue. It seems that more often women are forbidden to hunt because something exclusive has to be reserved for the men to make them feel special. Anthropologist Margaret Mead once claimed that men have to do something that women are not allowed to do,[1] supposedly because men do not have the powers of giving birth and producing milk. Whether women hunt or not, it is often they who keep the group alive, using a set of skills, a store of knowledge and such qualities as dexterity and shrewd observation to find this food.

There are gatherer/hunter women living today and some of them are more 'liberated' than most women in industrialised society. Many so-called primitive people are not worn down with overwork as so many peasants and urban workers are. A gathering and hunting community will search out the food they need for the present and then relax and play. They do not acquire surpluses, because they have the skills to find food whenever they need it and if they are nomadic there is a disadvantage in carrying too many stores. They may be vulnerable to accident, a snakebite or other hazards of nature, but as long as they can move freely in their accustomed environment their food is all around them and cannot be stolen by other people. Their food is also adapted to the environment and unlike most agricultural crops cannot be destroyed by drought or pest.

As for the reproductive functions of a gathering woman, she has some advantages that many other societies have lost. As we saw in Chapter 4, she would start menstruating and child-bearing later and stop earlier than women in other societies, and her children would rarely be less than three or four years apart. Her way of suckling inhibits ovulation and even if she is sexually active she is unlikely to get pregnant while she breastfeeds for the first few years of her child's life. The lactational infertility may be reinforced by the marginal nature of her diet.

She will rarely be plump and this may be the reason why she will start to menstruate later and stop earlier than most modern women.

THE ORIGINAL AFFLUENT SOCIETY

Gatherer/hunters, though sometimes slightly undernourished, are rarely malnourished; vitamin or other specific nutrient deficiencies are rare. The customary diet of the !Kung of the Kalahari desert consisted of eighty-five species of food plant, including thirty roots and bulbs, as well as fifty-four species of animals and they only needed to work a two-and-a-half-day week (of six hours work a day) to provide themselves with an excellent balanced diet.[2] If this is an example of desert dwellers, consider how bountiful was the environment and provision for those living in more fertile regions of the world, which were the very areas to be appropriated by colonial invaders. The nutritionist A. S. Truswell found that the !Kung were healthier than people in industrialised countries, with no dental caries, no high blood pressure, obesity or heart disease. Anaemia was rare and the majority, including the women, had adequate iron intakes. Anaemia is the scourge of women in both peasant and industrialised societies resulting in some cases in more or less permanent exhaustion, as well as poor growth and development in children. It is often perceived as an inevitable state for menstruating or pregnant women. A gatherer/hunter woman might be protected from anaemia by several factors. Firstly, her way of breastfeeding would prevent menstruation and the contraceptive effect would protect her from blood-depleting miscarriages as well as pregnancies. Secondly, her varied diet would provide many sources of iron which would be well absorbed because of the high doses of vitamin C she gained from all the fresh fruits and roots she ate. If she were nomadic, this mode of life would prevent faecally spread parasites like hookworm from invading her environment. Lastly, she would not drink tea, coffee or milk with food, which all significantly reduce the absorption of dietary iron. Of course all these factors are rapidly disappearing as contact with 'civilised man' dismantles these ways of life.

The low density population of gatherer/hunters, their nomadic habits and absence of domesticated animals meant that the common infections of settled group were absent or unusual. Tragically this has sometimes meant that the resistance to the many infections that invaders brought had never evolved. Truswell observed that diarrhoea (the biggest single killer worldwide of babies) was low amongst the !Kung. The prevalence of certain infections such as measles is linked to the density of population and to overcrowding; small nomadic groups rarely created the environment for the measles virus to flourish. Semi-nakedness and outdoor existence would ensure maximum vitamin D status so that poor bone development and pelvic deformities, suffered by many urban women because of chronic deficiency during their childhood, would not impede normal childbirth, nor would nomadic groups suffer from osteoporosis. The continuous physical exercise of hunting, gathering, walking and dancing would all have beneficial effects that frantic joggers and weight trainers are so eager to achieve in modern western society. Sahlins, in his book *Stone Age Economics*, has called these societies the 'original affluent society'.[3]

THE MYTH OF THE TRADITIONAL WOMAN

Two modern assumptions about 'traditional' female roles are conspicuously absent from many of these groups. Firstly, 'woman's place in the home' did not exist because no one had homes as we know them. A nomad who moves on and constructs a simple shelter at each encampment could not be described as 'domestic' or 'tied to the home' for her work was certainly outside in every sense of the word. Secondly, in many pre-agricultural groups, fertility is not revered in the way it is in many agricultural societies. There was no pressure on women to produce lots of children, which may have happened with the demands of the periods of intensive work needed in agriculture, and they rarely had more than five or six pregnancies in a lifetime. I want to draw attention to this lack of emphasis on maternity and fertility because I believe that the interpretation of woman as mother in western society is harmful because the role is perceived to be exclusive and excluding. To be a good mother a woman is supposed to devote herself entirely to her children (and often a dependent and childlike husband), and to do so she must be set apart from 'normal life' and consequently is separated from control over her economic survival and social independence. Though there might be a period of dependency on other women for food immediately after childbirth, during her everyday life a gatherer woman is self-sufficient and well able to support her own children. In most gatherer/hunter groups children are well cared for both physically and psychologically and are fully integrated into everyday life, unlike our own children who are segregated so carefully. Children may be breastfed and stay close to their mothers in the first two to three years, but after this phase they rapidly become very independent, learning all the skills necessary for survival and participation in their own society at a rate which puts our own ponderous educational methods to shame. For example, 4-year-olds in Papua New Guinea skilfully catch and roast insects which provide an important contribution to their diet.[4]

AN EXAMPLE OF EQUALITY: THE HADZA

One surviving tribe, the Hadza of Tanzania, live on marginal land and lead the sort of existence that many of our ancestors might have done. A Hadza woman gathers food for herself and eats most of it on the spot, her children quickly learning to do the same. She takes any extra back for the group to share out. The men do the same, only with meat, and there is no priority of eating or beholdenness in this sharing. She builds her own grass hut which her husband might share with her, but she owes him no service. She fetches water for herself and her children, she makes skin clothes for herself and her daughters only. The men are not especially saintly and are sometimes violent, but if this happens the women form a band and attack the man. If a husband hits his wife, she will leave him, and there is no social pressure to make her stay. It seems therefore that marriages are founded on a genuine attraction or mutual affection and companionship, as there is no economic or social reason to maintain the union. It is also quite normal for older women to marry younger men, which I believe is sign of a more equitable power structure between the sexes. It is common for marriages to last a lifetime; the anthropologists James and Lisa Woodburn have found that many Hadza couples are still together after twenty five years. It seems that Hadza men are not especially keen to have children, for they stay with a wife who does not bear them.[5]

I find their lifestyle of interest because this independence, command of skills and ability to resist male coercion through female solidarity it what some modern women in industrialised societies would like to achieve. Here are 'primitive' women who have all this and they are not overworked or exhausted with the effort. Also it is not a society where women are better off because the men are especially gentle and kind. The Hadza woman resists an ever-present potential male oppression through the strength of her female relationships. Because she is not in competition with men nor exploited by them she is quite free, when she has a baby, to care for it in the way she chooses. Lactation failure is unknown in Hadza society and breastfeeding is gradually supplemented by nutritious foods such as bone marrow, soft fat and ground baobab berries. When the baby develops teeth, mothers pre-chew meat for them, which may have an added advantage in that the salivary glands are linked into the immunological system, which may give further protection against disease. Hadza children are healthier than those in other societies where medical services are non-existent or inadequate. Derrick Jelliffe and his colleagues found few of the usual problems of rural and urban children in tropical countries. There was no kwashiorkor, marasmus, anaemia or other nutritional deficiency and no ascaris, the round worms which are so common in most 'poor' societies and which add to the risk of malnutrition.[6]

Childcare is a straightforward matter in this society and does not conflict with a woman 'earning' her living, indeed it is integrated effortlessly with the educational and economic system. Suckling a baby is easy when you can do it while you work or can pause whenever it suits you because you are the one in control of your own work, welfare and survival. This work pattern is also far more efficient than in societies where a supervisor is needed to ensure that work gets done. Power is control over resources and the Hadza woman has control over her own food supply and her baby's.

THE ARROGANCE OF MODERN RULE

There is no government in the world that fully respects nomads or other 'Stone Age' people. At best they are ignored, more usually there are clumsy attempts to 'integrate' or 'educate' them and often there is systematic harassment, persecution and even genocide. An unquestioning sense of superiority or patronage accompanies most decision making by those in authority. In the report *Our Common Future*, the World Commission on Environment and Development states that tribal and indigenous peoples have lifestyles that 'can offer modern societies many lessons in the management of resources in complex forest, mountain, and dryland ecosystems',[7] the destruction of breastfeeding has as devastating an effect on the ecosystem as overgrazing or excess tree felling and it is one more example of the modern defiance of nature with its damaging spin-off effects – such as accelerated population growth – which those who promoted the widespread use of substitutes and supplements never considered. We must learn from these groups who have breastfed so well for so long.

AGRICULTURE

Agriculture and the domestication of animals changed the relationship of humans with their environment and with one another. They led to the control of land and of women because men became dependent on both for their survival. Perhaps the chance dropping of wild grain seeds that then sprang up regularly and an awareness of the habitat of a particularly tasty and easily caught animal motivated people to return to the same spot again and again. If it is possible to get food without moving on, why bother to wander? The evidence that agriculture developed after the last ice age suggests that climatic changes reduced the food availability from gathering and hunting and those who had found ways of conserving their food supply had more chances of survival.

Cultivation requires periods of more intensive and sustained work than gathering; there is planting, weeding, pest removal, harvesting and processing to be done. Storage requires a lot of work in the construction of silos which are still never completely protective against vermin, fungi or decay. Pastoralism and stock rearing require constant supervision of the animals. The anthropologists Farb and Armelagos see the greater amounts of food available through agriculture and animal domestication as a cause of population rise. They claim that 'better nutrition' in the form of increased availability of energy from large quantities of grain or root crops meant lower infection rates, less death and hence more people. It is true that populations rose, but it was probably for other reasons. Evidence indicates that many gatherer/hunters had better-quality diets and a less pathogenic environment and enjoyed better health than agriculturalists. Historians look at the evolution of agriculture as though it only happened because it was a 'good thing'. This theory that all development or evolution is due to the purpose of the final cause is known as teleology. An example is the idea that giraffes developed long necks so that they could reach up to the high leaves. The non-teleological approach is to say that giraffes who happened to have long necks were lucky enough not to starve to death and so only long-necked giraffes and their offspring who inherited this trait survived. In our hierarchical mode of thinking, the idea of agriculture being 'superior' to gathering and hunting, and of course the idea of industrialisation being another step 'forward', is teleological. Just because it happened does not mean that it was necessarily advantageous, nor that it was entirely without benefits.

Farb and Armelagos argue that the main advantage of agriculture was that the denser population of a sedentary village allowed for greater protection against enemies and more cultural interaction. I disagree; running away and hiding from enemies, unhampered by possessions, may be a better strategy than collecting in one place and fighting them off. As for cultural interaction, many of the pre-agricultural peoples had complex and fascinating rituals and ceremonies which included the artistic impression that we so admire. The beauty of pre-historic rock paintings in Europe, Africa and Australia show that artistic skill is not a unique benefit of agriculture. The idea that some lesser human had to do all the work while the talented individuals sat around inventing 'culture' is belied by the fact that so many of the non-working groups actually spent their time quarrelling and devising rituals and rules to maintain their social status, while often it was the slaves who produced the art as well as the food. It was usually a minority of the elite who actually wrote, thought or produced works of art, but of course they had the power to define what was art and so their work was exalted. What agriculture seems to have spawned is the oppression of certain castes and groups who were coerced to do more than others, and women in most agricultural societies came under pressure to work harder and sometimes to bear more children. [8]

THE DISADVANTAGES OF SETTLEMENT

The dependency on particular crops and food stores would have made communities more vulnerable to theft, pests and weather. Guarding the stored food became a full-time job and more men may have devoted themselves to that task which is now seen as the very essence of masculinity, warfare. Women might have seen the need to conserve men's precarious strength for fighting and therefore increased their own share of ordinary work. Although men are seen as 'strong' because of their larger size and increased musculature, women have more stamina. If more men devoted themselves to warfare, more aggression and easily provoked conflict between neighbouring communities would have developed, and consequently more deaths and social pressure on women to bear more sons. The pattern of exalting and supporting motherhood after losses in a war has persisted right into the twentieth century (see Chapter 6, page 182).

With settlement came more infection from faecal contamination and regular contact with animals and parasites, and perhaps more infant death. The Hadza men did not mind whether the women bore children or not, but most agriculturalist men want children and women may yearn for many babies when they are an investment in future support. Women may have taken the first step on the slope to oppression via the domestication of plants and animals. Both practices are actually less energy-efficient than gathering and hunting, a fact recognised by groups like the Hadza who see that the dubious value of attempted food security is far outweighed by the exhausting work input required. Also, you cannot merely plant the foods you always gathered; it is a minority of plant and animal species that respond to this sort of control. Many a nutritious 'weed' will only grow under certain conditions that are impossible for humans to manipulate. For example, some seeds only grow after passing through the digestive system of a wild animal.

In seasonal climates, there is the need to plant, weed and harvest within a certain time scale, and as the principal foragers of vegetable foods it was probably women who stayed around one area to perform these tasks. In horticultural/hunting societies which represent an intermediate phase of change to agriculture, women usually grow the staple foods and men continue to hunt. If the crop needs frequent attention it is harder to leave and 'domestication' of the crops, the animals and the women is established simultaneously. Perhaps sustained periods of food abundance and therefore increased energy intake and a period of weight gain did make women more fertile, though it might not have improved the quality of nutrition. Populations have increased with the development of agriculture and pastoralism, but this may have occurred as a result of a deliberate plan to produce more children and perhaps a seasonal superabundance of energy sources that shortened the effect of lactational infertility. With the availability of non-human animal milk and supplies of starchy staples the earlier use of baby foods other than breastmilk, particularly during the periods of intensive work, might have interfered with the frequency of nipple stimulation that maintains anovulation. Some traditional societies use substitute baby foods earlier than is nutritionally necessary and the practice may be linked to intensive seasonal labour. The health compromise has been recognised, and many groups know that other foods given too early can make a baby ill, but the priority of food production for the whole group may compel them to take this risk.

WORKING MOTHERS: THE USINO OF PAPUA NEW GUINEA

When a woman has to work hard to produce food and at the same time care for her child, the balance between food provision for the whole group and for the baby through ready access to the breast becomes more delicate and the social priorities may change according to the circumstances. What is very clear when we look at agricultural or horticultural societies is that women have an acknowledged key economic role and that they breastfeed very successfully. The Usino in Papua New Guinea could not comprehend the idea of lactation failure, but the women did not live in a romantic cloud of idealised motherhood. They sometimes grumbled about the restrictions of the baby wanting to suckle while they were working on their sweet potato plots and as soon as they felt it could survive a few hours without breastmilk they might leave it with relatives, but everyone believed that a baby must never cry and breasts were as much used to comfort as to feed. In our own modern society women who want to breastfeed and earn a wage are often regarded as over-demanding and unrealistic. Babies are the investment in the future, but such is our obsession with the quick return and our ignorance of the real value of breastfeeding that we lack a truly social attitude to childcare, involving as it would compromises with other forms of productivity. Women in these societies are providers for the whole family and the compromises worked out to suit the baby, the mother's work and the group economy are as complex as any childminding arrangements made by the western mother who works outside the home, but breastfeeding lasts well into the second year or longer. [9]

Women in these societies would not have sacrificed the welfare of their children for the good of the group because children *were* the good of the group, so the women's role as principal food provider would not have been organised to conflict with breastfeeding. They may have shared breastfeeding for in many societies women have done and still do this, but usually the rhythm of work interwove with the rhythm of a baby's needs. There is more prolactin in a woman's bloodstream at night, indicating perhaps that babies have over the millennia derived more milk from their mothers at night than during the day. To this day, most African and Asian women sleep with their babies who soon learn to suckle freely without even waking their mothers, and our ancestors must have done this too.

NIGHT RULES

I have heard modern psychologists describe sleeping with the baby as a symptom of an 'overprotective' mother. As most human babies throughout history and millions in the twentieth century have nowhere else to sleep but in their mothers' arms, there must have been endemic 'overprotectiveness' since life began. There is a contemporary cultural resistance to the idea of a baby suckling at night. 'Sleeping through' in a separate bed as soon as possible is the aim of most parents, yet many other activities take place at night (to the detriment of our daytime productivity) without earning such disapproval. Sex, intellectual discussions, parties, as well as shift work in many sectors of the economy are all accepted as night-time activities. Most of us smile at a yawning colleague who spent time in nocturnal lovemaking, drinking or setting the world to rights, yet a mother and baby who suckle at night are objects of pity and concern. The mother is seen as a slave to her child and she is criticised for this, but slaving for other people during the day is taken for granted. Society is condemning of the 'demanding' baby who does not conform to social convention quickly, but admiring of the 'demanding' boss who gets his workers to exhaust themselves during the day.

SLAVERY

With the development of agriculture, pressure of work stimulated the strong to coerce the weak, for before the need for such intense work who would have bothered to force others to slave? Slavery is difficult to define because the modern concept of working for no pay is inadequate, as in the past monetary reward was often a minor part of economic survival. Slavery is as much about the psychological control of the master over the slave as of the physical domination, cruelty and exploitation which we associate with the word. Many waged workers have suffered and still suffer the last three and yet are not viewed as slaves. There have been cases of slavery in the modern United States where employers ruthlessly exploit immigrant workers. [10] There are also slaves in some West African countries who have strong personal bonds with their owners to the extent that they might even work in Europe and send money to their masters. Presumably the benefits of security attached to the relationship have outweighed the benefits of breaking the bond, or perhaps the idea of 'freedom' within the wage market system of racist Europe is too frightening.

Women have been slaves to men in much the same way. The unpaid housewife jokes about being a slave, but it is true. She works for the welfare of her husband and his household for no monetary reward and her status in the world is always lower than his, often in her own eyes. She is quite dependent on his whim and the fact that a number of men behave decently does not negate the unequal power structure. The fact that many men have abandoned their wives when the emotional or sexual bonds have altered makes many women's situations less secure than that of the traditional bond slaves of, for example, the Tuareg in Niger whose masters are obligated to them for life.

To justify the coercion of fellow humans, particular ideologies have developed. Most slavery is justified by ideas about superior and inferior groups and physical characteristics such as sex and skin colour make differentiation easy. Of course most slave ideologies sprang from the imaginations of the dominant group, but often the exploited group internalised the ideology and accepted their lot, because they knew no other way. In ancient

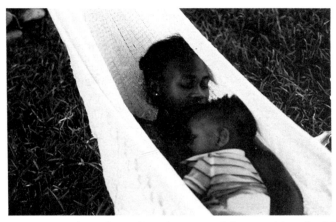

9 Margaret Kyenkya of UNICEF sleeping with her son Mugado (*Photo:* Gabrielle Palmer 1987)

Greece and Rome as many as 80 per cent of the people were slaves and did all the work, not only the manual but also the bureaucratic, clerical and artistic labour. To the great philosophers such as Plato and Aristotle, this was 'natural'. A slave was the property of his or her master as were all the women in his family, and it was argued that both slaves and women were born 'naturally' inferior. Western 'civilisation' has been based on the ideas of ancient Greece, where the concept of 'democracy' (government by the people) assumed that slaves and women should continue to be without political power. Similarly, modern 'democracies' assume that children cannot possibly participate in any decision making, though they are often more honest and altruistic than adults.

Slavery had a profound effect on childcare. Firstly, powerful women, who usually derived their power through being the wives or daughters of powerful men, could coerce other women to suckle their children for them. Secondly, the organisation of labour took priority over the welfare of a slave's baby.

THE CARIBBEAN EXAMPLE

I want to illustrate the manipulation of infant and mother relationships to suit the slave owner, rather than the couple, with an account of early nineteenth-century practices in the Caribbean, because the starkness of the example is reflected in the modern world. Social planners today claim to have the interests of babies at heart, but the organisation of 'wealth creation' takes priority and damages the lives of women and children. Slave trading has existed for centuries, but as European naval capacity expanded so did the trade, in response to the demand for labour in the newly established colonies. This phase in history produced some of the worst excesses of callousness about human life. At one stage, particularly in the route between Brazil and Africa, it was actually cheaper to bring new slaves rather than to provide even the most basic conditions for survival so that child rearing was considered unnecessary. In 1817 an observer in Jamaica, a Dr Williamson, noted that the rearing of children was not encouraged on some plantations: 'on account of the loss of labour incurred by the mother's confinement and the time afterwards required in raising the infant'.[11]

The idea of disallowing women to bear children just so as to use their labour strikes horror in the liberal soul, but it is still happening all over the world. In South Africa, companies demand that women present certificates of long-term hormonal contraceptive injections before they can be employed. In the Philippine Bataan Export Processing Zone, the Mattel Toy company offers prizes to those workers who undergo sterilisation.[12]

Dr Williamson, with the professional detachment of a pig farmer, thought it would be more efficient to breed slaves on the plantations rather than continually replace them with newly transported ones because 'a more vigorous set of labourers than the Africans generally become was brought forward in the course of time'.[13] To this end marriage should be promoted and inducements offered to encourage women to have babies. Women were excused certain tasks and given more free time for each child they managed to rear past infancy. The babies were to be breastfed by their mothers but to be kept in nurseries during their working hours. Mothers were allowed two one-hour periods for breastfeeding and if the baby needed food at other times the older women nursery workers gave panada (a mixture of bread, flour and sugar). Women were not allowed to suckle for longer than sixteen months and were separated from their children at this stage. The reason was that they must start breeding again and continuing lactation might prevent conception. This was quite contrary to a women's cultural customs. A Dr Collins, who in 1811 laid down his *Practical Rules for the Management and Medical Treatment of Negro Slaves in the Sugar Colonies,* stated,

> Negroes are universally fond of suckling their children for a long time. If you permit them, they will extend it to the third year . . . Their motives for this are habit, an idea of its necessity, the desire of being spared at their labour or perhaps the avoiding of another pregnancy; but from whichever of these motives they do it, your business is to counteract their designs, and to oblige them to wean their children as soon as they have attained their fourteenth or sixteenth month . . . If you neglect to do this, you not only lose some of the mother's labour, but you prevent their breeding so soon. [14]

THE CONTINUING COERCION

This assumption, that the control of fertility is something for the authorities to manipulate according to economic need, with no respect for the wishes and dignity of individuals, has not changed. We see this in many twentieth-century societies where demographic concerns influence the supply or withdrawal of contraceptive provision and information. It is black women in the US and Europe who have been most coerced into abortion, early sterilisation and unsafe contraception and discouraged from 'breeding'. In several countries where access to contraception and safe abortion had been established there has been a reversal of these policies on the demographic and racial grounds. In Romania, a free abortion policy was replaced by strict prohibition of all birth control. Women endured compulsory pregnancy tests and questioning if they were negative. This resulted in the huge number of Romanian 'orphans' placed in institutions because their mothers could not care for another unwanted baby. Women are the best judges of whether they can cope with a baby and unwanted childbearing always leads to more desperate acts of unsafe illegal abortion or abandonment. In France white couples were urged by a national advertising campaign, 'La France a besoin des enfants', to produce more citizens, whilst black immigrants have difficulty in obtaining the generous state benefits and fiscal incentives designed to encourage large families. In Singapore women with less formal education lose the chances of house loans and other benefits if their families increase while graduate couples are offered free holidays in romantic places in an attempt to induce them to breed, the authorities apparently believing that graduate status is an hereditary characteristic. [15] Many nineteenth- and twentieth-century health protagonists have been concerned with the tendency of the poor to breed too much. Presumably as they were no longer useful as slaves they should conveniently die out. The irony is that one of the most effective methods of birth control, lactation, was deliberately denied to the slave women in order to make them bear more children, yet now it is the fertility of black women that is viewed with alarm by the powerful white dominant groups. The modern international economy, which is principally controlled by the giant transnational companies and the governments who protect their interests, uses methods similar to the early slave traders. It is cheaper and more efficient to replace labour than to reproduce it sequentially by allowing women workers concessions for maternity leave and childcare. Unlike the earlier slave traders they do not have to ship human beings across the globe, but can move their workshops and plantations instead. As soon as workers attempt to ask for fairer wages and decent working conditions, they become 'uneconomic' and the company, with all the benefits of the microchip revolution and modern communications, can abandon a mobilising and rights-conscious workforce and move their production sites to a more 'pliable' community in a poorer country where people are too desperate to reject the lowest pay levels. It is commonly women who are utilised in this insecure trade pattern. Unlike the core workers who are usually men with some job security, women are hired and fired according to the needs of the company. In this precarious climate of employment, achieving basic health and safety standards in the workplace is hard enough; to ask for maternity leave and nursing breaks is to ask for the moon. The basic rights of maternity leave and nursing breaks established by the International Labour Organisation as long ago as 1919 are still ignored worldwide whenever there is no state commitment to them (see page 182).

It can be argued that there is no comparison between the conditions of an eighteenth- or nineteenth-century Jamaican slave and a modern woman worker. On one Jamaican estate the women slaves performed two-thirds of the agricultural work and did more basic labour than men. Women were reputed to be stronger and 'a better investment' than the men, living on average four or five years longer. Half the childless women and one-third of the mothers died in their twenties or thirties. This is a horrifying figure, but compare it with the fact that the expectation of life at birth in England in 1811 was 37.6 years (in 1976 this figure was 75.8 years).[16] This does not mean that all English women died at 37; in fact if they reached that age they had a reasonable chance of living another twenty years. Expectation of life at birth is calculated by making an average of everyone's age at death, including babies and children who are more vulnerable. The 1976 figure is as much a reflection of the decline in infant and child mortality as of the fact that more people live longer. The point is that modern medical skills, awareness of the ill-effects of poor hygiene and nutrition and the knowledge that germs can cause disease did not exist as they do now. The wife of the cruel plantation owner was as likely to die in childbirth or have her baby die as was a slave woman and her child. What is shameful is that with current knowledge of the effects of overwork, lack of health and safety standards, inadequate diet and poor or non-existent medical care we still accept a system that keeps so many workers in bad conditions, so as to maintain economic prosperity . . . for whom?

The Jamaican woman and others like her in all the colonies,

who slaved and bred more slaves for her masters, contributed to the economic prosperity of nineteenth-century Britain by producing the cotton, sugar, cocoa and tea upon which much of that wealth was founded. Among her descendants today are the black women of Britain and the United States who suffer discrimination in the allocation of education and jobs and are among the lowest paid of all workers. In the United States the black infant mortality rate is more than double that of whites. [17] Black women everywhere are more likely to be coerced into sterilisation or persuaded to use risky forms of contraception. In both Europe and the United States, black women are more vulnerable to the criticisms of the agents of welfare and may lose custody of their children because poverty and long working hours prevent them from bringing up their children in the way that is promoted as ideal.

WET NURSING AND ITS RELATION TO CLASS

Though the great majority of babies have been fed by their own mothers, wet nursing has been recorded since the pre-Christian era. The custom of shared suckling which has existed in many societies and still exists today is a quite different practice from that of hiring another woman to feed a baby. The first is an act of female solidarity and co-operation, but the second was carried out principally for reasons of social identification rather than for the benefit of the child or the mother. In some eras, when a noblewoman breastfed her own child she was seen as exceptional. Blanche of Castile, the mother of King (later Saint) Louis IX of France (1215-1270), was so committed to maternal breastfeeding that when a lady-in-waiting suckled her son when he was crying she made him vomit up the milk. [18] There was variation between individual women, households and regions, but it was certainly accepted for many centuries that important women often did not feed their own babies.

Why did the elite women not breastfeed? It was not because of participation in public life, for though a few women managed to wield some political power they were the exceptions to the rule.

Public suckling was accepted, so modesty was not the reason. It was unlikely to be for psychological reasons, for if a poor woman could breastfeed then a less overworked or hungry noblewoman should have no problems. There are several possible explanations.

Firstly, the noblewoman had the power to pay or coerce another woman to perform this task. Class structure is derived from the power relationships between people. The noblewoman was expected to delegate all physical labour to others in order to demonstrate her own and her family's high status. Just as today a wealthy businessman might insist that his wife takes the car to go shopping even if she dislikes driving, 'because what will people think of me if they see my wife carrying shopping bags on the bus', so some powerful families would not have tolerated the women members doing what every ordinary peasant woman had to do. Remember the tale of the princess and the pea, where the test of royal blood was proved by the fact that the strange visitor could feel even a tiny pea through twenty mattresses? I always thought she was dreadfully bad-mannered to complain about the bedding, but the story illustrates the belief in and admiration for noble 'delicacy'. As it became usual for the noble baby to be wet nursed, it probably became difficult for a mother to defy custom and if the exceptional woman insisted on feeding she may have had problems due to the social disapproval. Eventually the myth that noblewomen were too delicate and special to suckle would have provided a strong emotional inhibition; how could she know that she could feed if everyone assumed she could not?

In North America today there is a generation of women who bottle-fed their children, not because they chose to, but because the idea of feeding their children in any other way did not arise. They may have been dimly aware, from glimpses inside the *National Geographical Magazine*, that distant tribes fed their babies at the breast, but this would have reinforced, through the innate racism of industrialised society, that this was something only 'primitive' people did. Amongst many North Americans and Europeans in the 1960s and 1970s (and even today), a bottle and a baby were as natural partners as a car and a petrol pump. In hospital a new baby was bottle-fed and a mother routinely given lactation suppressants. If she ever considered the idea of breastfeeding there was an assault course of deterrents and her collapse at one of these would reinforce the common assumption that breastfeeding was difficult and inappropriate for the modern baby. So it would have been the same for many a noblewoman in the past; the idea of feeding her own child would have been as extraordinary as hoeing her own fields. However in one of those social double-binds that seem to beset women whatever they do, the upper-class woman was frequently criticised by medical writers for being an unloving mother because she did not breastfeed. The situation is exactly the same for many modern bottle-feeding women; their culture, the commercial pressure and the maintenance of misinformation makes it almost impossible for them to breastfeed, yet some health workers will criticise them for 'choosing' artificial feeding.

MUTILATING FASHIONS

Other factors emerged that made breastfeeding difficult even for the woman who considered it. In Europe until the fifteenth century, women's clothing was loose and relatively comfortable and evidence shows that maternal breastfeeding was more usual even by noblewomen during this era. By the sixteenth century fashionable women wore corsets of leather, bone or even metal which completely flattened the breast and the nipple. Grigori Kozintsev's film version of *Hamlet* made in 1964 has an evocative scene of Ophelia being laced into such a corset. If corsets could damage the internal organs or crack the ribs, which they did, then they certainly would have damaged developing breast tissue and restricted and harmed the nipples. In the twentieth century Dr Cicely Williams noted the same effect in upper-class Chinese women who wore very tight and completely flattening dresses and then found themselves unable to breastfeed. The breast seems to have gone in and out of favour as a marker of fashionable beauty. Until industrialisation poor women remained relatively unaffected by these trends and being fashionably dressed was confined to an elite who typically had to do extraordinary things to emphasise their eliteness.

Why women should suffer pain and damage their bodies to achieve a certain 'look' is a measure of the emphasis of their status as objects. The self-destructive pursuit of an entirely arbitrary standard of beauty has not died out with the abandonment of corsets. Since the 1960s millions of women have had cosmetic breast surgery. In the United States surgeons advertise without alluding to the pain and risk, charge huge sums and half their clients are low income women. Not only do most of these women jeopardise their ability to breastfeed their babies (though it is possible in some cases), but they also may lose the sexual and sensual feelings that they can experience through their breasts. If a nipple has been surgically repositioned, the delicate nerve structures leading to the hypothalmus and the complex endocrine system involved in arousal are unlikely to function as before. Imagine thousands of men having part of their body reshaped surgically and losing all function, just so it can be gazed upon and handled by women! The tragedy of fashion is that it changes so arbitrarily that a woman can lose the little illusion of power that she has paid for so dearly in both money and pain.

WOMEN OF BREEDING

There is a third significant reason for some of the elite women of history not breastfeeding. A noblewoman's principle function was to provide heirs and it was known that breastfeeding might prevent her from producing more children. A falsehood of history is the myth of the poor 'breeding like rabbits'. On the contrary, it was the aristocrats that deserved this comparison. In pre-industrial England eighteen pregnancies were not uncommon amongst the nobility. Ann Hatton, a wealthy seventeenth-century heiress, had thirty children: 'Five sons and eight daughters, besides 10 who died young and seven infants stillborn.'[20] In England, the poorer peasants and artisans married later than the aristocracy. Not only did women breastfeed their own babies, but they suckled others, both in the day-to-day sharing of childcare and as a waged job. This protected them from the excessive fertility of the noble lady whose baby was put out to nurse at birth. Evidence from seventeenth-century rural England shows an awareness of the contraceptive effect of lactation. Women took on another child after their own was off the breast or if their own child died. Country women rarely had more than seven children and this was not due to excessive mortality. Records show that birth spacing was greater among the poor than the rich and that their babies were more likely to survive.

Another pretext for wet nursing was the common belief that a breastfeeding woman must abstain from sexual relations, which persists in many countries to this day. Valerie Fildes, who has researched the history of infant feeding, does not think this was a widespread taboo in England, but Linda Pollock in her book *Forgotten Children* thinks this was the main reason for wet nursing, and she recounts the belief that semen was supposed to curdle the milk. [21] (This concept of semen entering the milk is not as ridiculous as it may seem, for as stimulation of the breasts may be followed by sensations in the pelvis and genitals the connection between the two areas of the body and the two white substances is an obvious one.)

For several hundred years before the eighteenth century, Roman Catholic doctrine advised wet nursing 'to provide for the frailty of the husband by paying the conjugal due'. [22] Presumably the conjugal needs of the nobleman (and the state of his immortal soul) were of greater importance than those of the wet nurse's husband or indeed the wet nurse. This conflict between sexual relations and breastfeeding persists to this day, as we have seen in Chapter 4. Many western women stop breastfeeding 'for the marriage's sake', often because their partners experience sexual jealousy of the baby's physical relationship with the mother. Health workers support this decision, for after all who is most important in our society, men, women or babies?

BEFORE THE INDUSTRIAL REVOLUTION

Wealthy women like Ann Hatton might not have had to worry about the harvest, but the vision of the endless cycle of pregnancy, childbirth and perhaps joyless sex acts evokes a picture of a life

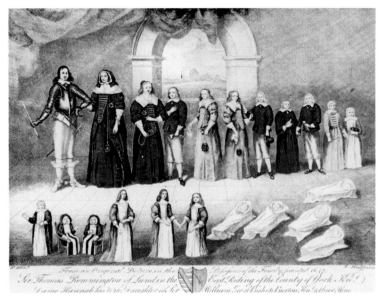

10 The typically oversized aristocratic family of Thomas Remmington of Lund, Yorkshire, including the deceased infants, 1647. (Courtesy of Mary Evans Picture Library)

similar to that of a queen termite whose sole purpose is procreation. The ordinary woman in pre-industrial society did not lead a carefree life, but her lot was not as bad as is sometimes assumed. There was variation between communities and of course suffering and oppression existed, but women had not yet been shoved into the cul-de-sac of the economically invisible 'home'.

There is enough evidence from the world of pre-industrial England to refute the common illusions of school textbook history. The myth of the little woman stirring a pot while her big strong man provided the means of their survival is one such myth. When people refer to the woman's place in the home they forget that before the Industrial Revolution everyone's place was in the home. The household was the production unit and every enterprise was inextricably bound up with the family. This did not mean that all the workers were family members, for in England most people went into some kind of service in another household. Wives and children were as vital a part of the whole production process as the workshops and manufacturing processes were, and as the latter were usually carried out in the same place as the living quarters, there was not the strong demarcation of 'home' and 'work' tasks that is taken for granted today. The wife who supervised or carried out the food preparation was both 'mother' and staff canteen lady. She was no more and no less economically dependent on her husband than he on her. It was as vital for a man to marry a wife in order to be a full member of society as it was for a woman to marry a husband. Unmarried men who stayed in service all their lives never achieved full economic participation and status and were seen to be as unfortunate as unmarried women. Women as well as men had worked, learned a set of skills and perhaps saved a little from their wages before they married. Because childhood ended early and marriage was late most men and women had at least ten years' working life before they established their own economic unit of a new household. The most unfortunate women were often from impoverished families of rank; they were prevented from doing manual labour, yet not provided with an education or a means of earning a living, and were supposed to be innately capable and desirous of attracting a husband to support them. However the majority of women were workers who participated fully in economic life in a way that was taken for granted.

Capitalism was already well established in England before the Industrial Revolution. For example, the wool and cloth industry was run by entrepreneurs who owned and controlled the raw materials and eventual sale of the finished products. The work was done in the countryside by cottagers, who were the great mass of ordinary people, and many women and children spun, carded and wove for the peripatetic controllers of their industry. This 'industrial' work was as important to their economic survival as work in the fields and the terrible rural poverty of late Victorian times was due partly to the disappearance of this type of employment. The countryside was not entirely concerned with the production of food, industry took place there and towns were more centres for trade and exchange than for manufacture. Though this society was patriarchal in the sense that men had the authority, women were active participants in economic life and the division of labour was not rigid. The historian Peter Laslett quotes an eighteenth-century observer of rural life who said, 'In the long winter evenings, the husband cobbles shoes, mends the family clothes and attends to the children while the wife spins.'[23] Girls became apprentices and women ran businesses in their own right, usually if their husband had died, but not always.

BABIES AND WORK

Because there was not the physical and mental divide between the workplace and the home, childrearing was, in the main, an integral part of the system. Young people left home and went into service in other households, and there they worked, ate, slept and loved or hated their fellow workers and employers. The intimacy of working relations might have kept a check on the excesses of the slave or factory owner. It would be uneconomic to ill-treat a woman in the neonatal period so that she or her baby died because both were part of the long-term production process. A factory owner could always replace a dead or worn-out worker, but a household production unit had a mutual interest in maintaining acceptable levels of welfare. Because marriage was linked with the setting up of a new household economic unit, so production was integrally connected with the activities that are considered now to be the housewife's. Breastfeeding the babies fitted into this system. It was simply another task that had to be done, like brewing the beer, making the bread, getting in the harvest or shoeing the horses. Until the time of the land enclosures during the seventeenth and eighteenth centuries, most harvesting had to be communal because different families farmed strips. One large field was shared between different households and co-operation was intrinsic to survival. The land enclosures took away the last shreds of self-sufficiency from poor people, and was done not only to facilitate more 'efficient' farming methods for the landowner but also to force people to hire out their labour. This taking away of people's land or access to land has been echoed around the world and is still happening. It is a guaranteed way of creating dependency and is paralleled in infant feeding. By taking away women's primordial right to sustain their own children with their own milk, through the destruction of traditional knowledge and the reorganisation of work processes, dependency on a powerful dominant group is created.

One school of thought argues that children were universally cruelly treated in pre-industrial times, with facts like the practice (not universal) of swaddled children being hung on hooks while people worked cited as evidence. It is impossible to know the whole truth, but I can see little difference between hanging babies on hooks and leaving them for hours in their cots, prams and playpens. Certainly I feel those of us who live in an age where it is estimated that one in five children is sexually abused by adults, as many again physically attacked, thousands taken away 'into care' from their parents or abandoned to endure the horrors of street survival in the hostile cities have little right to judge.[24] Linda Pollock paints a different picture and shows that tenderness to the young was prevalent in the past.[25] Certainly children were valued, not least for the economic contribution of their work. Though I want to guard against romanticising the exploitation of children, their integration into all the daily functions of an economic community meant that learning a whole series of jobs was not a separate process that began at the social recognition of adulthood, but was unconsciously absorbed by imitation and participation over many years. One of the bad effects of compulsory education is not merely that children are deprived of this integrated skill learning, but that women become more exploited and overworked. This happened throughout the late nineteenth and early twentieth centuries when mothers were condemned for keeping their children out of school, yet never given a new source of assistant labour. Today in developing countries, women work hard on the land to pay for schooling, only to be deprived of their children's much-needed help, and both boys and girls miss vital primary learning in domestic skills and childcare and this contributes to the marginalisation of these jobs.

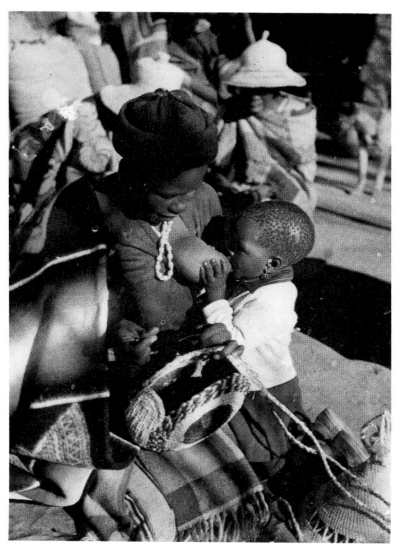

11 Lesotho mother and her school age child enjoying a breastfeed while she works. (*Photo:* Dirk Schwager *c.* 1970s; courtesy of Lesotho Cooperative Handicrafts, Maseru)

In pre-industrial Europe a child would have grown up seeing her mother both working and rearing babies. Most children would have handled and played with several babies before experiencing the responsibility of their own. A girl would have learned how to position the baby on the breast by seeing it done a thousand and one times, just as she learned how to stack a corn stook. By the time she had a child of her own she would have been as confident of mothering skills as she would of gleaning or spinning. Much of twentieth-century life consists of embarking on tasks for which we have an overload of theoretical knowledge and little practical experience. This does not matter in terms of production because so many tasks are divided into disparate components. An individual may be trained to make coat collars, but not to tailor a coat, to assemble microchips but not to create computers, to perform kidney surgery but be unable to help someone lead a healthier life. When modern western parents have a baby they may not only be holding a new human for the first time in their life, but may also never have experienced a truly multi-faceted job with total responsibility for the outcome, and yet they are assumed to be capable through books and the advice of strangers being the sole carers of the child. In pre-industrial societies both in the past and in the present, the opposite situation existed. A mother had learned throughout her life about the practicalities, rhythms, crises and overall management of the production process and also the same of childcare. Not being able to breastfeed a child or time the harvest would be as incredible as someone from our own society being unable to switch on a television.

WET NURSING AS AN ECONOMIC FUNCTION: THE EXAMPLE OF SEVENTEENTH-CENTURY ENGLAND

During this era, the integration between earning a living and the daily tasks of household life included breastfeeding because it too was part of economic production. Though most babies were breastfed by their mothers, throughout history writers on childcare debated maternal or wet nursing. As with so much history, the customs of the rich and powerful minority are better recorded than the common experience of the ordinary person, and for the most part these writers addressed the elite. The irrelevance of medical opinion to the great majority of childbearing women reflects the exact same attitudes of present-day paediatric writers. Most modern baby care information has a feeding section describing the relative merits of 'breast or bottle' as though this is a choice available to all women. The decision, which may involve hours of reading for the formally educated woman, is not part of most women's lives, just as for the peasant women of pre-industrial Europe the great debate of whether the mother or the nurse should feed the baby was irrelevant.

In the same way that some women in the modern world might choose a feeding method because social pressures outweigh the consideration of what is best for the baby's health, so in the past, in spite of writers urging maternal breastfeeding, some mothers still used wet nurses even though it was less good for the baby. Babies sent 'out to nurse' many miles from their birthplace would have had to withstand a new range of germs both on the journey and in the nurse's household. It was slightly safer if the nurse was from the same household as the mother for they would have had more chance of exposure to the same diseases, but a baby is born in tune with her mother's protection and the immunology of placental transference and suckling are geared to maternal breastfeeding (see page 67). Of course, in those days this knowledge did not exist, but it was observed that babies succumbed to disease while being sent out to nurse and that they did better if fed by their own mothers.

Wet nursing has been commonly viewed in two ways. One was that this was a terrible example of the exploitation of women and it is erroneously assumed that the nurse's baby was often deliberately left to die of neglect so that the woman could sell her milk to survive. The other was that the wet nurse was a drunken slut who neglected or even murdered her charges. Though there are grains of truth in both these stereotypes, the average situation was far less horrifying. The typical wet nurse before the Industrial

Revolution was a respectable married woman. Often her husband had a job which involved travel to and from a main urban centre and in this way the family had contact with the upper-class families who were seeking a wet nurse. Except in the case of royalty or the upper aristocracy, the baby was usually sent to live with the nurse so that her own household life was undisrupted. Pay was quite good and, what is more, the nurse could combine her sale of a commodity and service with a method of contraception.

One of the most remarkable wet-nurses of all time was surely Judith Waterford. In 1831 she was written up in both medical and lay papers. She celebrated her eighty-first birthday by demonstrating that she could still squeeze from her left breast, milk which was 'nice, sweet and not different from that of young and healthy mothers.' Judith was married at the age of twenty-two, and for the next fifty years supplied milk to babies. She fed six children of her own, eight nurslings, and many children of her friends and neighbours. In her prime she produced two quarts of breastmilk unfailing everyday, but admitted sorrowfully that after the age of seventy-five she could not have managed to breastfeed effectively more than one infant at a time. (From I. Digby and B. Mathias, *The Joy of the Baby*, 1969)

A DECENT JOB

Wet nursing was like the catering trade: your status was derived according to whom you fed. The chef at the Ritz has greater social prestige than the cook at a local transport café, though both may fill stomachs to their customers' satisfaction. Royal wet nurses were given pensions for life and sometimes a whole gaggle of noblewomen briefly suckled the royal infant just to gain this status. Resident wet nurses often had considerable power within the household. They were given the best food and were not to be upset, as people were aware that stress could impede lactation.

They believed that the nurse's temperament formed the baby's character. Quite illogically, one reason for discouraging noblewomen from feeding was that they supposedly lacked the desirable placid temperament that would be passed on to the baby through the milk. No one seemed to notice that they themselves may have been wet nursed by ordinary country women with supposedly placid natures. In spite of the obsession with lineage and 'blood', these noble biological parents apparently influenced only the positive attributes of the child and any adverse characteristics could be blamed on the wet nurse.

Country women were also probably healthier. Nowadays the concept of the tough rural woman is a distortion of the facts of health in many countries, but in seventeenth-century Britain it may have been true. As seventy five per cent of the nation lived in the countryside poverty was not exclusively rural, and right up to the twentieth century there were lower infant mortality rates in the agricultural regions than in the urban areas. Unless there was an exceptionally long, dark winter, the outdoor life of most rural working people would have protected them from vitamin D deficiency (see Chapter 3, Page 63) which could affect the health of both mother and infant. The rich woman lying on her couch in the drawing room and perhaps only venturing forth in a carriage, lest the sun freckle her lily-white complexion, might have been vitamin D-deficient. The working woman could not have afforded a doctor so she would have escaped the frequent bleedings which became a universal remedy for all ills, used during pregnancy and even as a treatment for perinatal haemorrhage. This exacerbated the chronic anaemia resulting from the cycle of miscarriages, pregnancies and menstruation of the non-lactating upper-class woman. Princess Charlotte (1796–1817), the daughter of the Prince Regent, died in childbirth because she had been attended throughout pregnancy by the 'best' doctors who had bled her regularly. A lot of wealthy women may have felt they were too ill and weak to breastfeed even if they had been able to, after these excessive medical attentions. Another important aspect of wet nursing is that maternal mortality rates were high, for although the proportion of childbirth complications was approximately equal to the modern rate, an obstructed labour was often unresolvable and fatal. Wet nurses were irreplaceable life savers in these circumstances.

The wet nurse was not only paid in money and goods such as sugar, tea and candles, but her connection with a wealthy baby could benefit her and her family. Influential connections still play a significant part in modern access to good jobs, positions of power and medical treatment. In the seventeenth and eighteenth centuries they were essential for advancement and openly accepted. Integrating yourself with a noble patron was a key to family security and if a woman had preserved the life and health of an important heir that family was rightly obligated to her. Some wet nurses did have a breastfeeding baby and would usually arrange for another lactating woman to suckle her. Sometimes a wet nurse paid as much as she herself was paid: 'Sir William Petre of Ingatestone Hall in Essex paid his son's wet nurse 10 pence a week in 1550, whilst her own child was nursed by another woman for 9 pence a week.'[26] Why should a woman breastfeed a strange child, denying herself the contact with her own for a penny a week? We only have to look at some modern families for an explanation. In England, average childminding costs use up half a mother's wages. This expenditure is universally perceived as her responsibility rather than the father's. Many better paid women hire cleaners (again seen as her delegation), buy more costly food and clothes and often a car, to ensure job success. Some English families use up the wife's entire salary to pay private school fees. Clearly a woman believes that she is gaining something worthwhile either in personal satisfaction, social prestige or benefit to her family if she makes no direct financial profit from her labour.

Many wet nurses earned good wages; one woman in 1650 earned 7s 9d (39p) a week (a labourer's wage was around 6s (30p)).[27] Many women continued to care for the babies after sevrage and if they fostered two or three children, as many did, they earned more money than their husbands. In sum, wet nursing was a good job for a woman, the life-saving properties of breastmilk and a good nurse were appreciated and the social boundaries were crossed, giving some women lifelong security or privilege.

CO-OPERATION AND EXPLOITATION:
DIFFERENT BABY MINDING CUSTOMS

In the seventeenth and eighteenth centuries, women were casual about suckling each other's children and we can compare this with some of the minding experiences of a modern bottle-fed child. Parents may hire a succession of nannies for daily care, use any available babysitter if they go out at night and the hotel baby minding service when on holiday. Though psychologists might be concerned about how this affects the infant's emotional development, the wide availability of these services indicates that some parents do not believe that their baby suffers from a haphazard selection of carers. In pre-industrial England, a baby may have been suckled by a relative or neighbour whenever a woman needed to leave him, but it was probably someone she knew and trusted well. [28]

The modern reaction to the hiring of a wet nurse often includes condemnation of the rich family who may have risked the nurse's child's welfare for their own baby's. I can see no difference between this and the fact that devoted middle-class parents in Europe and America use a whole range of consumer goods, from babygros to toys and rattles, which are produced in the low-wage economies of Korea, Taiwan or even the inner cities of Europe and the US by women workers who may have to neglect their own child in order to survive. Books recommending breastfeeding often suggest 'getting help with the housework so that you do not get overtired'. The help may be a Filipina woman who has had to leave her children in order to earn low but essential wages for her family. Many of the practical conveniences of our lives, from the washing machine to our knickers, are produced through the insecure and low-paid labour of women in the global economy. There is often an unthinking acceptance of injustice. A woman who breastfed her own children said to me, 'When we were in Bangladesh my servant did leave her baby to be bottle-fed while she worked for me, but it was better for her family as she could help them more with the wages she earned.' This woman did not feel that her wealth had any links with the Bangladeshi woman's poverty. The servant may have felt compelled to leave her baby, but in that society it was a terrible risk. Why should the poor baby be deprived of his mother's milk and cuddling so that the rich woman could suckle hers in more comfort? In most circumstances, babies could easily accompany their mothers to work, but the competition for jobs is so intense that no servant would dare request doing something which might cause minor inconvenience to her employer.

Perhaps the most extreme modern example of this situation exists in South Africa where white children are cared for by black nannies who are separated from their own children for years. The white parents are doing what they see is best for their child and the nanny's suffering is carefully disregarded or denied with such mental gymnastics as, 'They don't feel the same as we do, they are used to being separated from their kids.' I suspect that similar denial existed in some parents who hired wet nurses. It would have been physiologically possible for most healthy wet nurses to feed two children, their own and their charge, but this was uncommon in wealthy families. The benefits of the added stimulus of two babies were recognised by some doctors (particularly in the USA) and the wet nurse was encouraged to continue feeding her own child. However most wet nurses before the nineteenth century hired themselves out after their own child could be safely taken off the breast. This may have contributed to the earlier sevrage that became the norm in England. In many other pre-industrial societies women suckled their babies for a couple of years or more, yet by this time in England many babies were taken off the breast at around a year. It is important to add that there were wide differences between regions in infant feeding practices. In certain areas of Europe artificial feeding was already well established before the nineteenth century, yet in east Lincolnshire women were reported to suckle their children until they were 7 or 8 years old even in the 1820s.[29]

CONTEMPORARY ATTITUDES TO WET NURSING

Some modern mothers are horrified by the idea of shared breastfeeding. La Leche League's policy is that the mother's own milk is the most biologically appropriate for the child (they are right) and that the special breastfeeding relationship is best when it is exclusive. One woman even made the comparison with adultery when I asked her about allowing another woman to feed her baby. This demonstrates the wide range of attitudes to baby care where in the same society a bottle may be handed to anyone who is around to feed the baby. Most hospitals, nurseries and day care centres cannot ensure that babies are fed by the same one or perhaps two people, and consequently these babies cannot experience their first relationship as one of a developing interaction of sensitivity between two people. The tragedy is that while we discuss these pros and cons, hundreds of babies are simply 'bottle propped', left alone with their bottles, some being manufactured with handles for this purpose. My own feeling is that shared breastfeeding is a unique opportunity for solidarity and friendship among women. My sister and I regret that we did not co-ordinate our childbearing so as to be able to do this. I recently heard of four women in London who all work outside the home and share breastfeeding. There have also been breastfeeding circles within babysitting circles. The existence of HIV infection has led to the official discouragement of wet-nursing in industrialised countries. However, in much of the world it is still the safest alternative to maternal feeding (see page 77).

Women I have talked to who have shared breastfeeding, usually temporarily, have felt very happy about it. Often it is fathers who have expressed reservations about 'their' baby being fed by 'another woman'. It seems that male feelings of ownership and possessiveness cut through women's solidarity in this as in many respects. While many women in the world are overburdened by too much childbearing, other women in industrialised society sadly refrain from having children because their male partners do not want them. If more women supported one another to bear children this would undermine the weighted economic control that enables men to direct women's fertility. Mothers, sisters and close friends could elect to support a child economically just as a father might and women who may not want to experience childbirth or breastfeeding could participate in the emotional satisfaction of parenthood. Of course this already happens in many areas of the world when women are abandoned by the fathers of their children. The idea of shared breastfeeding for lesbian mothers seems so obvious, yet I can see that worldwide prejudice against lesbians, especially lesbian mothers, would muster forces to prevent any such movement. Women sharing childcare, and indeed their whole lives, in such an intimate way threatens the stability of male social control.

OTHER ASPECTS OF WET NURSING

In England, before the Industrial Revolution, illegitimacy and abandonment were less common than on the continent of Europe. In France wet nursing was more usual and had been under state control since the twelfth century. Perhaps market forces played a part in this, for the more readily available a product, the more likely people are to use it. Shop-bought bread replaces the home-made product when it is cheap and widely available. In Spain, Italy and France, high illegitimacy rates led to the establishment of vast foundling hospitals with a revolving container (*tour*) in the door where the baby was placed and the parent and child guaranteed anonymity. If the social set-up prohibited an unmarried mother from rearing her child, at least it allowed her to utilise one result of this pregnancy, the milk, and this could not only enable the woman to earn a living, but perhaps also protect her from a further pregnancy. The plentiful supply of wet nurses might have then induced more women to hire them just as the use of domestic servants always tallies with their availability and cheapness. Why there should be fewer unwanted pregnancies in England before the Industrial Revolution than on the continent is a fascinating subject beyond the scope of this book. What is likely is that because there was more maternal suckling in England and less wet nursing which involved the abandonment of the nurse's own child, there were lower infant mortality rates.

In eighteenth-century England one source of wet nurses was the new lying-in hospitals which were founded through a combination of medical ambition and philanthropy. Only respectable poor women with references could deliver there and demand exceeded provision. Later some of these hospitals were to become centres of infection and a feared cause of mother and child death, but when they opened the chance of a couple of weeks of free food, rest and assistance in labour was attractive to the ordinary woman. They also became centres where families could seek a wet nurse. The very wealthy made these arrangements privately before the birth and would deliberately select a woman who already had a thriving baby, as proof of her quality. However many people had to seek out a wet nurse in a hurry, because a mother had died in childbirth or the original wet nurse proved unsatisfactory, and they would go to the lying-in hospitals where a mother whose baby had died could hire herself out. Women were also hired by the managers of foundling hospitals. Although some people express revulsion at the idea of a newly bereaved mother having to feed a strange baby, this might have been a positive benefit.

A friend of mine who miscarried after seven months of pregnancy started to lactate and experienced an overwhelming need to hold a baby. She asked the hospital staff if she could 'borrow' a baby to cuddle in her arms, but they refused and she felt deprived of a means of comfort and relief from the agony of bereavement. These feelings are not unusual, and whether the baby is dead or removed for all the other cultural or medical reasons, many women have suffered because they have not been allowed to hold either their own or any other baby. Much of the sorrow of the bereaved mothers might have been soothed by the task of breastfeeding and caring for another baby, so that being a wet nurse in these circumstances could have been a consoling job. The contact with the child did not end with sevrage; many adults cared for the welfare of their nurses until they died and loved them as though they were their mothers, which in a way they were. The bonding effects of the suckling relationship are often stronger than the effect of the act of giving birth. In 1986 two Irish babies were accidently given to the wrong parents, one mother breastfed the 'wrong' child and when the mistake was discovered and the babies exchanged she was devastated. She felt closer to the suckled child than to her biological baby.[30]

Towards the latter part of the eighteenth century a fashion for maternal breastfeeding swept through aristocratic circles due to the influence of William Cadogan (see Chapter 3, page 40). Whereas in earlier eras maternal feeding was advocated for the baby's sake, it was now advocated to benefit the mother. Early feeding prevents engorgement, mastitis and abscesses. It may also help expel any fragments of retained placenta through stimulating the uterus to contract. If infection occurred, which was a risk with all these conditions, in those days septicaemia and death could result, so these theories were indeed sound.

THE DECLINE OF WET NURSING

As the class of respectable country women diminished because of the changes wrought by the Industrial Revolution, wet nurses were drawn from a different group of women and their quality and status diminished. A Victorian wet nurse was more likely to be a younger unmarried mother who had sent her own child to a less caring minder, possibly one of the notorious 'baby farmers', and she would have been less respectable, less experienced and maybe even less proficient at the techniques of baby care than her typical predecessor. Married wet nurses were viewed with suspicion, supposedly because they only took the job after 'family disturbances' and might prove greedy and hard. I suspect it was actually because they may have been less subservient than the young, socially-ostracised unmarried girl.

Unlike many of her predecessors, the wet nurse had to live in and be completely separated from her offspring in case she was tempted to feed it. This attitude displays an ignorance about breastfeeding physiology, for with the majority of healthy women, two babies would actually maintain a more copious supply, as Judith Waterford's record showed (see pages 95 and 160). Most of the babies of these later wet nurses were separated very early from their mothers and usually died. There was a change in general attitude to wet nurses. A Dr Haden said in 1827, 'wet nurses are unfortunately a necessary evil,' but they formed 'one of the conveniences which money can command'. Some wet nurses were part-time prostitutes, and 'undoubted authority proved that the moral taint was transmitted through the milk'. Also, 'Fallen women proved by their very condition, that they possessed uncontrollable, ill-disposed emotions,' which affected the quality of their milk which was even supposed to convey cancer.[31] This ambivalence towards the nurturers of their children, which had been less prevalent when the death of the nurse's baby had not been part of the process, could have been a projection of guilt by the upper towards the exploited classes. By focusing on the nurse's inferiority the rich could avoid confronting the moral dilemma of their complicity in the death of her infant. It also led to the search for artificial foods.

The same attitudes are reflected in so many human situations. The modern quest for technology has been motivated by the aim of avoiding the just treatment of workers and profit sharing. Cows and machines are easier to deal with, because they do not ask for justice. What is important about wet nursing is that before technology and milk surpluses launched the mass production of artificial baby foods, this was the only viable alternative to a mother feeding. As with so many other autonomous skills, this means of economic survival was destroyed by mechanisation and industrialisation. As wet nursing declined, women who formerly would have hired out their services in this way, and could be self-supporting right into old age, had to resort to the poorest-paid menial tasks or prostitution and their health and well-being were damaged as a result. Over the course of the nineteenth century a means of employment unique to women disappeared, and both doctors and commerce paid a key role in this redundancy.

ARTIFICIAL FEEDING BEFORE THE TWENTIETH CENTURY

The fear of Syphilis

Wet nurses were believed to be routes of transmission of syphilis. They themselves also feared being infected by infants with the disease. Syphilis was not transmitted through the milk, but through lack of hygiene and contact with sores (chancres) or lesions on the baby or the nurse. The fear of syphilis may have been on the same level as the current fear of HIV infection. The evidence seems to indicate that wet nursing was only an indirect route of transmission of syphilis and there were many other ways of catching it. It must have been convenient in some cases either for the family to cite the wet nurse or for the wet nurse to cite the baby as the transmittor of infection rather than admit to some sexual transgression. Syphilis is easier to catch than HIV, for the bacterium that transmits it is tougher than the 'AIDS' virus. The problem of syphilis is thought to have motivated the various attempts at artificial feeding, known as 'dry nursing', which included direct suckling of animals, particularly goats, by the baby.[32]

Though a few stalwart individuals, like the beer-swilling baby mentioned in Chapter 3 (page 85), survived attempts at artificial feeding, this was exceptional and 'dry nursing' as it was called was usually lethal. In 1829, the Dublin Foundling Hospital was closed down because 99.6 per cent of the babies died. They were fed artificially and not wet nursed.

The Swinish and Filthy Habit

There were a few areas where, for no apparent reason, artificial feeding became customary. In southern Germany, there was a tradition, which dated as far back as the fifteenth century, of rearing babies on 'meal pap' (flour and water or milk) and animal milk. There were clear regional differences which were much stronger than any difference between rural and urban life. A nineteenth-century writer reported that in the district of Oberbayern,

> A woman who came from northern Germany and wanted according to the customs of her homeland to nurse her infant herself was openly called swinish and filthy by the local women. Her husband threatened he would no longer eat anything she prepared, if she did not give up this disgusting habit.[33]

Not surprisingly, about 50 per cent of the babies died. As late as 1889 a comparative report in the *British Medical Journal* on infant mortality showed certain areas of southern Germany to have rates of death in the first year of life reaching over 400 per 1,000, four times the Norwegian rate. The reporter commented that 'German nurslings are either particularly delicate or particularly unfortunate in their mode of their bringing up [*sic*]. The difference can hardly be due to climate.'[34] Climate probably played a part in the survival in some infants. In the twentieth century in the Punjab, Indian infants artificially fed with animal milks had a mortality rate of 950 per 1,000.[35] Valerie Fildes has argued that artificial feeding only ever became a custom in cold, dry climates where animal milk was plentiful and did not become contaminated so quickly. Also she suggests that because it was the custom, people might have become more adept at preparing the food with some cleanliness.

The neglected babies of Nedertorneå

Hygiene and fresh milk were not notable in another part of Europe where artificial feeding had become customary. In Nedertorneå near the Finnish/Swedish border, a Doctor Carl Wretholm arrived in 1836 and reported,

> I have never seen children so lovelessly treated as those of the Finns. All day they scream in the cradle, skinless due to uncleanliness and vermin. Nobody takes care of them. Instead they are fed with thick and viscous soured milk, given through unclean nipples, which are never washed.[36]

'Artificial nipples' were usually made of an actual cows' teat and the feeding bottle was a horn. In her book *Breasts, Bottles and Babies*, Valerie Fildes has an illustration of a Finnish cradle with a horn in a holder suspended over it, perhaps the original 'propped bottle'.[37] The main cause of death was diarrhoea, and Wretholm employed a midwife to conduct a breastfeeding campaign. By 1851 the infant mortality rate which had been around 400 per 1,000, had halved as 'almost every mother in the town now breastfeeds her children'.[38]

No one has found out exactly why these Finnish women did not breastfeed. In other areas with the same pattern of life and labour, women suckled their babies, so it was not because of their work. However many women said that they did not feed because their own mothers never breastfed them and also that they were considered lazy when breastfeeding. These undramatic reasons make perfect sense to me. Most of us do things because they were normal in the household where we grew up. A family friend used to boil the spinach in three changes of water and serve up a splodge so horrifying in taste and texture it put me off this vegetable for years. When asked why she prepared it this way she replied that that was how her mother had done it. I expect if she had cooked it lightly or even served it raw she would have been called lazy. The overcooking of vegetables is a traditional English custom which carries no nutritional or culinary benefit, but was done because no one thought there was any other way to cook until foreign travel broadened the palates of the middle classes. As with bottle-feeding, those of us who survived it can say, 'Well it never did me any harm!' The mothers in Nedertorneå had grown used to horn feeding; perhaps it had been used years before for an orphan, seemed convenient and caught on. Frequent diarrhoea was probably accepted as a normal part of infancy and because not every baby died the custom continued. However as soon as someone explained that their babies were less likely to die or get ill if they breastfed (and presumably helped them to do it), they changed to the safer method of feeding. How could these communities have accepted such a high infant death rate when the solution seemed so obvious? Perhaps, having lost the knowledge of lactational infertility, some parents saw frequent infant death as a way, however painful, of limiting their families. Perhaps in these regions pasturage was so good that there was surplus milk and putting it into babies was less work than producing more butter and cheese. The baby milk industry was to evolve because there was plenty of spare cows' milk around, and modern health workers dole out excess supplies of baby milk dumped by the companies to breastfeeding mothers because they do not like to 'waste it'.

These communities may not have assumed a cause and effect between feeding method and death; after all if your baby dies, you do not necessarily perceive that this is part of a regional trend. It seems appalling that the Finnish community could bring babies into the world and then treat them so dreadfully, yet in modern Europe we invest vast resources into the maintenance of the lives of low birth weight babies (who might only be small because of their mothers' social disadvantages), yet those and other babies might get ill later because their families are poor or from an avoidable accident. Some of the doctors who use technology to save the lives of very tiny babies sincerely feel that these other aspects of the society which kill or hurt these children are not their responsibility. Health services may save many babies, but it is the same society that allows thousands of youngsters to die on the roads or from alcohol and other drugs, simply because the high prevalence of cars and drink is 'good for the economy'. Future historians may ask how our society could have been so callous about the young and be baffled by our contradictory values.

The most common cause of death for youth ages 15 to 24 in all developed countries is motor vehicle accidents, and the USA follows Australia with the highest death rate for young men from this cause. *(The Wall Street Journal, Oct. 2, 1990. People Patterns)*

The Industrial Revolution in Britain: The Era of Progress?

CHANGES IN ENGLAND

Once more I must refer to the deficiencies of my own education which I share with so many of my generation. I was given the following version: 'The Industrial Revolution was something that happened in the nineteenth century when George Stevenson invented his steam engine "The Rocket". Suddenly everyone built machines, people dropped their pitchforks, rushed to work in the town factories and so much wealth was created that Britain became prosperous and commanded much respect worldwide. This was all due to the inventive English mind and the stable English values, endorsed by Queen Victoria's stolid personality and the discipline of the Church of England. The Industrial Revolution was "copied" by the other leading nations as everyone wanted to be like us. We helped a bit by sending red-faced young men to the colonies to teach the natives how to be "civilised". This was known as "the white man's burden".' One of Margaret Thatcher's most memorable statements was her desire for a return to Victorian values. I suspect her history education was as appalling as mine.

The real facts are less easy to assimilate. Technological change had never stopped since before the Iron Age. There had been other industrial revolutions earlier, such as that of the development of wind and water power in the Middle Ages. The nineteenth-century period of accelerated change was the culmination of many processes reaching a stage of development where they could cross-fertilise. Sailing ships, water pumps, mills and looms had existed

for thousands of years and had been improved and refined over
centuries of trial and error and experience. This is often forgotten
when rapid industrialisation is seen as the key to development.
The internal combustion engine was a major breakthrough, but
the development of the motor car utilised hundreds of years of
experience of wheel and bodywork construction, from cart and
carriage production. Industrialisation was a culmination, not a
beginning, and so many of the 'benefits' that were exported have
been more than just a failure, they have been a disaster. Millions
of dollars have been wasted on the import of motor vehicles which
have been entirely inappropriate for the tracks, climate and
economies of poor tropical countries. Similarly, the para-
phernalia of artificial feeding has contributed to the damage of
babies and national economies. We are only just beginning to
realise what the costs of industrialisation are for our own society;
what has happened in poor countries is devastating.

The original desire of rulers for gold and treasure as wealth to
prop up their dynasties led to the colonisation of the regions
which provided them. As more imported commodities enriched
European economies, it became advantageous to influence their
production at the source and eventually to seize territorial and
political control. Tea, cocoa, sugar, minerals and numerous other
products, produced by slaves and, later, by indentured labourers,
could be acquired in low-priced abundance. As the home markets
became saturated, exports increased and eventually the producers
of the raw materials were purchasing the manufactured goods.
Indians who had hitherto developed the finest fabrics were now
wearing English cloth made of their exported raw cotton. The
management of estates producing plentiful supplies of raw
materials made the colonies a vast storehouse for the development
of British industry. The technological breakthroughs were
significant, but steam power might have been ignored if there had
not been the motive to rush the raw materials to the factories and
the finished goods out of them. The ordinary people did not flock
to the towns because of the thrill of the night life. As machines
were developed to cope with the new abundance of raw materials,
there was no advantage for the capitalist owners in continuing to
distribute wool and flax for spinning, weaving and dyeing in the

rural areas where they had been produced. A centre of manufacture in the form of a factory, built near to the reception sites of the new imported raw materials, was more profitable. Without the economic supplement of the capitalist's outwork, rural poverty (established by the land enclosures) increased, and the only way to survive was to go to the towns. As a generalisation, whenever a comparison is made between rural and urban poverty, in the post-industrialised setting the country dweller is worse off than the city dweller. This is often used as an argument to state that rural life was always terrible and that urbanisation is in itself a good thing. What is forgotten is that the very process of urbanisation impoverishes the countryside because it removes production from the rural areas to the towns. For example industries such as lace making and straw plaiting were thriving in the seventeenth and eighteenth centuries and were women's trades. A woman could combine a range of horticultural and domestic tasks with other skilled work. When the eggs had to be collected, the beer brewed or the baby fed she did not have to ask an overseer permission to stop work. For example, lace making requires a small cushion and pins and patient dexterity. Experience would increase a woman's speed and ability so that her earning potential would rise over the years, only to decline with her eyesight by which time she had trained her daughters. A lacemaker would have been proud of her skill, but when lace making machines were invented, demand for her handmade product fell and her lifetime's development of a unique skill became worthless. We know about the Luddites breaking the machines that destroyed their livelihoods; there must have been many a woman with a broken heart left to an old age of increasing poverty, her very identity as a craftswoman dissolved in the tidal wave of 'progress'. People had no choice but to go off to the towns to seek work, and when women came to have children the new organisation of labour did not allow for childbirth and breastfeeding. Because an urban woman could not produce food, she was entirely dependent on her own or her husband's wages to stay alive. Excluded from more and more occupations, as the ideology of the 'home' became established, women became increasingly dependent on men for their means of survival and this altered the power structure of the household. A rural woman had access to the food available, a husband could not easily hide the eggs or forbid the consumption of potatoes from their shared ground. Money paid only to the husband could be hidden or spent before the woman had access to it. Her survival now depended on fate providing her with a partner who earned enough for a family and felt responsible for their welfare. Women without children gained more independence with the rise of available employment, but married women were increasingly under pressure to stop work, and if they did and had a mean or drunken husband they had to resort to demeaning tactics with which to persuade the wage earner to share out his money. In the latter part of the nineteenth century wages rose, but as is so often the case women, especially mothers were the last beneficiaries of economic growth.

INCREASING MOTHER AND CHILD DEATHS

This first phase of change from household to industrialised production was not good for mothers or babies. Rural conditions had not been healthy by modern standards, but urban conditions were horrific. Density of population increases cross-infection and diseases of faecal contamination are more common when hundreds use one privy as was common in the factories and overcrowded slums of the expanding cities. Maternal mortality rose sharply as the century drew to a close and puerperal fever, associated with overcrowding and cross-infection, was a leading cause of death. Infant mortality had always been worse in the towns than the country. An average figure of 150 deaths per 1,000 live births is judged by the historian Peter Laslett to be typical of the rural parishes of the sixteenth, seventeenth and eighteenth centuries. Compare this with the 235 per 1,000 for Central Bradford between 1891 and 1895. Diarrhoeal deaths rose steadily, doubling as a percentage of infant mortality causes in the last fifteen years of the century. Infant mortality started to fall after 1905, but diarrhoea still accounted for 28 per cent of infant deaths in 1911. [1]

An increase in medical knowledge and skill and a greater availability of food supplies is usually associated with a fall in the infant mortality rate, but the reverse was happening. England had become a wealthy and powerful nation, but little of the wealth reached the mass of mothers and babies; the structure of their lives had disintegrated as the nation's prosperity increased.

THE 'UNOCCUPIED' WOMAN

I do not want to argue that everything was rosy until Victorian times, for it was not and certainly thousands of women and children had suffered poverty, sickness and oppression in the previous centuries. What is important is that during the process of industrialisation, advances were made in technology, understanding and medical knowledge that could physically improve the quality of people's lives. The construction of sewers and safe water provision, the mass production of soap and the rise in food availability, as well as the discoveries of bacteria, pasteurisation and the importance of hygiene, should all in theory have made everyone's lives more comfortable. They did not and women were left behind in the march of progress. Jane Lewis describes the political framework in *Women in England*:

> As the workplace became separated from the home, so a private, domestic sphere was created for women, divorced from the public world of work, office and citizenship. Moreover, during the early period of industrialisation this separation of spheres between the public and the private was given legal sanction: married women were not permitted to own property or make contracts in their own names. They were thus shut out from the world of business. Furthermore, the 1832 Reform Bill made their exclusion from political citizenship explicit for the first time.

In spite of the lip service paid to 'domestic duties', in 1881 the Census excluded women's household chores from the category of productive work and for the first time housewives were classified as unoccupied. Before these changes in policy, the economic activity rates for both men and women had been recorded as equal at about 98 per cent, now only 42 per cent of women were perceived officially to be contributing to the economy.[2]

TWO APPROACHES: DR REID AND MRS GREENWOOD

By the end of the century, some doctors wanted to forbid married women by law from going out to work. In 1901 a Dr George Reid, concerned about the discrepancy between the decline in the general death rate and the high infant mortality rate, saw women's employment as the cause of the problem and echoed the sentiments of many doctors when he stated,

> Now it is perfectly true that we cannot legislate as to how mothers shall feed their children, but surely we may reasonably expect the State to exercise some control in the case of those mothers who sometimes from necessity, *but more frequently from inclination, neglect their home duties and go to work in the factories.* (my italics)[3]

The blaming of mothers for earning their living and 'neglecting their duties' became a well-established principle that survives today. The fact that women had earned their living and supported their families since human life began remained unacknowledged, as it still does. The fact that these women were contributing to the wealth of the nation and to the pockets of many of the stockholding rich, including no doubt some of the very doctors who exclaimed against them, was ignored then, as it is today. If employers take on a particular section of the labour force it is not out of philanthropy. The pottery owners, for example, employed married women because they could realise more profits from such a skilled workforce by paying them lower wages than men.

There were a few people who saw beyond the 'neglect of duties' argument. Mrs Greenwood, a sanitary inspector in Sheffield who published a pamphlet for the Freedom of Labour Defence, pointed out that 'such reasons as the love of work and desire for a higher standard of living, or for greater comforts than the husband's wages afford, influence some of the best women of the working class, who are industrious, self-respecting and thrifty, and whose homes are models of cleanliness and order'. Mrs Greenwood was also aware of the sexual politics of the issue: 'Moreover, to prevent women from earning after marriage would be to place them entirely in the power of their husbands, be they good, bad or indifferent, and would practically repeal for many of them the Married Woman's Property Act.' (This Act had been passed in 1870 to give women control over their earnings.) Mrs Greenwood also foresaw another aspect of discrimination: 'Employers would hesitate to teach girls trades they might not continue in when proficient, and women themselves would not enter industries which would be practically closed to them after marriage.'[4]

But Dr Reid was not so analytical and he clearly thought mothers were stupid: 'If by some means the simple fact could be brought home to mothers that milk, and preferably human milk, is the only permissible diet for infants . . .'[5] He assumed it was innate ignorance that made mothers abandon breastfeeding. Most working mothers realised that breastfeeding was better and did it when they could. During the Lancashire cotton famine in England (1861–65), women breastfed their babies and the infant mortality rate dropped.[6] The changes in the organisation of production had never been challenged by the doctors, though to be fair there were a few calls for crèches and breastfeeding breaks, but this never developed into effective political action on their part. Where mothers were not under the intense pressures of urban poverty, breastfeeding could flourish. In *Lark Rise to Candleford,* an autobiographical account of rural life in the 1880's, the author, Flora Thompson, records how all babies were breastfed: 'When the hamlet babies arrived they found . . . the best of all nourishment nature's own . . . No milk was taken and yet their milk supply was abundant.' Not taking milk may have been an advantage as its consumption by the mother is linked with colic in the breastfed baby. The increase in adult milk consumption has paralleled the twentieth-century decline in breastfeeding and may have contributed to feeding problems. A bottle-fed baby brought on a visit to the hamlet had its bottle held up as a curiosity. Babies were breastfed casually and publicly, including in church: '. . . or to see Clerk Tom's young wife suckling her baby. She wore a fur tippet in winter and her breast hung like a white heather bell between the soft blackness until it was covered up with a white handkerchief, "for modesty".'[7] This 'modesty' was not shame and it was taken for granted that breastfeeding in church was normal.

Whereas religious duty and baby nurture could be combined, factory production made such human compromises difficult. Factories were not like churches; they were noisy, dirty, dangerous places. Mothers who might have quite naturally taken their child with them to the fields or to a small, non-mechanised workshop would be loath to bring their babies into these 'satanic mills'. They were not fit for the workers, let alone their infants. Dr Reid, who felt so strongly about women going to work, did actually suggest crèches and an extension of the compulsory (and unpaid) maternity leave from one month to three months. He wanted mothers only to be allowed back to work if they could show 'that satisfactory provision had been made for the care of their infants'. The onus was definitely on the mothers and not the employers, yet it was the health of the nation, not individual suffering, which was his primary interest. Dr Reid admitted that his concern about infant mortality was not wholly a humanitarian question: 'in the face of the decline in the birth rate of the country during recent years it may assume, if it has not already assumed a serious economic aspect.'[8]

THE MOTIVE FOR CONCERN: BREEDING THE SOLDIERS AND MALE WORKERS

The survival of 'the race' became this era's obsession. Concern about the rising infant mortality rate was motivated by the goals of populating the colonies with white people and providing an army. At the time of the Boer War (1899–1902), it was found that 60 per cent of the recruits were too small and too unfit for military service.[9] The horrified authorities attributed the phenomenon of the shrinking Englishman to a deterioration in long-term nutrition. (Though it has been commented that hers was an unusually prosperous area, it is of interest that Flora Thompson records that there was not a single maternal death in Candleford during the whole ten-year period she describes, and she also notes that the country people were all taller than the town people).

Women had to breed more surviving workers, colonisers and soldiers, but not only were they not paid for this contribution to the economy, they were also impeded from access to it themselves and blamed if they needed to work in the environment that neglected the primary needs of the future workers. To this day telling mothers what to do is seen as a vital part of the maintenance of infant health, but attempts to organise society to accommodate those who actually perpetuate and preserve the health of the human race are denied and derided. The 1919 International Labour Organisation convention giving nursing mothers the right to two half-hour breaks a day without loss of pay had been ratified by eighteen countries by 1951 and many more by 1975. This is more honoured in the breach, for in most of the free market economies few women dare demand these rights from employers who are only too eager to show women as unsuitable employees. In the US women's groups have rejected moves for better maternity protection on the grounds that this will lead to further discrimination.[10] Much female employment is in the fringe economy anyway and workers may be laid off at the slightest show of assertiveness. For the same reason few unions, not even the predominantly female ones, have made this right a priority issue as they are more concerned to prove that 'women are as "good" as men'. Scandinavia and some Eastern European countries have had a better record, but the situation is by no means perfect. Paid maternity leave and nursing breaks are often seen as luxuries for women which many rich countries do not implement as a universal right. Enabling mothers and babies to fulfil this brief period of vital nurture is not a favour to a woman, it is a contribution to the whole of society.

Many companies 'invest' their profits in works of art, sponsorship of cultural events, political donations and grants and scholarships to academic institutions. They also spend vast sums on prestigious buildings, furnishings and entertainment as well as large, well-publicised gifts to 'charity', often rewarded by generous tax concessions. Yet an economist told me that business could not possibly 'afford' to give a little time off for their employees to breastfeed their babies or provide a simple crèche for mothers who wish to feed their babies at work.

THE APARTHEID OF MOTHERS

The movement of production from the home to the factory changed the situation for women for ever. The separation of 'work' and 'motherhood' was established and the family unit became a group of consumers rather than producers. 'Work' became something that men did outside in the big wide world. If women wanted to participate, their roles as mothers and partners to men were of no concern to the employer. Workers still needed someone to prepare their food, wash their clothes and clean the house, so it was in the interests of profits that these duties fell upon an unpaid mate. Reproducing the workers was necessary, but if one woman lost all her babies because she went back to work too early or the conditions of her work discouraged the possibility of a breastfeeding baby accompanying her, it did not affect the economic unit of the large factory. Within a household economic unit, poor health and dead babies hindered production, with industrialised production workers are replace-able and the employer has no economic motive to concern himself with the welfare of the workers. This situation persists to this day and improvements in welfare have only evolved because of many decades of struggle through painstaking and painful organisation and solidarity. The strength for the worker in the new system was in numbers and many men and women resisted, organised, suffered and died to achieve the few basic standards of decency which exist in some parts of the world today. Women's part in the development of trade unions has been significant and under-recognised but men have dominated the movement, especially in the early twentieth century when even ardent trade unionists began to internalise and accept the idea of the 'normality' of women's role in the home. Mothers were not dominant in the trade union movement, principally because their second job left them with no time to participate.

Gradually, the idea of motherhood being something that happens behind closed doors, in the private, seraglio-like home, became taken for granted. This attitude still exists and the integration of mothers and babies into public life is universally viewed with ridicule and alarm in industrialised society. It is worth remembering that this same attitude existed towards any woman until relatively recently (and still does in many quarters). Winston Churchill was horrified at the thought of a woman in the House of Commons, claiming that it was like having a woman in his bathroom (though why he should be so upset by a woman in his bathroom has always baffled me). The excuses for female exclusion *per se* are strikingly parallel to those for breastfeeding couples. Women are 'shrill'/babies are noisy; women need special provision such as separate toilets and sanitary towels/babies need their nappies changing; women distract attention by their looks/babies distract people by their gurgling and charm; women arouse men and make them feel uncomfortable/babies irritate people and are out of place.

, Everyone believes that their environment is the normal one. In fact industrialised society is so new and so rapidly changing that it is distinctly abnormal when viewed across the panorama of human existence. In much of the world, women do not perceive a contradiction or conflict between their economic participation and their childrearing, even though colonialism and 'development' has done its best to change things.

MISERY AND ISOLATION

After the Industrial Revolution the sexual and social division of labour crystallised. No longer could the husband mind the children and mend the clothes while his wife span. In the factories there was no equivalent of the harvest when even the grandest might roll up their sleeves and muck in. Different tasks were allotted to different groups and there was less intermingling of the sexes in the same jobs. The pretexts for this were not just traditional concepts of the division of labour, but an increasing obsession with the control of women's sexuality. Women were barred from heavy manual wage earning labour, only to carry out unpaid heavy physical work at home. The zeal with which Victorian reformers worked to 'protect' women from such jobs as mining was more a concern for the effect of sexual opportunity on their souls than for the effect of heavy work on their health. Little provision was made for alternative employment when industries were barred to women and many were angry at being deprived of their livelihoods. Women had worked at heavy jobs for centuries alongside men.

An urban worker about to give birth was often without support. Though this varied from region to region, family and neighbour support structures were hard to maintain when the factory hours ruled. Tasks like washing and food preparation had to be done and increasingly a woman had to pay someone to do them. The cities were filthy with the grime of factory and household chimneys so there was far more washing and cleaning to be done. Children were now in factories (and later on the schools), so they were at the beck and call of the mill owners rather than helping their immediate family. Even if female relatives or friends were available they could not leave their waged labour during the set hours to help. The old country midwives helped with the washing and household tasks and could always be paid in kind and future favours, but in the cities there was a scale of fees and everything cost money.

THE 'MATERNITY' LETTERS

Maternity: Letters from Working Women edited by Margaret Llewellyn Davies depicts the lives of some women at the turn of the twentieth century. As literate women and members of the Women's Co-operative Guild, they were acutely aware that they

were better off than many others. The fact that most of them had
led lives of unceasing pain and humiliation makes the experience
of the other nineteenth century British working women all the
more horrifying. There are statues dedicated to the unknown
soldier and plaques listing the military casualties of war in most
towns and villages. There are no memorials to the thousands of
women who worked or served the male workers who created the
wealth and consequent power of Europe and the United States.
There are no statues commemorating the unknown baby who
died because progress made life too hard for her mother.

Maternity reveals that a life of bad health, overwork, under-
nutrition and sexual exploitation was the lot of most women.
They were unprepared, ignorant and anxious and they were aware
of this:

> Owing to the worry connected with this misfortune [her baby
> had died], also having to be up so soon after the confinement
> and for want of rest. I felt my health giving way, and being in
> a weak condition, I became an easy prey to sexual intercourse,
> and thus once more became a mother in fourteen months.

During this era the missionaries and other colonisers were doing
their best to civilise the 'savages' in places such as the colonised
areas of Africa. In several African socities, as in many other parts
of the world, both prolonged lactation and codes of sexual
abstinence protected both the mother and child from the risks of
closely spaced pregnancies. Polygyny was one way of confining
sexuality to a prescribed system which prevented such gross
exploitation of women's bodies, but this was energetically
discouraged by Christian missionaries. Meanwhile back in
'civilised' society, Christian marriage allowed a man complete
access to his wife's body regardless of her feelings or the effects
on her own and her baby's health. Women 'submitted' just to
deter their husbands from adultery, but though having more
than one wife was seen as unchristian, many women were
raped within monogamous marriage with complete social
compliance. Female submission to male conjugal rights was
intrinsic to marriage and to this day many legal systems do

not yet recognise the concept of rape within marriage.

The women who wrote these letters condemned their own ignorance and regretted the fact that they were far from their mothers or intimate female support at the time of birth which they knew was a crucial factor for the woman's and baby's welfare. This is quite a different picture from the seventeeth century where women often went home to their mother's house for several months when they had their first babies, just as many women in Africa and India still do today. There was no written information, body functions were taboo in everyday conversation and a town woman may never have had the opportunity to watch an animal giving birth. My own grandmother, who at the beginning of this century lived in London lodgings with strangers, was completely ignorant of how babies were born when she was pregnant with her first child.

Women tolerated appalling discomforts because they did not know whether they were normal or not. The accounts of prolapsed wombs, burst varicose veins, piles, protracted labour and doctor's hands groping for retained placentas without any anaesthetic makes the modern reader wince. What is most poignant in the book is how grateful women are just for brief periods of health or if their husband was 'good', that is, if he did not rape them. Miscarriages distressed them more profoundly than the pain of childbirth and they were acutely aware that 'nerves' and worry were detrimental to their own and their baby's health. If they wanted medical help during childbirth they had to save money and going without food was the only way they could do this, which itself would have reduced their chances of a straightforward labour and a healthy baby. If they did go out to work it was taken for granted that all the domestic duties were theirs alone.

Margaret Llewellyn Davies comments,

> Writers on infant mortality and the decline of the birth rate never tire of justly pointing to the evils which come from the strain of manual labour in factories for expectant mothers. Very little is ever said about the same evils which come from the incessant drudgery of domestic labour.

The 'Maternity' letters reveal that women were only too aware that breastfeeding was best;

> From the second day [after the confinement] I had to have my other child with me, undress him and see to all his wants, and was often left six hours without a bite of food, the fire out and no light, the time January, and the snow lain on the ground two weeks . . . When I got up after ten days my life was a perfect burden to me. I lost my milk and ultimately my baby.

This writer goes on to describe profound depression and adds, 'Can we any longer wonder why so many married working women are in the lunatic asylums today? Can we wonder that so many women take drugs, hoping to get rid of the expected child?' All she asks for is some rest and relief from overwork. It is now so well established medically that stress, overwork and poor nutrition are detrimental to the health of mothers and babies that we forget that this had not been 'scientifically' established. Though the medical world continued to emphasise the ignorance of mothers, the mothers' letter in *Maternity* show women's awareness of the needs of mothers and babies. Most mothers did breastfeed and took a shy pride in this fact. When they failed to breastfeed this was yet another sorrow to add to the endless account of misery. They knew that artificial feeding was dangerous and also that stress exacerbated physical problems even though this was not acknowledged 'scientifically': 'After my second [child], I was very ill with my breasts, but, of course, I put that down to my husband's lack of work.'

What is emphasised more than the physical hardship is the anxiety, their 'nerves', the consciousness that their state is never-ending and that they were always fearful of death. The very anxiety that they might not be able to breastfeed would have increased the risk of lactation failure. A woman who had to get out of bed before she had recuperated from the birth simply to do the washing and cooking and cleaning and who lived in dread of her husband's sexual advances was in a state of dread and fear that could easily inhibit her let-down reflex: 'Before three weeks I had to go out cleaning and so lost my milk and began with the bottle.'[11] Unlike most of the 'savage' societies of the empire, there was no compulsory, socially supported rest period for newly delivered mothers.

The milk companies have argued that their products kept children alive for all the mothers who could not breastfeed and there was a 'demand'. The fact that the new organisation and stresses of industrialised society created so many of the burdens for women that prevented them from breastfeeding meant that the companies themselves were creating the conditions which ensured that their product would be needed.

I have described urbanising Britain because the pattern of change for women's lives and the effect of this on infant feeding has been repeated around the world. The process of industrialised urbanisation appears to cut women off from their support systems and expose them to stresses, both emotional and physiological, which make it more difficult for them to breastfeed. Hard work itself does not impede lactation, as clear evidence from so many rural societies indicates, nor does living in a city, as thousands of privileged Europeans and North Americans have proved in the 1980s. An increase in fertility often accompanies urbanisation and this may be connected with changing breastfeeding patterns. Milk companies and doctors are always claiming that women do not want to breastfeed. This seems exceedingly rare in the rural situation, but does occur in the urban. I suspect that when women are producing more children than they want, this burden may prompt them to turn away from breastfeeding as an expression of their excessive and scorned fertility. They may not know how to limit conception, but they may try to limit this next phase of motherhood as an attempt to salvage some autonomy. The introduction of damaging practices makes breastfeeding failure likely and a mother who experienced difficulties is bound to discourage her daughter. Several of the letters in *Maternity* describe the experience of a 'gathered breast' (i.e. mastitis) or an abscess. This indicates that they were probably not feeding the baby frequently in the early days after the birth and this early restriction is often linked with later lactation failure. During this era health workers were advising 'regularity' and restriction. The concept of lactation being a drain on the mother was widely accepted, so women may have restricted feeds to try to conserve their strength.

There are so many changes which accompany the process of industrialisation that it is an oversimplification to pinpoint one as a cause of decline in breastfeeding. Among these conditions were a loss of intimate knowledge and support, an intrusion of erroneous medical supervision into a personal relationship and the widespread availability of products which were promoted as adequate breastmilk substitutes. The new methods of production which made life more difficult for breastfeeding women and increased the numbers of dead babies were producing hundreds of products which were widely advertised with extravagant and misleading claims and were making a good profit for their manufacturers.

FOR INFANTS AND INVALIDS

The widespread marketing of condensed milk worried the medical authorities. In 1911, an official report was able to collect no less than 100 varieties of machine-skimmed and forty brands of full-cream condensed milk, and this was not an exhaustive collection. Dr F. J. H. Coutts who produced the report explained the nutritional inadequacies of the product, particularly the skimmed variety. As the techniques for machine skimming improved, more and more fat was removed from the milk, but in 1899 a government regulation had demanded large and legible

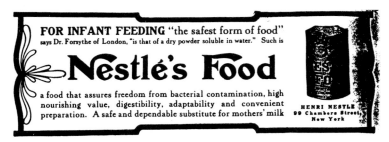

FOR INFANT FEEDING "the safest form of food" says Dr. Forsythe of London, "is that of a dry powder soluble in water." Such is

Nestlé's Food

a food that assures freedom from bacterial contamination, high nourishing value, digestibility, adaptability and convenient preparation. A safe and dependable substitute for mothers' milk

HENRI NESTLÉ
89 Chambers Street,
New York

12 Advertisement for Nestlé's Food in the *Journal of the American Medical Association*, 1912

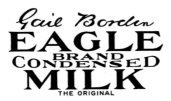

A SUCCESSFUL INFANT FOOD MUST BE NEITHER TOO WEAK FOR PERFECT NUTRITION, NOR TOO HEAVY FOR COMPLETE DIGESTION

Gail Borden

EAGLE
BRAND
CONDENSED
MILK
THE ORIGINAL

is a safe, satisfying and wholesome food, which in the most stubborn case is easily and completely assimilated.

Samples and Feeding Charts, printed in any language desired, sent upon request.

BORDEN'S CONDENSED MILK CO.
"Leaders of Quality"
Est. 1857   NEW YORK

13 Advertisement for Borden's Condensed Milk in the *Journal of the American Medical Association,* 1914

labelling and the production of skimmed condensed milk declined until it virtually disappeared. All the advertisements claimed the milks to be perfect substitutes for mothers' milk. One product which under government regulations had to say 'unsuitable for infants' did so in minute print, but in huge letters claimed to be for 'INFANTS AND INVALIDS'. In addition to their nutritional inadequacies, the milks' claim to 'purity' and sterility proved unfounded; one analyst discovered every brand he tested to contain microbes. The report did not mention brand names routinely and discreetly described each one by a letter of the alphabet. [12]

The technique of condensing milk, patented by Gail Borden in the USA in 1865, was introduced to Europe by Charles Page, a former correspondent of the *New York Tribune.* At the end of the American Civil War he became US consul in Switzerland and together with his brother formed the Anglo-Swiss Condensed Milk Company in 1856, which later (1905) merged with a local company called Nestlé. Page's fusion of business interests and political duties was a model for the future of the baby milk business. [13]

ORIGINS OF THE SUBSTITUTE MILKS

During the 1860s a German chemist, Justus von Liebig, the 'father of modern nutrition', invented the 'perfect infant food'. It was made of wheat flour, cows' milk, malt flour and bicarbonate of potash. It was patented and commercialised and delivered in liquid form, but did not sell very well. Then a powder form was developed and some of the cows' milk replaced by pea flour. Liebig was considerably annoyed by the doctors who reported that this food was indigestible or who doubted that it was the counterpart of mother's milk. One of his admirers argued,

> For instance, if we were to say that this preparation does not agree with newborn babies, such a statement could not be supported on theoretical grounds, since in the food they get the very same ingredients as in mother's milk. As therefore this milk agrees with them I cannot understand why they should be unable to digest Liebig's food. [14]

These cussed babies were the first of several generations of naughty infants who refused to digest a whole series of foods which devoted nutritionists constructed as exact counterparts of mother's milk, which of course we all know is rich in pea flour and bicarbonate of potash. Some of these babies even had the cheek to die after being fed these perfect products.

This spirit of concern for babies was not easily dampened and another German, Henri Nestlé, a dealer in mustard, grains and oil lamps, claimed to have saved the life of a baby who, having allegedly rejected his mother's milk and all other food, accepted Nestlé's *'farine lactée'* (Nestlé's Milk Food). By 1873, Nestlé were selling 500,000 boxes of *'farine lactée'* per year in Europe, the United States, Argentina, Mexico and the Dutch East Indies. The wondrousness of *'farine lactée'* did not prompt them, however, to adjust the marketing of condensed milk for infants when they merged with the Anglo-Swiss Condensed Milk Company in 1905. Delivering milk to babies began to be a large-scale task for these philanthropists and was seen as a noble, life-saving one. It also happened to be extremely profitable, for as efficiency in the dairy industry increased and transport communication improved, cows' milk became cheaper and more readily available. In Britain, with the introduction of frozen and chilled meat imports, meat prices for the home-grown product began to fall to such an extent that many farmers turned to dairying as an alternative to fatstock raising and to supplying the liquid milk market which they found buoyant when other products had to compete with cheap imported food. Another group of people had been philanthropically delivering milk to infants for over a million years, but they were women, and as every nineteenth-century scientist knew, they were not to be trusted to do things properly.[15]

THE MILK DEPOTS

The spread of substitute feeding was not engineered entirely by the commercial manufacturers of patent baby foods. At the turn of the century the 'milk depots' were established in France, Britain and the United States with the declared aim of providing uncontaminated milk for babies. They were also a good way of monitoring the babies and their mothers. Their founder, Dr Budin, tried to encourage breastfeeding, but like so many of his contemporaries he dreaded overfeeding and steps to avoid this ruined breastfeeding for many women. These depots were the forerunners of health clinics all over the world where a cheap or free product is used to tempt mothers to come and submit to the vigilant eyes of those who know best. The decline of breastfeeding has paralleled the spread of these institutions.

Many have argued that the milk depots saved lives, and certainly it must have been a relief for mothers whose milk was failing, because the skill to re-establish lactation had been lost and the change in social relations deterred them from feeding one another's babies, to know that they could get a supply of cheap milk for their babies. However there was no proof that the depots had any effect on the infant mortality rate which began to fall after 1905. The Medical Research Committee noted in 1917 that the drop in the infant death rate was the same in widely separated towns, some of which had milk depots and some not. What the milk depots established was the link between artificial milk distribution and the health centres which persists to this day, the world over.[16]

KEEPING MILK SAFE:
THE MOTHER'S RESPONSIBILITY

The widespread use of factory and household refrigeration has made many people forget what a risky product milk has been even in industrialised countries until relatively recently. Outbreaks of epidemics of infections in 1929 and 1936 were milkborne, according to the British Medical Association who issued warnings in the national press. At that time 2,000 deaths a year were due to bovine tuberculosis. When mothers bought their week's supply of pasteurised or sterilised milk from the milk depots, it still had to be kept fresh. Sterilised milk kept better, but in fact the process destroys more nutrients than pasteurisation. Mothers also used sweetened condensed milk, either whole or skimmed depending on what they could afford, but the tin had to be opened in the shop and somehow kept uncontaminated in the home. One investigator found that diluted Nestlé's condensed milk, incubated at 37 degrees centigrade, contained 11 million bacteria after twenty-four hours. Dr Coutts's report (see page 190) found most samples of infant foods already contaminated before use. Hygiene was impossible in the average overcrowded, ill-equipped home. Only the rich had water closets, and working-class people in most urban areas had middens which were large, leaky, uncovered receptacles, sunk below ground level, or ash privies which were cemented at the bottom and above ground level and had ash thrown in at the front and the contents removed from the back. These facilities were often shared by several families. In the Yorkshire city of Hull between 1918 and 1939, 79 per cent of infant deaths due to diarrhoea were in houses with privies or pail closets. [17]

THE BLISS OF RURAL IGNORANCE

Poor mothers all tried to breastfeed and attempted it even if they were told not to, but in spite of continual railing against those unworthy mothers who did not suckle their babies there was little interest or research into breastfeeding difficulties and no training of medical students in the subject. What advice there was actually contributed to the breastfeeding failure and the lucky ones were those who escaped the erroneous advice of the health workers. Rural women who did not have access to the milk depots had quite different problems.

> 'We didn't have no bottle for our children. Fed them all ourselves. Every one. All nine. Till they were three years old, some of them. You'd be standing there washing, and they'd hang on to you and want a teat. I didn't know see. I tried to wean them several times, but then they'd get in again and have another drop. I had no end of trouble weaning my children.'

This woman was desperately poor, often hungry and overworked, but she had no problems with her milk supply. She lived close to her mother and relatives but had never learned about 'overfeeding', scrubbing her nipples or the importance of routines: 'I didn't know see.' She lived in such a remote part of the country that she was beyond the ministrations of health visitors so she stayed obliviously certain that breastfeeding worked: 'I had so much milk, I didn't know what to do with it. Drip? It used to run away so, I had no end of milk. But you couldn't afford to bring your baby up any other way.' [18]

She was also deprived of the widespread advertising of baby foods. The common advertising style of the day was the personal testimonial:

'Doris until three months old had nothing but the breast: she then weighed only eight pounds and seemed to be wasting away from malnutrition. Then we tried your Frame Food, and she immediately commenced to pick up, until today from a puny mite she has grown to be a *fine strong girl* with vitality and stamina that is simply wonderful.' Mr Polwin, Stanley Stores, PO, Southend on Sea.[19]

In Laurie Lee's autobiographical novel *Cider With Rosie*, he recounts how his mother used to spend hours writing fictional testimonials (for things she never used) to manufacturers in the hope of earning a few shillings, but they often used them without paying.[20]

Frame Food, like many baby food manufacturers, offered a free sample tin and was advertised in the *Nursing Times*. Baby food adverts also appeared in the medical journals as well as newspapers, magazines, cookery books and even children's books such as the *Infant's Magazine Annual* (1913) where Neave's Food, recommended from birth and used in the Russian Imperial Nursery, was advertised opposite the title page.[21] As it happened Neave's Food could not save the members of the Russian Imperial Nursery from more powerful forces.

Political changes in other places stimulated the marketing tactics of the companies:

Glaxo, makers of a patent baby food, ask for the attention of welfare workers aware of the terrible obstacle of ignorant mothers (perhaps the chief contributing cause of infant mortality), point out how war work means more babies have to be artificially fed and name some of the many official bodies using Glaxo.[22]

The advertisment opposite was published in *Maternity and Child Welfare* in 1917 when many doctors were still blaming mothers for allegedly 'refusing' to breastfeed. The Glaxo advertisement boasted that six city health departments, corporations and a 'School for mothers' had used a total 354,000 pounds' weight (778,800 kilos) of their dried milk powder.[23] These boasted

Saving the Babies.

The Importance of Diet.

Every worker in the cause of saving infant lives has come face to face with the great obstacle of ignorance on the part of so many mothers. This ignorance is one of the tallest barriers which the welfare-worker has to surmount—and perhaps the chief contributing cause of infant mortality.

As in matters of cleanliness and clothing, so does this ignorance wreak great harm upon the infant in the vitally important matter of diet. Welfare-workers know only too well how many infants languish for want of sufficient, correct, and regular nutriment. Particularly is this true in the case of infants whose mothers are prevented from looking to the feeding of their children by occupations other than domestic. With so many women engaged in war work, this difficulty has been vastly aggravated.

For years Corporations of the Midlands, such as Sheffield, Lincoln, and Rotherham, have grappled with the task of conserving infant life. The officials and the welfare-workers have had to face the feeding difficulties in countless cases. Earnest and sincere, these workers have patiently striven to overcome the ignorance of mothers, and have brought knowledge and practical advice to many a hard-worked and worried woman who did not know how to care for her child, scarcely had time to do so even if she knew.

We are proud to say that the diet difficulty has been largely solved in so many of these cases by the use of Glaxo.

Glaxo contains nothing that is foreign to milk. At the source of supply, before any chemical change has taken place, this milk is dried to a powder. The Glaxo process makes the powdered milk germ-free, and prevents the curd subsequently forming a dense clot. Glaxo is packed in closed vessels and is prepared for use by merely adding boiling water. An infant can, by taking Glaxo, obtain a continuous supply of germ-free milk.

Among the many Official Bodies continuously using Glaxo may be mentioned the following :

	lb.
Sheffield Corporation have purchased	137,000
Manchester School for Mothers, over	60,000
Rotherham Corporation, over	65,000
Bradford Health Department, over	50,000
Lincoln Health Department, over	25,000
Birmingham Health Department, over	17,000

Glaxo is specially packed and sold at a special rate to Official Bodies, Crèches, Mothers' Welcomes, and Schools for Mothers.

The address of Glaxo is : Dept. 71, 155, Great Portland Street, London, W.

The Proprietors of Glaxo are: Joseph Nathan & Co., Ltd., London, and Wellington, N.Z.

14 Advertisement from *Maternity and Child Welfare* (Jan. 1917) cited in Anna Davin, 'Imperialism and Motherhood', *History Workshop* no. 5, 1978.

quantities indicate that there was not much attempt to control or restrict sales. Mothers still had to pay for the milk in spite of their patriotic war work. British commerce was thriving on the alleged ignorance of mothers, but across the Atlantic industry was creating an even stronger base with the help of the doctors.

Markets are
Not Created by God

Markets are not created by God, nature or economic forces, but by businessmen . . . There may have been no customer want at all until business created it – by advertising, by salesmanship, or by inventing something new. In every case it is business action that creates the customer. (Peter Drucker, business and management theoretician, *Management*, New York, Harper & Row, 1974, p. 61)

THE ESTABLISHMENT OF THE US MARKET: IDEAL CONDITIONS

A baby milk market was created in the late nineteenth and early twentieth centuries, and was conceived through the mutual attraction of the manufacturers and the doctors. This love affair developed into an enduring and stable marriage which has lasted to this day. Though European industry was playing a significant role, the conditions in the United States were ideal for this relationship to blossom. Several factors contributed to the change from breast to artificial feeding which have echoed across the world. The United States was industrialising and urbanising rapidly. Any shortfall in workforce numbers could be quickly made up by immigration, and poor Europeans flooded into the United States with little choice but to accept the conditions and wages of the host country, which were little better than those in Europe. The majority of rural women continued to breastfeed, but increasingly urban workers were forcibly separated from their babies and replacement feeds became necessary and available. There continued to be family unit labour, as in the oyster canning industry where mothers still brought breastfed infants to work, but increasingly the pressures of industrialised production led to babies being left at home. Besides the changes in production methods, other factors which accompany industrialisation affected infant feeding. The Fall River study of infant mortality in a textile manufacturing town in 1908 cited artificial feeding as a significant cause of the excessive number of deaths from diarrhoea, but it was observed that a proportion of mothers who stayed at home were also bottle-feeding. The authors of this study claimed that the main factors in a high infant mortality rate were a high proportion of 'foreign-born' mothers, high female illiteracy and a high birth rate. The stress of rapid change, the absence of supportive female relatives and the attempt to adjust to an alien way of life seem to disturb important cultural practices which protect mothers and babies. It is difficult to discover the exact reasons why a mother stopped breastfeeding, but contemporary experience shows that the availability and promotion of alternative foods usually has a demoralising influence on both individual and social confidence in breastfeeding. If mothers believed that alternative infant foods were good and no-one said they were dangerous, what reason was there not to use them? If absorption into a new society leads to the abandonment of customs as culturally important as dress, it is not surprising if infant feeding practices change. If replacement feeds were used a womans' breastmilk supply might decrease and her need for the substitute foods become established. This would also make her more likely to become pregnant and more closely spaced births would lower the chances of survival of her babies. In the country as a whole 58 per cent of babies were still breastfed at twelve months in 1911, but the urban rate was lower than the rural.[1]

'GO FOR THE BEST': HOSPITAL CHILDBIRTH

It was not only the poor urban workers who were breastfeeding less, but also increasing numbers of the expanding middle-classes.

Doctors were taking over the birth process and hospital deliveries increased as the twentieth century progressed. Hospital practices destroyed breastfeeding, as they still do. It could be argued that this was a small price to pay for an improvement in mother and child health. However, between 1915 and 1930 in the US, maternal mortality did not decline and deaths of babies from birth injuries actually increased. Hospitals advertised widely, urging mothers to 'go for the best', so that women believed they were getting just that when they paid the high prices. Midwives were gradually outlawed, although poor women continued to use them. The denial of orthodoxy and eventual disappearance of the profession of midwifery in the US led to the loss of a set of skills which survived in Europe, where midwives (not without a struggle) increased their status during the same period. Midwives were a little more knowledgeable about breastfeeding than doctors because most of them had actually done it. Also, their role was always to assist nature whereas a doctor was trained to seek out its defects and remedy them. The majority of doctors then, as now, were woefully ignorant of the practicalities of breastfeeding. Sadly they managed to convince the maternity nurses of the rightness of their ideas.[2]

'THE SENSITIVE ORGANISATION OF THE MOTHER': THE CULT OF FEMALE FRAILTY

The major nineteenth-century discoveries, such as the role of bacteria in infection, had generated a new optimism about the conquest of disease. It was perhaps inevitable that a reverence for all things 'scientific' should be accompanied by a scorn for 'natural' processes. Improved living standards and public health measures, such as safe water provision, contributed more to the decline in death rates and killer diseases, such as tuberculosis, than medical knowledge. But this knowledge was increasing, and doctors communicated their own faith in their new skills to the general public. In the US, the 'specialist' was coming into vogue and paediatrics was a speciality gaining in reputation.

The wealth of the rising middle and ruling classes changed the role of woman from producer to consumer. The joke of the wife spending her husband's hard-earned money persists to this day. What is forgotten is that the cult of excessive expenditure by the rich was and is necessary for continued economic growth when workers' low wages restrict their purchasing power. Someone had to be buying the products, and the wealthy wife devoting her life to the selection of household goods, clothes and other status symbols was an important cog in the capitalist wheel. Her conspicuous consumption reflected her husband's financial success and helped retain confidence in his market skills. A breastfeeding wife might be as demeaning to a successful industrialist as a wife who reared chickens. Why do it yourself when you can afford to buy the 'latest' product? Besides, the rich, fashionable lady was seen to be a fragile creature:

> It was as if there were two different species of females. Affluent women were seen as inherently sick, too weak and delicate for anything but the mildest pastimes, while working-class women were believed to be inherently healthy and robust. The reality was very different. Working-class women, who put in long hours of work and who received inadequate rest and nutrition, suffered far more than wealthy women from contagious diseases and complications of childbirth. [3]

While women workers were struggling to keep their children fed and alive, their leisured sisters were being convinced by male doctors that they were too delicate to do anything, let alone feed babies. In the past, rich women had frequently delegated childcare, usually to a wet nurse, and as artificial feeding became less lethal, this practice could be abandoned. A bottle would be less of a rival for the child's affections. Though they advocated the superiority of breastmilk, doctors did not believe that upper-class women were able to breastfeed and they despised the lower-class wet nurse: 'the physical defects of the bottle we can understand pretty well, and can to a great extent, guard against them. Its moral qualifications compared with those of the wet nurse, are simply sublime.'[4] The great problem with breastmilk was, in the minds of the doctors, that it came out of women's bodies, and Dr Rotch's ambiguous attitude was typical of a common medical attitude which persists to this day:

> Also the mere fact of the milk being obtained from the human breast does not preclude many dangers which arise from it as a food, owing to the highly sensitive organisation of the mother allowing the mechanism of the mammary gland to be interfered with. When this mechanism is interfered with good milk may also become a poison to the infant . . . It is evident, therefore, that there is nothing ideal about breastmilk.

Whereas, of course, Dr Rotch considered his own formulae ideal.[5]

TECHNOLOGY AND THE NEW PRODUCTS

During this era, technological innovations were welcomed and 'modern' methods of feeding paralleled the railway, the motor car and plumbing as the way to a comfortable future. Women could be relieved of the burdens of nature through the wonders of modern science, and many of them welcomed this liberation. Improved dairy farming led to milk surpluses in the industrialising countries and new methods of preservation were invented. Condensed milk was first developed in 1853 and evaporated milk in 1885. The Walker-Gordon Milk Laboratory was set up by Dr Thomas Morgan Rotch in 1891 where cows' milk was modified, after which it was delivered directly to the consumer. For the first time in history a baby could be fed cows' milk without the family having direct access to a cow. In the milk-producing countries, improvements in dairy production led to whey surpluses that prompted the search for a market outlet. Whey became the base for artificial baby milk as it is today, not because research proved it to be the most suitable food, but because it was there and it was cheap. New materials and production methods also developed the feeding bottles and teats, which became widely available. In 1897 a bottle was patented that could be suspended over the cot for the baby to feed alone, and another had short legs so that it could stand on a baby's chest. These, together with a wide variety of foods advertised as ideal for infants, were put on the market. [6]

THE 'FORMULA' CULT

Doctors were in the market too. The focus on the 'problems' of the rich was more profitable and less distressing than trying to tackle the insurmountable troubles of the poor. The cult of the uniquely frail infant digestion was less of a fraud than the cult of female frailty for, deprived of breastmilk, a baby certainly did need close medical supervision. As knowledge about the constituents of human and cows' milk increased, doctors devised recipes for imitating human milk. They experimented with different proportions of ingredients and, because rigorous exactitude was a part of scientific respectability, they presented their recipes in the form of complex mathematical and chemical formulae. A successful cake is also a complex chemical reaction depending on precise proportions of ingredients, but cake is not called formula whereas artificial baby milk is, to this day, in the US and the countries under its cultural influence. It is a ridiculous term reminiscent of the pseudo-science of those doctors.

$$M = \frac{Qb - bC}{b} \qquad C = \frac{L(b^1 F - a^1 P)}{ab^1 - a^1 b} \qquad C = (2F + S + P) \times 1\tfrac{1}{4}Q$$

15 Highly-complicated formula used in infant feeding (Cited in Jelliffe, *Human Milk in the Modern World*)

At first each baby (and of course it was only the rich who could afford this service) would have an individual 'formula' made up to suit its particular digestion. This was seen as a matter of life and death, as Charles Warrington Earle stated at a meeting of the American Medical Association in 1888: 'One food nourished [*sic*] a given baby well, but may, if administered persistently, kill the next baby.'[7] A variation of 0.1 per cent of an ingredient was thought to be crucial. The mother had to return every few weeks to have the formula adjusted. However when this cult of individuality became commercially inconvenient to the doctors it rapidly went out of fashion.

ETHICAL MARKETING: A BRIEF TUSSLE AND A LONG HAPPY TRUCE

While doctors were preaching the dogma of a custom-made preparation, more mothers were buying commercial infant foods over the counter. They were widely advertised in newspapers, domestic magazines and medical journals and were easier to prepare than the paediatricians' formulae. Nestlé's Milk Food (the life-saving *'farine lactée'*) and Horlicks's Malted Milk only needed to be mixed with hot water. The doctors objected to the commercial foods, supposedly on nutritional grounds, but it was also a fact that the mother who could buy her baby food ready-made was less likely to visit the doctor, which meant a loss of income. It was also a loss of prestige. In 1893 Dr Rotch wrote,

The proper authority for establishing rules for substitute feeding should emanate from the medical profession, and not from non-medical capitalists. Yet when we study the history of substitute feeding as it is represented all over the world, the part which the family physician plays, in comparison with numberless patent and proprietory foods administered by the nurses, is a humiliating one, and one which should no longer be tolerated.[8]

The manufacturers realised that conflict with such an influential body as the doctors was not in their interests. They began to court the doctors who actually found the formula making difficult and who realised it would be more advantageous to form an alliance with the manufacturers. One doctor negotiated with a representative of an infant food manufacturer, Mead Johnson, to produce a product he favoured, Dextri-Maltose, and it was tested in 1911 at the Babies' Ward of the New York Post-Graduate Hospital. The development of the infant food industry has depended on the repeated testing of unproven products on unsuspecting consumers without their informed consent. If a scientific team wanted to set up today the experiment that has been carried out on babies over the past hundred years, the most lax ethical committee would throw out such a proposal.

Doctors began to recommend certain commercial foods. They did not prescribe them like a drug, but by agreement with the manufacturers, no directions were put on the package and the mother was instructed to consult her doctor before using the product. This was 'ethical' marketing, but the infant foods were still widely available and there was no attempt to control their sale to only those women who could afford a doctor. Mead Johnson provided doctors with feeding calculators and other items which made 'it easier for the general practitioner to obtain better co-operation from the mothers',[9] Mead Johnson advertised publicly, but they boosted the doctor's position: 'When Dextri-Maltose is used as the added carbohydrate of the baby's food, the physician himself controls the feeding problem.'[10] For the doctor to flourish, feeding did indeed need to be a problem, for if it were not, why should the mother visit him? In the days before immunisation, antibiotics and rehydration methods, there was little a doctor could do for a sick baby. However with carefully supervised artificial feeding the doctor could maintain the illusion, to himself as well as the mother, that he was useful. Perhaps a good side-effect of the reverential 'formula' making was that better hygiene was maintained. A doctor's control had to be skilled, the baby must not die, but nor should it be wholly without feeding 'problems'. Mead Johnson could boast with all honesty in 1923 that their 'ethical' marketing policy was 'responsible in large measure for the advancement of the profession of paediatrics in this country because it brought control to infant feeding under the direction of the medical profession'.[11]

Other companies followed suit, 'Simulated milk adaptation' was launched at a meeting of the American Pediatric Society in 1915 and tested on another batch of babies conveniently ready for experiment in the Babies' Dispensary and Hospital, Cleveland. The advertisements in the lay journals directed the consumer to a physician; in the medical press they extolled the ease of preparation which 'rouses the parents' enthusiasm and adds to the prestige of the physician'. The commercial success of this approach convinced the other companies that this relationship between doctors and manufacturers could be a happy one. Nestlé had been advertising directly to the public for decades offering free samples and booklets, but in 1924 it launched Lactogen which was to be sold in the US 'only on the prescription or recommendation of a physician. No feeding instructions appear on the trade package.'[12] Horlicks launched their new milk modifier with the same message. The fact that poor mothers could not afford both the product and a physician's fee did not appear to be a matter of concern. Many paediatricians continued to advocate breastfeeding and were uncomfortable with the relationship with commerce. The Philadelphia Pediatric Society believed that advertising through medical channels implied 'recommendation by the members of the AMA [American Medical Association]' and undid the doctors' work of trying to educate the public 'to the fact that infants cannot be fed in this indiscriminate manner'.[13]

In 1924 the AMA set up a committee to investigate the question of infant food advertising. By now the use of commercial foods was so well established that it seemed impossible to recommend their withdrawal. The benefits of breastfeeding and the dangers of 'unsupervised' artificial feeding were reiterated, but the committee applauded the 'disposition on the part of many manufacturers of proprietory foods to cooperate with the medical profession and its medical journals'.[14] The scruples of the Philadelphia paediatricians could not withstand the force of commercial interests. However the balance of power did not weigh solely in favour of the industry. When Horlicks refused to change their labels and advertising of Malted Milk, 'for infants from one week to 12 months',[15] they were no longer allowed to advertise in the medical journals and Horlicks lost their place in the infant foods market.

By this time the AMA's Committee on Foods controlled the acceptance of advertising copy. Mead Johnson described the economic benefits of cooperation with the medical profession with disarming candour:

> When mothers in America feed their babies by lay advice, the control of your paediatric cases passes out of your hands, Doctor. Our interest in this *important phase of medical economics* springs, not from any motives of altruism, philanthropy or paternalism, but rather from a spirit of enlightened self-interest and cooperation because [our] infant diet materials are advertised only to you, never to the public. (my italics)[16]

When I was researching this material I looked for the original advertisements in the journals and could not find them. Many libraries discarded and destroyed advertising material in order to lower the binding costs. Thus the evidence of this medical/ commercial liaison is not visually apparent to the historical/ medical investigator. This acts as another screen for the medical profession from the long history of their more questionable activities. If you are confronted with the old advertisements interspersed throughout the medical text, you realise that the medical profession shamefully endorsed a load of old rubbish that did more to relieve patients of their money than of their suffering. (The librarians' part in this censorship is, I believe, innocent but outrageous. They are like amateur archaeologists who destroy the ancient cooking pots because they believe that only the jewelled swords are important.)

DOCTORS AND DIAGNOSIS

This medical/commercial relationship in the US became a model for similar relationships the world over and has undermined breastfeeding wherever it has been established. Companies will capitulate over direct advertising to the public if they are pressured, but they fight tooth and nail if they are kept apart from their beloved doctors. The evidence for the advantages of breastfeeding is discovered repeatedly but, just as in the early part of the century, this evidence is put on one side if it disturbs the harmony between industry and the established medical hierarchy. When Cicely Williams was imprisoned in a Japanese internment camp in Malaya during the Second World War, there were twenty babies born to twenty British women; all were breastfed and all survived and were healthy. Their mothers suffered physical and mental stress, but they had Cicely Williams's support, and with her experience of ordinary African and Asian mothers, she knew that breastfeeding worked. Her faith in the process was the only supplement needed. Women need confidence in their bodies, not products which destroy this.

The proportion of women suffering serious complication in childbirth is the same now as it was in eighteenth-century England, yet in the supposedly advanced world most women are treated as if they were medical cases when they give birth. The very process of medicalisation destroys both general and individual confidence in the body's ability to function and consequently disturbs the hormones involved in childbirth, making the fears into self-fulfilling prophecies. With breastfeeding, failure is even more unlikely than with childbirth, yet in the modern world milk insufficiency is awaited eagerly. What women should remember is that doctors and milk manufacturers need us for their daily bread and in the case of infant feeding we would need them only rarely if society were not organised to maintain the structures of dependence. When I asked a Swedish midwife how she and her colleagues coped with the complications in her small maternity unit, she replied, 'We don't have any.' Skilled ante-natal care could predict potentially difficult births and these took place at the main hospital. This illustrates the key medical skill, diagnosis – not only of illness, but also of its absence. Because so much training involves seeking out disease, doctors can forget about health. When women say they have too little milk, health workers often suggest a substitute before they have investigated the problem.

In the early part of the twentieth century, the infant food industry expanded as doctors proved how risky artificial feeding was. A study in Boston in 1910 found that bottle-fed babies were six times more likely to die than those that were breastfed. Another study of infant mortality rates in eight US cities, carried out between 1911 and 1916, found the same sixfold risk for babies in low-income families and a fourfold risk in high-income families. These high mortality rates were not just due to diarrhoea which is associated with poor hygiene, but also to pneumonia, measles, whooping cough and other communicable diseases. Bottle-feeding does not merely put the child at risk from a contaminated bottle, but also deprives her of the immunological factors in breastmilk. All these illnesses are more likely to be fatal if the baby is born into a poor family which is badly housed, uneducated and unable to get medical help quickly. The plain fact is that poverty causes suffering and death, which is why breastfeeding is such a fantastic phenomenon; the poorest child has a better chance of survival if her mother is not a victim of the political, economic and cultural forces which deprive her of the ability to feed her own child. [17]

The situation is the same today even with all the advances of modern medicine; a study from an urban area in southern Brazil carried out in 1985 shows that bottle-fed babies are four times more likely to die from a respiratory infection and fourteen times more likely to die from diarrhoea than those exclusively breastfed. [18]

Even as late as 1924, when medical knowledge, public health and living conditions were improving, a study in Chicago revealed the same pattern of mortality. This study of 20,000 infants, all from poor families and under the supervision of the health care of local welfare clinics, discovered that at nine months of age the bottle-fed infants were fifty times more likely to die than those who were still breastfeeding. The custom was noted of 'trying to make the baby regain its birth weight by ten days old. To do this the child was bottle-fed in addition to breastfeeding. It is difficult to insist on breastfeeding because *nurses and physicians are eager to have the infant show the greatest possible gain.*' (my emphasis) [19] It was the medical staff, not the mothers, whom it was so difficult to convince that breastfeeding worked. (Later, in the 1970s, Dr Natividad Clavano found in the Philippines that persuading the medical staff of the importance of exclusive breastfeeding was far harder than convincing the mothers.) Babies freely fed in the neonatal period usually gain weight rapidly, but routines and supplementary feeds make it hard for mothers to establish an adequate supply. Of course a baby will not take in enough breastmilk if she is not allowed near her mother's breast. These destructive practices continue all over the world today, because health workers are still ignorant about breastfeeding and the medical/commercial relationship needs to keep it that way. [20]

In the 1920s, any well-informed paediatrician must have known about these studies, yet there was no effective body of protest against the companies' activities. Throughout this era most articles about infant feeding started with the ritual praise for breastfeeding, like the prayer of grace before a meal, before the author launched enthusiastically into a discussion of the various merits of different artificial foods. As in Europe, there were few attempts to discover the causes of breastfeeding problems or failure, though there was criticism of women who refused to breastfeed. The arbitrary, irrational rules of the maternity wards were rarely questioned and the doctors' authority was absolute.

Most pioneer women in the United States (and of course every native North American) had not only breastfed but had also provided most of the food and necessities for the household, spending only a few dollars a year in the market economy. The wealthy industrialist's wife depended on her husband economically, was beholden to another man, her doctor, for the skill to keep her child alive and to an industrialised product to replace her banished breastmilk. The enforced uselessness of her existence often led her into a cycle of depression and psychogenic ill-health which, along with damaging management of early breastfeeding, led to inevitable lactation failure. For the poor women who contributed through their work to the wealth creation of the US, heavy labour in home and factory, poor nutrition and bad living conditions precipitated greater rates of birth complications, stillbirths and smaller, more sickly babies. Many mothers would have needed special encouragement and nurture to establish and maintain lactation and this was just what urbanisation destroyed. Breastfeeding failure, infrequent feeding and early supplementation would have meant a greater likelihood of closely spaced pregnancies, thus burdening women more. Commercial baby foods were acknowledged to be dangerous when used without instruction, yet neither doctors nor manufacturers attempted to restrict or control their distribution. Ignorance was a mother's crime; as long as she was able to buy a doctor's knowledge she would be absolved, but most mothers could not afford this means of absolution.

EXPANDING THE MARKETS

Eventually better living standards, education and medical care in Europe and the United States offset the more lethal effects of artificial feeding. After the Second World War immunisation was developed and became available in the industrialised countries, conquering epidemic childhood diseases such as polio and diphtheria. Measles, still a major killer in Africa, became preventable. Antibiotics came into widespread use and a minor respiratory infection could be treated immediately and the risk of pneumonia avoided. Almost all mothers could read feeding instructions and an expanding army of health workers taught them how to prepare bottles safely. There were still risks in bottle-feeding, but resulting problems could usually be dealt with by the medical services at hand. The economic costs of this vast medical back-up are often ignored. In 1979, in a middle class US suburb, medical costs for bottle-fed babies were 15 times that for breastfed babies (US$68,684, US$4,460). In 1991, in an English town, the costs of treatment for 150 bottle-fed babies who were hospitalised for gastroenteritis was estimated to be £225,000 (US$382,500). Hospitalisation for gastroenteritis is almost unknown for exclusively breastfed babies. [21]

As industrialised society created a healthier environment, mother and babies could now contribute to the prosperity of the baby food manufacturers without having to sacrifice so many infant lives. However there is an illusory complacency about the effects of bottle-feeding in post-war Europe. At many a conference some academic will say confidently 'Most of us here were bottle- fed and we are all healthy!' I have a personal interest in this statement because according to my mother I developed gastroenteritis during an epidemic in 1947. Diarrhoea was still a problem of artificially fed infants and there were outbreaks of gastroenteritis throughout the 1930s and 1940s in Great Britain, Ireland and the United States. The disease was linked with bottle-feeding, though in the United States scientific comparisons were invalidated by the universal practice of supplementary feeding. Research comparisons of breast and bottle-fed babies have been obscured by the fact that until recently there were so few exclusively breastfed babies in industrialised societies. I was lucky enough to survive artificial feeding because my mother could call a doctor quickly, but when blasé academics point to our universal health, I suspect they pass over many petty histories of distressed parents and babies whose fortunate outcome means they do not hit the statistics. It is rarely the medical researchers who are wiping the sore bottoms and washing out the soiled sheets in between anxious attention to the miserable, wailing child. My mother, like most women, had wanted to breastfeed but a helpful doctor, a family friend, had told her that she had insufficient milk and must put me on the bottle. I was three weeks old, a time when most women still need support to establish breastfeeding, but my mother had no one to encourage her and like her doctor friend she was ignorant of how breastfeeding worked, though as she breastfed her fourth child, she was evidently able to produce enough milk. [22]

If the bottle-fed child was more prone to illness than the breastfed, at least medical skills were improving apace and this meant the doctors were becoming increasingly important fixtures in infant life. So there were more jobs, more careers and more sales of drugs, even though public health measures should have decreased the dependency on medicine. Defenders of our society may say that all this was worthwhile as now the appalling nineteenth-century contrasts of misery and wealth have been eliminated. But they have not; the extremes of poverty have now discreetly moved to remoter places and there are more horrifying contrasts than ever before. The international organisation of labour and capital echoes the social and economic differentials of nineteenth-century Manchester or New York; so do the urban squalor, the inadequate public hygiene and the commercial morals. The foundations of this system were consolidated during the days of colonial expansion.

EMPIRE BABIES

The British Empire was founded on commercial interests. Not only were the colonies sources of cheap raw materials and labour, they also formed new markets for the sale of British products. In the late 1920s the Empire Marketing Board (EMB) boasted that the Empire overseas purchased almost one half of British manufactured goods. An EMB poster in 1927 claimed 'Jungles today are gold mines tomorrow,' and under a drawing of two traditionally dressed black men was the statement, 'Growing markets for our goods.' In 1910 Britain sold just over £8 million worth of goods to the African colonies and imported £5 million worth. By 1925 these figures were £24 million and £20 million respectively. Artificial milk was taken along with the Christianity, the tinned fish and the plantation managers to forge the economic links that were the principal goals of colonisation. [23]

THE EXAMPLE OF THE BABY MILK MARKET IN COLONIAL MALAYSIA

Malaysia had been a British colony since 1826 and one of the principal products was rubber, produced on large estates where women worked long hours. Profitability was dependent on low production costs through low wages. Later in the century one rubber product was the bottle teat which, besides being marketed in Europe, could be sold to the rubber tappers for their babies. [24]

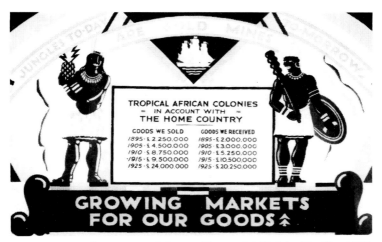

16 Empire Marketing Board Poster (*Poster:* McKnight Kauffer 1927; courtesy of Public Records Office, London)

Just as the organisation of factory labour in Britain had disrupted breastfeeding, so did plantation employment. Traditionally, suckling continued for two to four years and babies were carried on their mothers' backs with constant free access to the breast. Plantation labour changed this and to this day women rubber tappers are underpaid and overworked. In a 1983 study in Penang, estate women said they felt too exhausted to breastfeed after a normal 5.30 a.m. to 4.00 p.m. day, tapping 600 to 700 trees. Work burdens have actually increased during this century, for older women report that intensive methods with more trees to be tapped did not occur in the old days.[25]

The colonial administration set up infant welfare clinics and British nurses energetically converted mothers to the idea of the clock. In a 1925 report on infant feeding there was the regretful statement that 'some mothers had not even seen a clock and those who had, could not understand what it had to do with the feeding of an infant'.[26] The zealous British nurses soon remedied this deficiency and by 1926 'the majority of mothers understand the clock and feed their children regularly by it and the boat-shaped bottle is accepted in most homes'.[27] The devotion to strict routines in nursing practice had sprung from the establishment of the profession by Florence Nightingale during the Crimean War, so that army conventions influenced the running of hospitals and clinics outside the military sphere. This was and is disastrous for mothers and babies because flexibility, spontaneity and a relaxed environment are vital for breastfeeding. Unlike traditional midwives, few of the British nurses who bossed the local Malaysians had themselves experienced breastfeeding and their training had instilled in them an unquestioning acceptance of disastrous 'rules of management'. Most of the British administrators' wives had been subject to this medical sabotage, so wherever they took their infants, there was a demand for a supply of milk. The companies were only too glad to use this to stimulate a local market and were aided by the ingenious assistance of the misguided infant welfare nurses. In Malaysia, the *Straits Times* was carrying advertisements for tinned milk from the mid-1880s onwards and by 1900 there were four brands available. From 1896 Mellin's Infant Food – the 'perfect substitute for Mother's milk' – was advertised weekly and by the start of the First World War Allenbury's, Nestlé's Milk Food, Milkmaid, Infantina and Fussell's were being advertised as specifically for infants. Glaxo joined them in 1915 and competitive advertising continued throughout the war. Feeding bottles and teats were also promoted and by the 1920s these six brands were still among the eighteen different brands featured in the thirty to forty advertisements per month in the *Straits Times*. These were originally aimed at the colonial elite, but the move to local language advertising started towards the end of the 1920s.[28]

THE NUTRITIONAL VALUE OF THE SUBSTITUTES: THE CASE OF SWEETENED CONDENSED MILK

Even though mothers having been going 'out to work' for thousands of years, the milk companies have claimed that mothers were giving their babies other and perhaps less appropriate breastmilk substitutes because they 'had to go out to

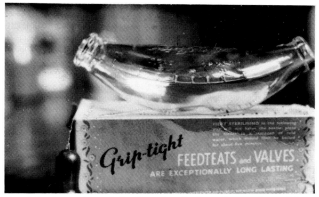

17 Grip-tight boat-shaped feeding bottle found on sale in Nairobi in 1984 (*Photo:* 1984 courtesy of Baby Milk Action)

work' (separation from their babies being an incidental act of God), and that therefore the marketing of commercial baby milks was a useful and good thing to do. Did the companies really have the babies' nutritional interests at heart? It had long been recognised in Europe and the United States that there were more cases of diarrhoea and more resultant deaths among artificially fed children during the summer than during the winter, and it was well known that tropical climates were riskier for infants. This did not deter the manufacturers, who advertised their products without warnings whatever the environment. Besides the added contamination risk of the bottles, teats and milk, some of the milk sold for babies was a nutritional disaster. Sweetened condensed milk has a high sugar content (about 45 per cent by weight) which reduces the concentration of important nutrients and makes the milk highly unsuitable for infants and young children. Some modern sweetened condensed milks are fortified with vitamins A and D, but those used before the Second World War lacked these vitamins. In Malaysia, sweetened condensed milk was highly recommended by doctors and manufacturers and was widely used as a breastmilk substitute, even though in Britain by 1911, doctors had recommended to the government that a warning label should be put on the tin advising against its use as an infant food. The reports (see pages 190 and 191) were published in England, and as the companies' European activities were affected by the reports' statements, they would have been well aware of their contents. Of twenty-one babies with rickets seen by Cicely Williams in Singapore, twenty had been fed on sweetened condensed milk. Vitamin A is vital for the health of the eyes and some babies fed on sweetened condensed milk have gone blind. Vitamin A had been finally identified and named in 1915, yet in 1936 Nestlé circulated in south-east Asia a diary for doctors with two pages of recommendations from infant feeding experts for sweetened condensed milk as an infant milk, with statements such as, 'Sweetened condensed milk is the food par excellence for delicate infants.'[29] The British government controls indicated that knowledge of the harmful effects was widespread so that this marketing was cynical and callous in the extreme. It was the effect of sweetened condensed milk that prompted Dr Cicely Williams to deliver her speech 'Milk and Murder' to the Singapore Rotary Club in 1939, where she said,

> If you are legal purists you may wish me to change the title of this address to Milk and Manslaughter. But if your lives were embittered as mine is, by seeing day after day this massacre of the innocents by unsuitable feeding, then I believe you would feel as I do that misguided propaganda on infant feeding should be punished as the most miserable form of sedition, and that these deaths should be regarded as murder . . .
> Anyone who, ignorantly or lightly, causes a baby to be fed on unsuitable milk, may be guilty of that child's death.[30]

In spite of the burgeoning knowledge about infant nutrient needs (a field in which baby milk manufacturers claim to be experts), marketing of Nestlé's sweetened condensed milk as an infant food continued right up until 1977. After that date label instructions for infant feeding were supposed to be removed, though tins with these labels continued to be found in developing countries for years after that date. As far as I can discover a warning about its unsuitability as a baby food is still not put on this product. The problem is not just one of illiterate mothers in developing countries. In the UK in 1982-83, health visitors discovered that some mothers still bottle-fed sweetened condensed milk to their babies (as their grannies and mothers had done), believing it to be safe as there is no warning on the label (unlike dried skimmed milk). On the advice of the Department of Health, the Health Visitors' Association contacted Nestlé and was told that 'the incidence of use of condensed milk for infant feeding is so low that there would seem to be as little justification for this move as there would be for a similar statement to appear on "doorstep milk".[31]

Besides, sweetened condensed milk was not covered by British government labelling regulations. As 6 per cent of UK mothers in 1980 were bottle-feeding unmodified milk (such as sweetened condensed milk, evaporated or 'doorstep'), some babies were at risk. Nestlé has a reputation for giving large sums for nutrition research, especially in the field of infant feeding, yet in 1983 it refused to spend the small sum needed to protect babies at risk from a product marketed zealously for decades as the infant food *par excellence*. Health visitors were advised by the Department of Health to explain to mothers individually that sweetened condensed milk was unsuitable. Health workers paid by the British National Health Service are not only expected to promote baby milks for no extra pay, but are also required to debrief the customer who follows a dangerous practice instigated by the marketing tactics of a previous generation.

In Malaysia, advertising of all milks continued to increase until the Second World War when breastfeeding rates went up because of the unavailability of artificial milk. The infant mortality rate dropped during this time of 'hardship', but when the British administration resumed control they saw a 'need' for large-scale imports of milk and intensive advertising was resumed. Whenever manufacturers claim to be responding to a 'need', it seems that people have to be reminded through advertising in case they have forgotten what it was they craved so desperately. The inheritance of the colonialists' medical ignorance and harmful marketing practices deprived both the Malaysian and Singaporean babies of breastmilk to this day. An article by a leading paediatrician in

Singapore states, 'Feeding a baby from the breast is never an easy thing and the mother must prepare for it before and during pregnancy.'[32] Millions of ordinary rural women would roar with laughter if they had that statement translated for them, yet I am convinced of the doctor's sincerity because breastfeeding is still mismanaged in Singapore maternity wards and I am sure that most of the women he knows have had difficulties (see illustration on page 80).

AFTER THE SECOND WORLD WAR

During the period after the Second World War bottle-feeding became the ordinary method of baby feeding in the United States and to a lesser extent in Europe. The neonatal breastfeeding rate fell by half between 1946 and 1956 and by 1967 only 25 per cent of American babies were breastfed on leaving hospital. Damaging hospital practices made breastfeeding a near-impossible procedure and only women with alternative sources of support and knowledge were able to do it. It became common to administer routine lactation suppressant injections (at a risk to the mother's health) immediately after birth.[33] By the 1960s and 1970s, bottle-feeding had become the 'normal' way of feeding a baby. Doctors trained in this ambience and with little knowledge of normal lactation were among the 'experts' who went to help the newly independent countries establish their health services. Until this time, the majority of rural mothers in these regions were continuing to breastfeed; they knew no other way and, unlike European and North American women, they had few lactation problems. Western-style maternity services were unavailable to them, so they avoided the sabotage of breastfeeding that the medical milieu provided. The standards of living in most of these countries were not rising as they had done in the west and the salesmen arrived with all the tricks of their trade ahead of the sewer construction, the water treatment and the comprehensive medical services which had alleviated some of the risks of their products at home.

Commercial skills were not inhibited by the absence of a

modern infrastructure and salesmanship quickly adapted to a new situation. Newly independent countries were attempting to 'develop' and as the colonial administrators withdrew, the business negotiators moved in, though sometimes they were the same people. The potential markets were irresistible to the companies, whose home markets were reaching saturation point. 'The high birth rates permit a rapid expansion in the domain of infant nutrition,' wrote Nestlé in 1970 when planning marketing in Thailand.[34] Growth and expansion were sacred words in commerce and with improving communications and transport, the new shop counter could stretch round the globe.

MILK AND CHARITY

Technological advances in dairy processing and transport all served to make dried cows' milk a convenient food to distribute. From the end of the nineteenth century onwards, the expanding dairy industries of Europe, the United States and New Zealand produced surpluses of skimmed milk, and contemporary nutritional theories tied in nicely with ideas about using up this abundant product.

In 1932, Cicely Williams described and identified kwashiorkor, the disease which means in one Ghanaian language 'the illness the child gets when the next baby is born'. It is the disease of the child who has been displaced from the breast. Unlike the form of malnutrition called marasmus, when a child is thin and hungry, the child with kwashiorkor is swollen and has no appetite. Dr Williams (who spent her later years trying to debunk the protein/kwashiorkor theory) found that milk could have a valuable therapeutic effect on feeding a child with this illness and she speculated that 'some amino acid or protein deficiency cannot be excluded' from all the possible causes. To this day no one is certain of the specific cause of kwashiorkor. There are many theories ranging from the effect of moulds (aflatoxins) in the diet to psychological influences. In spite of this uncertainty, kwashiorkor is still described as a 'protein deficiency' disease in textbooks. Like most manifestations of malnutrition, kwashiorkor is prevented by adequate food intake and is, in most cases, a disease of poverty. However fascinating might be its biochemical pattern to the research scientist, it need not be widespread at all.

Nowadays most marasmus and kwashiorkor and the combination of the two are called protein/energy malnutrition (PEM). The medical management of PEM involves the careful refeeding of the child with low-protein, high-energy food mix, usually composed of milk powder, oil and sugar, because they are the cheapest and most readily available ingredients. This mix could be made of other multi-nutrient foods besides milk, for it is the energy density of the food that is the important factor. Ironically many of the children who needed this treatment developed PEM because they were bottle-fed and the same product, milk powder, that was implicated in their disease was used to try to save them.

Back in the 1930s and 1940s the idea of protein deficiency was convincing, and kwashiorkor was common where cows' milk was not a significant part of the diet and appeared to be cured or prevented by its consumption. So the concept of milk being a 'protein food' and the answer to malnutrition became well established. Milk is actually a multi-nutrient food, so it was rather arbitrary that 'protein' was seen as the magic ingredient rather than calcium, zinc, various vitamins or indeed energy. However, protein had been a long term favourite of nutritionists and here was a dramatic vindication of their faith in its powers. Anyone dealing with children in the 1930s and 1940s worshipped cows' milk and was sincerely convinced that it was the answer to most nutritional problems – and it happened that there was a lot of it about.

After the Second World War, dried, skimmed milk was 'a fortunate by-product of a domestic surplus-disposal problem'. It was more satisfactory in every respect to dump it in developing countries than to have to bury it, which was contemplated by the US Department of Agriculture at one point. Besides the planning of dried skimmed milk distribution, elaborate plans and committees were formed to manufacture 'protein-rich' food supplements from dried skimmed milk, but in the end they proved to be commercial failures so were abandoned. During these post-war years an obsession with the 'world protein gap' and the 'impending protein crisis' led to the allocation of resources into ways of combating this 'problem'. Then nutritionists thought a bit more, redid their calculations and, oops, they discovered that the problem was not there. Almost overnight the 'protein gap' ceased to exist and became the 'great protein fiasco'.[35] It is still hard to convince people that it is actually quite difficult to become protein-deficient if you get enough to eat. Most foods contain some protein and you would have to subsist on boiled sweets and cooking oil to meet your energy needs and be protein-deficient. Malnourished children are deficient in all nutrients and particularly energy. The so-called 'high-protein' foods such as meat, milk and eggs are also high in fat, vitamins and minerals. High-protein diets may even have negative effects; a high-protein supplement given to pregnant women resulted in an increased rate of premature delivery.[36] The amount of protein utilised in the body depends on the amount of energy in the diet, so giving protein without extra energy is a waste of effort. Putting a teaspoon of oil in a child's traditional grain porridge may increase the protein in her diet more effectively (and cheaply) than if you replace that porridge with a lower-energy portion of 'protein-rich' food.

It was during the phase of the imaginary 'protein gap' that the international agencies embarked on distributing tons of dried skimmed milk around the world. The attitude of the nutritional establishment was this:

Largely through the good offices of UNICEF, many thousands of tons of DSM have been distributed to children in countries which are *short of dairy cattle*. The improvement in health of children receiving this milk has been demonstrated in controlled experiments and vast numbers of children have benefited.[37] (my italics)

As I explained in Chapter 2, milk, though a useful product, is not an indispensible food, and after infancy children stay healthy on diets without it. In poor countries, many children do not get enough food and any 'controlled' experiment where children were given more to eat would show improvement in health. The idea of countries being 'short of dairy cattle' illustrates the ethnocentric bias of nutritional scientists many of whom have strong links with the food production system of the industrialised world. Avocado pears are a useful food crop in tropical climates, producing a high-energy, vitamin-rich food supplement, yet there are no vested interest groups persuading industrialised cold countries to invest in expensive technology because we are 'short of avocado trees'. It was cheap dried skimmed milk, though, not the whole dried milk that was favoured for worldwide distribution, because there were non-nutritional advantages: 'We aim not only at improving the standard of nutrition but also, as a necessary corollary, at expanding the market for milk.'[38] In Nigeria, where Fulani women had always bartered milk for grain (and still do, though their livelihood is threatened by 'development'), the British residents became interested in organising milk collection when their butter supplies from Europe were cut off during the Second World War ('Cynthia, I'll be damned if I'll have my omelette cooked in palm oil, we'll just have to teach these natives to churn'). The buttermilk was discarded and in 1954 UNICEF recommended that it should be roller-dried and distributed via the medical service. This milk obsession went hand in hand with scorn for breastmilk. A World Health Organisation consultant who visited Nigeria in 1955 referred to mothers' 'impoverished milk', and as mothers were confronted by health workers and told to reduce the number of breastfeeds, they were encouraged to supplement with substitute milks.[39]

In the Caribbean, mothers had been positively discouraged from prolonged breastfeeding (called 'over-nursing') by the Colonial Health Administration for years:

> their mothers keep them at it for sixteen to eighteen months, during the last seven or eight months the children draw an abundant supply of a highly unnutritious fluid from the breast . . . No amount of advice will prevent the women from carrying on this deadly habit.[40]

This was written in 1917, but the attitude was still around in 1952 when clinic nurses were advising mothers that seven to nine months was the desirable length of time for breastfeeding. Nurses also instructed mothers not to let their babies fondle their breasts.[41] Fortunately for British sensibilities, UNICEF dried skimmed milk was soon to put a stop to all this fondling.

By the early 1960s UNICEF was distributing 900,000 kilos of milk annually; this was going to babies as well as mothers and children all over the world and was frankly used as a means of enticing mothers to clinics, just as the infant milk depots had been used in Europe. In Sarawak in 1954, dried skimmed milk donated by UNICEF and government-supplied evaporated milk was seen by health workers as 'bait' to attract mothers to the clinics. In Singapore, 22,590 kilos of free powdered milk were given out by clinics in 1959.[42]

Dried skimmed milk is high in protein and calcium, but unless it is artificially fortified it lacks the fat soluble A and D vitamins. Rickets is not a widespread problem in sunny countries but vitamin A deficiency is probably the most widespread and serious nutritional problem of poverty. Its occurrence is linked with frequency of diarrhoea, which itself is more likely with the use of dried skimmed milk. Xerophthalmia (eye damage leading to blindness due to vitamin A deficiency) is reported in seventy-three countries and in Bangladesh alone 30,000 children a year go totally blind because of vitamin A deficiency.[43] Although vitamins A and D may be added to dried skimmed milk, these can deteriorate in storage. In 1991 the EC produced 40 per cent of the world supply of dried skimmed milk and sent out 83,500 tonnes as food aid.[44] Many children who suffer from periods of marginal malnutrition recover and go through a phase of catch-up growth with no long-term ill-effects; eyesight has no comparable recovery. With all food aid it is notorious that any donated food inevitably replaces home meals. In many areas of the world where dried skimmed milk was distributed, the traditional diet included leaves, fruits and oil seeds (avocado is an ideal source of vitamin A as the oil facilitates absorption) which were high in vitamin A, and by zealously promoting this 'protein' supplement there might have been an accompanying reduction of other important dietary components such as vitamin A.

Dried skimmed milk was distributed in countries where the use of milk after sevrage was not customary. As many children were suckled by their mothers for three or four years, they were not deprived of a balance of nutrients. In many societies any non-human milk is perceived as a replacement for breastmilk and donation is interpreted as a health message to give this to a baby instead of suckling, an idea often endorsed by the resident foreigners' custom of giving non-human milk to their own babies. Since the Second World War the 'normal' practice in most industrialised, milk producing countries has been for any breastfeeding to last for a token three to six months and then replacement by either whole or modified cows' milk. Health workers and milk distributors spread this pattern all over the world, to the delight of the baby milk industry who could then persuade mothers to replace the inferior dried skimmed milk with their expensive products. UNICEF is now energetically promoting breastfeeding; sadly this is part of undoing its own terrible mistake made in the name of nutrition. They were not the only misguided organisations; all major charities, church missions and other relief agencies did untold damage to breastfeeding and to the economic and health independence of newly independent countries through energetic milk promotion. This practice persists to this day in refugee camps and other focal points of international aid which become sinks for dumping milk. This depresses local food production and purchase, discourages breastfeeding and appropriate local dietary habits, creates a need for imported products and often a black market, and generally accelerates the economic and social breakdown which may have precipitated the refugee problem in the first place.

Most health ministries still see milk as a vital part of child nutrition and people feel deprived if they cannot get cheap milk for their children. Governments now have to spend scarce foreign exchange (often earned through selling their own high-quality food products) importing a product that they did well without for thousands of years. Peru, for example, has a policy of providing a daily cup of milk for every child. They import whole dried milk from the UK which means that Peru is spending hard currency on a feeding programme that is fixing the idea that cows' milk is essential for child health. It may be useful in the short term if parents are too poor to buy enough local food, but in the long term it is a policy which creates dependency, both of the Peruvian families on their government and also of Peru (a highly indebted country) on the industrialised nations. This makes it harder for the government to resist international interference in internal decisions. Though health education informs parents not to use cows' milk to replace breastmilk, it has had this effect. When countries import dried milk on a large scale, local dairying is depressed as a result and the local products are rejected in favour of the multinationals' glamorous tins. When the baby milk industry protests that they are not wholly responsible for the decline in breastfeeding they are right; the aid agencies as well as medical misinformation prepared the market by helping to create a need. By the 1960s the marketing campaigns of Nestlé, Cow & Gate, Wyeth, Bristol Myers and others were advancing all over a developing world where charity had helped map out the roads.

· 8 ·

The Lure of
the Global Market

SELLING TO THE SHACK AS WELL
AS THE MANSION

The companies who boasted about their 'ethical' instruction 'To be used only under the direction of a physician', in the US, abandoned this directive when they expanded their promotion into the Third World. They used every method they knew to persuade mothers to use their product: billboards, radio and newspaper advertising and 'milk nurses'. These were saleswomen: 'Nestlé nurses, these girls dressed as nurses, dragging a good lactating breast out of the baby's mouth and pouring in baby milks.'[1] Milk nurses were sometimes trained nurses, but whether they were qualified or not was irrelevant because they were employed by the infant food companies to visit new mothers in the hospitals or at home in order to sell them baby milk. The recruitment of qualified nurses drained emerging health services of badly needed staff. They were usually paid on a commission basis and they earned more than any trained nurse in the health service, and they still carried the prestige of a qualified health worker. An investigation in Nigeria in the early 1970s showed that 87 per cent of mothers used artificial milk because they believed they had been advised to do so by hospital staff who in reality had been milk nurses allowed into the hospital.[2]

These messages undermined faith in the rival product. 'When breastmilk fails, choose Lactogen . . .' Like a bad spell the words put the idea of failure into a mother's mind where it had never

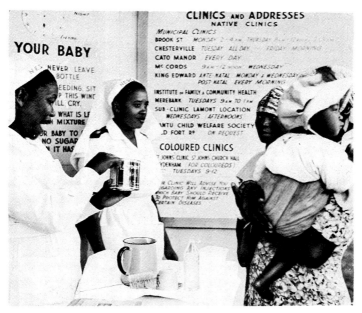

18 Nestlé milk nurses in South Africa in the 1950s (*Photo:* from *Nestlé in Profile*)

existed before, and could inhibit her let-down reflex and decrease her milk. The radio was a good way to reach the illiterate. In August 1974, in Sierra Leone, 135 thirty-second advertisements for Lactogen (Nestlé) were broadcast over the Sierra Leone Broadcasting Service. In December 1974, there were forty-five thirty-second ads for Cow & Gate (Unigate) and sixty-six for Similac (Abbott-Ross). On one day, fourteen separate advertisements were broadcast (three Similac, four Cow & Gate, and seven Lactogen). The language was principally the local Creole: 'Now Lactogen a better food cos it don get more protein and iron, all the important things dat go make pikin strong and well. Lactogen Full Protein now get more cream taste and Nestlé den guarantee um . . . . Lactogen and Love.'[3] Ironically, more protein and iron were just what was harmful for an infant's body. Research showed that the ads were effective: 'Depth interviews brought out very clearly the mother's positive attitude to bottle-feeding.'[4] Many mothers were convinced that artificial milk was a sort of medicine, especially as it was endorsed and distributed through channels of health care. The fact that it was an imported product and was already used by the colonial elite added to its status.

No single baby milk company had a monopoly on immoral promotion, but the giant food company Nestlé was the world leader in baby milk sales and had been the boastful innovator of some of the most effective techniques:

> The advent of television as a universal means of communicating with the shack as well as the mansion permits the standardisation to an increasing extent of advertising and promotion. Nestlé uses the medium extensively wherever it can. Where it still can't, the company relies on newspapers, colour magazines, billboards and other outdoor displays.

> In less developed countries, the best form of promoting baby food formulas may well be the clinics which the company sponsors, at which nurses and doctors in its employ offer child-care guidance service.

> In the less developed countries, effective distribution may call for unusual, imaginative techniques.[5]

These claims were made in 1970 and were not confined to baby milk. During that year, mothers in the Ivory Coast were giving Nescafé to their toddlers because a radio advertisment proclaimed, 'Nescafé makes men stronger, women more joyful and children more intelligent.'[6] Nestlé had already been informed of the dire effects of baby milks in the developing countries. Many health workers wrote to Nestlé during the 1960s and 1970s explaining the problems. The complaints were usually ignored unless adverse publicity was threatened such as newspaper coverage or questions in Parliament, as happened in Jamaica in 1965.[7] Many doctors expressed anxiety at the increasing numbers of younger infants arriving at the hospitals with diarrhoea and

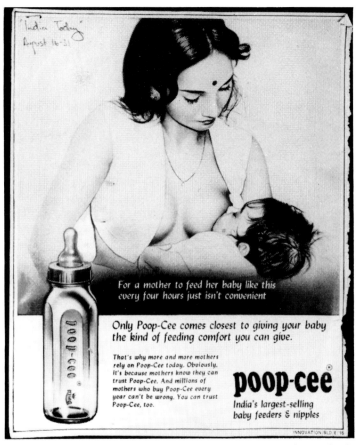

For a mother to feed her baby like this every four hours just isn't convenient

Only Poop-Cee comes closest to giving your baby the kind of feeding comfort you can give.

That's why more and more mothers rely on Poop-Cee today. Obviously, it's because mothers know they can trust Poop-Cee. And millions of mothers who buy Poop-Cee every year can't be wrong. You can trust Poop-Cee, too.

poop-cee®

India's largest-selling baby feeders & nipples

19 Advertisement for Poop-Cee feeding bottles and teats (from Charles Madawar, *Insult or Injury,* Social Audit Ltd., London, 1979)

malnutrition. 'Bottle-baby disease' was increasing in areas where the only real breastfeeding problem was death of the mother and in those cases a foster mother was usually willing to feed. In a tactful article, 'Commerciogenic Malnutrition', Derrick Jelliffe pointed out the inappropriateness of the promotion of their products in developing countries and suggested a dialogue between the industry and the doctors about this issue. Catherine Wennen described the problem in Nigeria where she worked during the 1960s. While trying to cope with the increasing numbers of babies sick from bottle-feeding, she was confronted with the widespread, aggressive publicity. She noticed the radio slogans, the giant billboards from which huge, healthy cardboard babies smiled down, the 'milk nurses' and the brochures and posters. She knew that this could not be attributed to lack of awareness of the risks for, as she noted, the companies had initially refrained from promoting to the 'unsophisticated market'. She became aware of the excellent public relations between the companies and top figures in the medical profession, the free baby milk for doctors and gifts to the hospitals. She approached the Nestlé manager in Lagos 'to point out the sad consequences of their indiscriminate sales promotion', but he did not want to talk.[8]

There were many doctors witnessing the same practices around the world and their increasing concern led to a meeting of the UN Protein Advisory Group *ad hoc* Working Group (its name a reflection of the protein obsession described in Chapter 7) in 1970 where paediatricians, industry and UN agency representatives discusses the problem. The proceedings were never made public, but it is known that the industry would not accept that the promotion and availability of baby milk had any impact on the decline of breastfeeding.

This is one of the great feats of double think in business. While marketeers and advertisers attribute rising sales to their strategies, if industry is challenged over their harmful effects, it quivers with innocence and protests that people never buy anything they do not need. Some public relations men have even claimed that their advertising had no affect, though why a company should profligately waste millions of dollars of its investors' money is difficult to understand.

Further Protein Advisory Group meetings which, needless to say, no breastfeeding women from developing countries attended, resulted in a sort of marketing declaration for artificial milk: 'In any country lacking breastmilk substitutes, it is urgent that infant formulas be developed and introduced . . .' Governments should support investment, promotion and measures which disseminated the use of these products. From industry's viewpoint the meeting had gone well. By 1979, a World Health Organisation survey found that fifty brands and 200 varieties of infant feeding substitutes were being distributed across 100 countries. About half the companies had established factories in developing countries and their distribution networks were spaced across a broad economic spectrum.[9]

THE BABY KILLER

The Protein Advisory Group's meetings' results echoed those of the American Medical Association's meeting in 1924 with the infant food industry. You cannot expect the representatives of business to accept damage to their sales without a struggle; if a squeamish employee resigns on a moral issue there is always a new delegate to fight for the company's interests. One company (Abbott-Ross) did call for 'restrained promotional practices' but they were not yet so big in the developing world so they had less to lose. While these discussions were continuing, the ordinary woman or man in the streets of the industrialised countries knew nothing about the problem. If there had been an earthquake, hurricane or war, pictures would have reached most newspapers and TV networks and emergency funds would have been set up. The child victims of the Nigerian Civil War (1967–70) had aroused widespread compassion, but this other quiet slaughter was unreported. Then in 1973 the magazine *New Internationalist* published an interview with two paediatricians with long experience in Africa, David Morley and Ralph Hendrikse, who described the problem in everyday language. This was followed in 1974 by a publication called *The Baby Killer*, produced by the British charity War on Want. It explained the issue in clear and simple language, and had pictures of the daily conditions of African life as well as of the promotion and its appalling results. The cover design conveyed the pain and the problem in the powerful visual message of a marasmic baby inside a feeding bottle. This was how I first learned about the issue. Twenty thousand copies of *The Baby Killer* in English were distributed and it was widely translated. [10]

In response, a British company criticised in *The Baby Killer*, Cow & Gate, sent an investigative team to both Asia and Africa and offered to withdraw its products from these areas, but government authorities and paediatric experts advised against this, claiming that 'better techniques of education and better controls on promotional activities were required'. [11] This decision is understandable when you consider the identity of 'government authorities and paediatric experts'. They were the elite, who had a lot to lose from company withdrawal. They were the recipients of gifts of equipment and grants for hospitals and medical schools, and their standards of living enabled their children to be more safely bottle-fed than poor children with the free milk the companies gave them. The cultural influence of the retreating colonials survived among some elite families, who eschewed 'peasant style' breastfeeding. The Jelliffes have pointed out that bottle-feeding is associated with authority, and breastfeeding with oppression, in the ex-colonies. The paediatric 'experts' were usually western-trained and consequently ignorant about breastfeeding. Many might genuinely believe that artificial milk filled a 'breastmilk gap', but a withdrawal of this and bottles and teats would have saved many lives.

THE NESTLÉ TRIAL

Within two months of publication, *The Baby Killer* had been translated by the Third World Action Group in Berne, Switzerland (AgDW, Arbeitsgruppe Dritte Welt), as *Nestlé Totet Babys* which means 'Nestlé Kills Babies', and Nestlé filed a libel suit against the group. In Switzerland the company was known for product quality and paternalistic fairness. To say they killed babies was akin to accusing the little red hen of laying poisoned eggs. In fact the image was carefully nurtured and they had already been taken to court themselves as defendants concerning questionable practices. In 1948, they had been convicted in Swiss courts of false labelling of condensed milk sold to the Red Cross and of a chicory/coffee product, Nescore. [12] During the preparation of

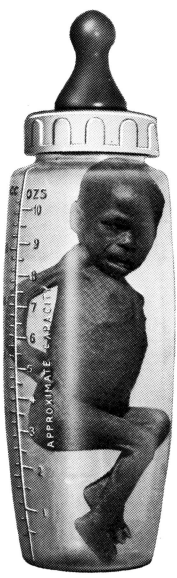

20 Logo used on the cover of
The Baby Killer (Andy
Chetley/War on Want, 1974:
Courtesy of War on Want)

their libel suit, Nestlé offered to settle out of court if the AgDW apologised, destroyed the report and paid all costs. AgDW refused and the case proceeded. Nestlé had originally issued proceedings on four counts, namely: the title, the charge of immoral and unethical practices, of responsibility for the death or damage of babies through its sales promotion policy, and of dressing their saleswomen as nurses to give a false scientific credibility. However before the final hearing, Nestlé withdrew the last three charges. The judge found the AgDW members guilty of libel in the title because:

> The adequate causal connection between the sale or any other type of distribution of powdered milk and the death of infants fed with such products is interrupted by the action of third parties, for which the complainant, in terms of criminal law, cannot be held responsible. In this sense, there is no negligent or even intentional killing.

The defendants were fined 300 Swiss francs (US$150) each, but the judge took the opportunity to state that Nestlé's advertising in developing countries went considerably further than in industrialised countries:

> The need ensues for the Nestlé company fundamentally to rethink its advertising practices in developing countries concerning bottle-feeding, for its advertising practice up to now can transform a life-saving product into one that is dangerous and life-destroying. If the complainant in future wants to be spared the accusation of immoral and unethical conduct, he will have to change advertising practices. [13]

If Nestlé had accepted the spirit of the judge's verdict, acknowledged its mistakes and changed its marketing of baby milk immediately, it would have been a coup for the defenders of big business and a rebuke to those who claim that transnational companies are inevitably immoral. Instead they refused to admit to unethical practices. The managing director stated, 'I was able to see that they (the advertising practices) were normal and usual advertising methods, used by manufacturers of such products all over the world,' and, 'We must affirm that we have full confidence in the ethical basis of our actions.'[14]

Yet Nestlé themselves had after 1924 proudly adopted a policy in the USA (where conditions were better than in poor countries in the 1970s) of selling Lactogen 'only on the prescription or recommendation of a physician' (see page 207). Baby milk accounted for a small percentage of the overall sales of Nestlé, the second largest food company in the world. They were advised at one stage by an advertising agency to pull out of the baby milk market because it was damaging their public image.[15] Who knows what motivated which individuals to resist change so obdurately? There was conflict between the company's diehards and those who were genuinely shocked to discover the extent and the effects of their promotional practices. The fact, as they had stated, was that they only did what was normal for all companies. Why should they adopt a commercially disadvantageous strategy and stop what everyone else would continue to do anyway?

'Well, as we were about to leave, one of the Sisters said, "Tell me, if you stop selling to people who are too poor to use the product safely, will you still make a profit?"

There was absolute silence. It must have been a full minute. Finally one of the corporate executives picked it up and said, "That is the crux of the problem." '

(Exchange at a meeting between the Sisters of Mercy and Abbott-Ross in Chicago. Reported in *The Bottle Baby Scandal: Milking the Third World For All It's Worth* by Barbara Garson, *Mother Jones,* December 1977.)

The Protein Advisory Group meetings brought the companies together and enabled them to form the International Council for Infant Food Industries (ICIFI), a group of nine companies including Nestlé. As though galvanised by the publicity from the Nestlé trial, the ICIFI proposed a code of ethics and published it just before the end of the first hearing. This code was so weak regarding advertising in the Third World that one company Abbott-Ross decided not to consolidate its ICIFI membership.

AN ATTEMPT AT SHAREHOLDER PRESSURE

In 1975 a group of Catholic nuns, the Sisters of the Precious Blood, filed a suit against Bristol Myers, an American company, charging them with 'making misstatements in its proxy statement'; in plain English, lying. When the nuns, as shareholders, had challenged the company to provide detailed information about its promotional practices abroad, they were informed that there was no promotion where chronic poverty or ignorance could lead to product misuse. Bristol Myers marketed in Latin America, in countries such as Guatemala where only 51 per cent of the population have access to drinking water. Forty per cent of Enfamil (a Bristol Myers baby milk) sales were outside the US and in 1974 advertising and promotion had cost them $296 million, almost three times as much as they spent on research and development.[16] Other investors could see the contradictions between the evidence found by the Interfaith Centre for Corporate Responsibility (ICCR), an organisation set up to monitor church investments, and the Bristol Myers statements, but the company refused discussion. The nuns, together with the ICCR, collected evidence from eighteen different countries which proved the falseness of Bristol Myers statements. However, the judge dismissed the case because the nuns had not suffered irreparable harm from the company's statement, implying that only malnourished babies themselves could bring a suit and that companies were free to lie if it did not hurt their shareholders. The sisters gathered support from other shareholders and appealed. They also had the backing of the US Securities and Exchange Commission, the statutory body which governs shareholder transactions. Eventually Bristol Myers decided to settle out of court, and agreed to send shareholders a report of the nuns' evidence and to halt direct consumer advertising and the use of 'milk nurses'.[17]

THE NESTLÉ BOYCOTT

In spite of the publicity and the lawsuits, the companies, including Nestlé, continued their widespread promotion. Then

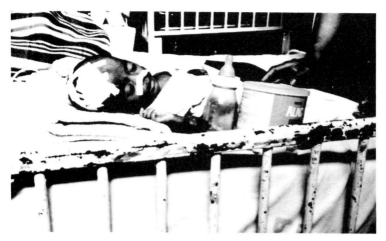

21 Sick Filipino baby with bottle and tin of Mead Johnson (Bristol Myers) 'Alacta' (*Photo: Action for Corporate Accountability*)

the release of Peter Krieg's film *Bottle Babies* in 1975 made a profound impact. Many people, having read descriptions of the problem, have explained that they never really felt involved until they saw the shot of the woman scooping water up from a visibly filthy pool with which to mix her baby's milk, or the wasted baby screaming as a drip was placed through a vein in her head.[18] This film was shown to hundreds of study groups and organisations concerned with world poverty, who felt exasperated by the companies' indifference. From the country where some of the most energetic marketing methods had evolved, the US, came the commitment and the ideas to challenge them. Whenever *Bottle Babies* was shown, a spontaneous reaction was a declaration to boycott Nestlé products. In Minneapolis, a group had formed who had called themselves the Infant Formula Action Coalition (INFACT) and in response to these avowals, they decided to co-ordinate a boycott which was launched in July 1977. It was one of the few actions they could take, for at that time only Swiss nationals could own shares (a Nestlé shareholder group did in fact try to bring about changes in marketing), US citizens could not use investor influence. The mainstream support for the Nestlé boycott in the US came from the churches, many of whom had direct contact with the developing countries through their missionary work and could verify the facts of the marketing abuses. INFACT's demand to Nestlé was that it should halt all promotion of baby milk. This meant no milk nurses, no free samples and no direct advertising. The boycott spread to Europe, New Zealand and Canada.[19]

A TALE OF THREE BABIES

In 1979 two American babies, Ben and Bradley, were rushed into hospital suffering from alkalosis, a condition where the body's alkali/acid balance goes awry and which if untreated may be fatal. Their condition was caused by their food, two infant formulas (Neo-Mull-Soy and Cho-free) deficient in chloride made by Syntex. Their parents, Carol and Alan Laskin and Lynn and Larry Pilot, turned to the Food and Drug Administration to discover whether there had been other reports of the disease linked to use of these products. They discovered that there were no requirements for infant formula manufacture except that they must be manufactured under sanitary conditions and that the label must state the ingredients. Syntex made some attempt to recall the formula from its retail outlets, but months later there was still tins on sale. The Laskins and the Pilots then contacted the press and the politicians and, as a result of the ensuing publicity received 60,000 queries. Congressional hearings were instigated, a parents' pressure group, FORMULA was established and by 1980, legislation was drafted setting nutrient standards for infant formula, requiring routine testing by manufacturers, as well as immediate notification of any problems which might present a health risk. Is this tale an accolade to the US system, its principles of freedom and the power of the individual?

There are some more details to this story: Carol Laskin is a health care management consultant, Alan Laskin is a management consultant with contacts in the media; Lynn Pilot is an attorney with experience in Congress and Larry Pilot an attorney employed by the Food and Drug Administration who specialises in food and drug law. In spite of Ben and Bradley having a hand-picked team of experts for parents, it was still hard for the Laskins and the Pilots to influence powerful bodies and formula 'mistakes' are still occurring (see Appendix 1). A Congressional subcommittee asked the Justice Department to prosecute the company for their poor recall of the dangerous formula, but by 1984 this had not happened, because the Justice Department argued that criminal prosecution was not necessary to prevent similar incidents in the future. As Maureen Minchin says, would you decline to prosecute a burglar because he had lost his ability to steal?[20]

The 1980 Infant Formula Act could be seen as a step forward for the protection of infants, but its power was yet to be established. The manufacturers agreed to the act in principle, but when the Food and Drug Administration drafted stringent recall procedures they disagreed. The Food and Drug Administration has no powers of coercion and in the drafting of consumer protection laws there is always the hazardous journey between proposal and final draft, where the vested interest groups are waiting at every turn to influence the wording. We are talking about potentially lethal products which might kill babies, yet the makers were trying to evade the responsibility of maintaining safe standards.

The companies complained about the regulation proposals in the first draft of the law and were supported by the American Medical Association who saw no need for regulation because the doctors felt that the industry should and could regulate itself. The Syntex company had removed salt (sodium chloride) due, they claimed, to 'consumer pressure' because of a theoretical link between dietary salt and high blood pressure, even though this meant that the chloride content was one-fifth of the amount recommended by the American Academy of Pediatrics. Here is an example of nutritional 'fashion' influencing the content of a baby milk.

I do not know how the AMA explained away the fact that the companies had repeatedly proved themselves incapable of self-regulation, but once more the doctors and the industry were found in cahoots. The American Academy of Pediatrics, supported industry too, because 'regulations might make formula unaffordable and reduce the number of specialised formulae *available to doctors*' (my italics).[21] The American Academy of Pediatrics, an organisation supposedly concerned with child health, thinks quality control an extravagance, whilst millions of dollars are spent by the formula industry every year on advertising and all other forms of promotion such as free lunches, conferences and services to doctors. In the early 1980s, the American Academy of Pediatrics received a renewable annual grant of $1 million.[22]

The Food and Drug Administration was still in the process of drafting the regulations (and being chivvied by the Reagan administration to weaken them) in 1982, when it announced publicly that another company, Wyeth, were recalling half a million cans of 'Nursoy Concentrate' and 'Ready-to-Feed' as they lacked vitamin B6 and contained excessive vitamin B1. A week later they recalled half a million cans of the brand SMA, but only after debate with the Food and Drug Administration. Deficiency of B6 can cause irritability, convulsions and even brain damage. When asked by the press why they did not pre-test the formula to ensure content and quality, Wyeth replied that they were not required by law to do so. Another move in the great tradition of 'ethical' marketing.

By 1982 the Food and Drug Administration had published its quality control regulations, which were a compromise between the original strong control proposals and the companies' vested interests. FORMULA and other parents' groups have filed a lawsuit charging that the Reagan administration has violated the Infant Formula Act of 1980 by leaving the specifics of quality control up to the manufacturers. Lynn Pilot commented that the supposedly explicit regulations did not even rise to the level of the Food and Drug Administration's rules for cold remedies, yet were dealing with an infant's sole source of nutrition. Thousands of babies had received the chloride-free formula. Perhaps we can say this was all a sad mistake, that modern medical skill saved the babies' lives and that all ended well. It did not. Lynn Pilot and Carol Laskin investigated the thousands of cases that parents reported to them. Children suffered from slow motor development, speech delay, kidney problems, reduced muscle tension (hypotonia), convulsions and dental problems. Learning difficulties and intellectual impairment were linked with the use of the product. One study showed that the longer the child had received the formula, the lower the score in an intellectual measurement test. An estimated 20,000 to 50,000 children had received the formula in 1978 and 1979. Such was Syntex's concern for infant health that they applied to the authorities for permission to 'donate' for export the batches of the formula that had damaged so many American babies. Just so that you do not collapse into complete cynicism about the state of US commercial morals, you may be relieved to know that permission was refused.[23]

This is just a sample of the long list of cases of defective products which have been marketed for infants, and they are only the ones we know about (see Appendix 1).

In 1982, a Filipina baby, Debbie, was taken to the public hospital were she had been born six weeks earlier. She had a high fever and had not responded to the antibiotics and antipyretics which a private doctor had prescribed. An upper respiratory infection was diagnosed and she was prescribed four further types of medicine for fever, colds and oral eruptions. Because there were no vacant beds she could not be admitted, so her mother, Cely, took her home.

Debbie had been delivered by caesarian section and weighed 3 kilograms, an adequate birth weight. Though Cely had planned to breastfeed, Debbie was put in the nursery and bottle-fed, the normal practice in the Philippines where hospital practices have followed the United States model. Debbie was discharged a day ahead of her mother and cared for by her grandmother who was told to feed the baby on infant formula until Cely joined them, which she did the next day. Cely's parents lived in four rooms in a congested area with poor ventilation and no ceiling under the metal roof which made it extremely hot. Their water source was a public tap outside and the toilet and bathroom were shared by three other families who lived in the same house. Cely, her toddler daughter and the baby slept in one room, her parents and two sisters in another. Her husband stayed in their own flat in another part of the city, but visited often. Cely attempted breastfeeding, but because her breasts softened quickly during a feed she believed she had insufficient milk, brought about, she decided, by the drugs used during her surgery. She fed Debbie formula and cleaned the bottles and teats with salt and water and boiled them for two minutes.

After her baptism at one month Debbie became ill and after the initial consultations, she got worse. Cely took her to the private hospital where she was admitted and given oxygen and dextrose. Tests showed that she might be suffering from salmonella septicaemia with concurrent meningitis and she was put in intensive care. She died and because her parents did not allow an autopsy the exact cause of death will never be known. Debbie 'lay in state' for a week before she was buried and Cely suffered from engorged breasts during this time. The money that her god-parents had given at the baptism paid for her funeral expenses.

This account is a shortened version of Debbie's history related in *Seven Infant Deaths* by Lorna P. Makil and Mayling Simpson. They analyse the reasons for Debbie's death and note that the family and hospitals did everything in their power to save her. She may have died from an infection or the side-effect of a drug, but the crux of the matter is that if she had been exclusively breastfed it is highly unlikely that such a well sized baby would have caught an infection so early. The early bottle-feeding in hospital conveyed the idea that it was a safe feeding method. It also prevented Cely's milk being properly stimulated by Debbie. If a baby is strong enough to suck at a bottle she can breastfeed. Debbie was a good birth weight so it would have been safe to give her nothing at all until Cely came round from the anaesthetic. If she had been 'roomed in' with her mother they would not only have established a good milk supply together, but saved money and staff time on feeding babies in the nursery, which could be devoted to other sick babies. The hospital was too overcrowded to admit Debbie when she was ill later; it was doubtless dealing with the problems of other babies whom they had started on bottle-feeding. Cely had never been told that giving bottles and formula would reduce her own milk supply and when the hospital discharged Debbie a day before Cely, indicating that separating a newborn from her mother was an acceptable practice, they even advised infant formula.[24]

WHO DUPES WHOM?

Ben, Bradley and Debbie suffered because their parents had trusted that a commercial product could be as good as the real thing. Skilful marketing and medical complicity had created that trust. Millions of other parents believed in the images projected by the baby food companies and endorsed by the medical profession. Lynne Pilot breastfed Ben for three and a half months, which is longer than average in the US and is recommended as sufficient by many paediatricians. If she had weaned her baby on to dilute fresh cows' milk and mashed family food, he would have been at less risk of damage, but for years paediatricians have recommended new products with unquestioning faith in the competence and integrity of industry. They are as duped by the companies as any poor illiterate woman. How many doctors and paediatricians actually get their free samples tested and give them thorough 'scientific assessment'? The American Academy of Pediatrics' guidelines (1976) recommended twenty-nine millilitres per litre for chloride, yet when tested the Syntex formulas contained nil to two millilitres per litre. It had been this low since 1978, yet as far as I can discover, no pediatrician had publicly discussed the possible risks that such a drastic change in ingredient proportion might entail. It always needs a sick baby to bring any fault to light. In *Nelson: Textbook of Pediatrics*[25] there is a chart of commercial food composition, but a footnote states that data are supplied by the companies, who have shown themselves to be consistently prone to error (see Appendix 1). If paediatricians are not alert to these problems and their source of facts comes from the fallible companies, where is accurate, relevant information to be found?

In the case of Ben and Bradley, it took the concerned and, as it happened, highly trained parents to confront a company and the official bodies with the links between a product and a serious illness. In the case of Debbie, her parents had neither the skills nor the access to information that would have made them realise the culpability of a product disseminated through the health system in their daughter's death. If paediatricians had been doing their job properly they would have tested the Syntex formulae and questioned the advisability of low chloride levels by checking through all the available evidence long before these tragedies occurred. In the hospital where Debbie was born, responsible paediatricians should not have allowed commercial baby milk to be used except in special circumstances. Doctors, however, are just as vulnerable to marketing tactics as the rest of us; companies merely use different methods to seduce them.

In the United States, women who need or wish to return to their employment after childbirth find it difficult to arrange breastfeeding. The same country that has such weak regulations (and they are among the best in the world) on the sale or composition of artificial milk has some of the most restrictive laws and customs against breastfeeding. The United States has no federal legislation concerning maternity protection, let alone nursing breaks, and there are many cases of women being forbidden to feed their babies at work or even being arrested for feeding their babies in public. The Syntex managers were never arrested for distributing a product that proved poisonous (many poisons work by depriving the body of an essential nutrient) for many babies.[26]

Cely came from a country which had formerly been a colony of the United States and, just as in the case of British-controlled Malaysia, so the Philippines had taken aboard the appalling breastfeeding management of her former rulers. In 1909, the US had forced a 'free' trade arrangement on the country which gave an advantage to the US, restricted the Philippines' international trading relations and stifled self-sufficient development. This legacy allows freedom of marketing to the baby milk companies, a policy which conveys no economic benefit, even when milk is produced in the country, for all the raw materials are imported and the profits go back to foreign companies (see Appendix 2). Over half the Filipino population live below the absolute poverty level and to feed a two-month-old on Nestlé's Nan infant formula costs over a third of the minimum wage. A bottle-fed Filipino baby is 40 times more likely to die, yet in 1988 only 22 per cent of one-month-olds were exclusively breastfed.[27]

But Debbie died in 1982, a year after the WHO/UNICEF Code of Marketing of Breastmilk Substitutes had been adopted and voted for by the Philippines. This should have changed things. Let's go back to the 1970s and pick up the story.

A PUBLIC HEARING

As more people in the industrialised world learned about the needless illness and deaths of infants in poor countries, they joined the groups who had discovered that Nestlé continued to lead the baby milk market and engage in aggressive promotion. According to *Fortune* magazine, Nestlé was probably the most profitable food company in the world in 1977, superseding both Unilever and General Foods. Nestlé could still have afforded to pull out of the baby milk market, but as the boycott grew, rather than reform their marketing methods they invested more resources in public relations. Nestlé claimed that the boycott did not affect them economically, but the Swiss journalist Jean-Claude Buffle has estimated that the boycott cost Nestlé just over US$1,070 million. For example, they paid a $1 million fee to the public relations firm Hill & Knowlton, who sent 300,000 glossy booklets to the clergy and religious bodies, explaining that Nestlé was not aggressively marketing the baby milk in the Third World. This was how many of the churches learned about the issue for the first time.[28]

As concern grew, Edward Kennedy, chairman of the Senate Sub-Committee on Health and Scientific Research, proposed and set up a hearing on the promotion and use of infant formula in developing countries and this brought the issue into the public spotlight. Representatives from industry, the health field and non-governmental organisations (NGOs) gave evidence. Oswaldo Ballerin, President of Nestlé Brazil, was questioned by Kennedy as to whether his company should market a product in areas without clean water and where people were illiterate. Ballerin evaded the question by reciting the nostrum that all the instructions were on the tin, but Kennedy persisted and Ballerin stated, 'But . . . we cannot be responsible for that.' Kennedy asked if Nestlé were able to investigate the use of their products in poor areas and Ballerin agreed that it was, but that they had not. Then Ballerin declared, 'The US Nestlé Company has advised me that their research indicates that this [the boycott] is actually an indirect attack on the free world's economic system.' This statement provoked laughter and Kennedy explained that a boycott was 'a recognised tool in a free democratic society'. [29] In their own report, Nestlé claimed that Kennedy 'was able to overwhelm the inexperienced witness new to the spotlight'. Few of the other testifiers were practiced witnesses and no one else there had reached such a pinnacle of power and wealth, yet Nestlé's account depicts Ballerin as a poor little chap and regrets that they overlooked Kennedy's 'lack of sympathy for big business and his commitment to the economically disadvantaged'. [30] Why should big business, which prides itself on strength, competence and public relations skills, be in need of 'sympathy'? As for the commitment to the economically disadvantaged, Nestlé claim to share this: 'I hardly need to emphasise that we are all equally distressed by this sad situation and we are also equally anxious to help in finding a solution,' proclaimed Carl Angst, General Manager of Nestlé, in a keynote speech at the thirteenth International Congress of Nutrition in 1985, referring to Third World poverty. [31] The concept of the Nestlé boycott being an anti-capitalist conspiracy was laughable. The boycotters included nuns, clergymen, business people and lawyers, parents and childless people, teachers, health workers and students all having different individual political and philosophical opinions. It was an issue which drew together many strange bedfellows, and as the boycott spread to other industrialised countries, it attracted support from many shades of political opinion.

GOOD CAPITALISM: THE PARADOXES
OF US SOCIETY

As a European I was interested by the strong and active commitment to the boycott among so many US citizens who were neither Marxists nor socialists, and through this I learned something about the paradoxes in the United States society. Although the United States embodies capitalism, there is in fact a long-established tradition of resistance to the big corporation when it behaves badly. One of the bulwarks of the power of the giant corporations in the United States is the Fourteenth Amendment to the US Constitution. The original aim of the 1866 Civil Rights Act had been to give equal rights to blacks; 'citizens of every race and color were to have equal rights to make contracts, to sue, and enjoy full and equal benefit of all laws and proceedings for the security of person and property.'[32] The effect of this legislation was not to change the position of the black Americans who were excluded from basic political participation in society until the 1960s and are still economically and socially oppressed by white racism. Instead, the corporations were able to increase their power by claiming the same rights as an individual citizen. Whenever a state government tried to curb, through laws, corporate action which hurt people, the federal courts invalidated any legislation by citing the 'due process' clause of the Fourteenth Amendment which prohibited a state government from depriving 'any person of life, liberty or property, without due process of law'. In the eyes of the US law, a legal entity such as a corporation is treated as a person, so that any attempt at restriction of company activity was interpreted as taking away the 'life, liberty and property' of the anthropomorphised corporation.

The idea of government interference contradicts the US concept of liberty, yet such was, (and is) the power of the companies that their interests and the government's are the same, for in spite of the myth that any US citizen can become President, only those who have the backing of the possessors of capital can get into politics. Corporations possess capital because the development of the law has provided the fiscal advantages that enable them to accumulate wealth while avoiding punitive taxation. This is one of the reasons why so many US companies have been able to grow so large and why the US has come to dominate the world economy. US citizens take these Goliaths for granted, but they have always loved their Davids and the dynamic between the two is fundamental to United States life. It was a faith in the possibility of 'good' capitalism that motivated many activists. The very name of one group, the Interfaith Centre for Corporate Responsibility, indicated that many US citizens believed sincerely that the large-scale capitalist enterprise could be induced to act morally. Nevertheless it was a fusion of corporate and political interests which was to override these moral considerations when the US government came to a decision on the World Health Organisation Baby Milk Code.

THE INVOLVEMENT OF THE INTERNATIONAL HEALTH AGENCIES

The aftermath of the Kennedy hearing was the involvement of the World Health Organisation and the United Nations Children's Fund, and the convening of the WHO/UNICEF Meeting on Infant and Young Child Feeding in October 1979. This was welcomed by everyone involved in the controversy. Of course mothers in poor countries, for whom, little had changed, remained unaware of all this activity on their behalf and they continued to take home their free samples and to cope with the diarrhoea, the debt and the funerals.

The baby food industries were put out that some of the participants at the WHO/UNICEF meeting besides themselves were from the very groups (the Berne Third World Group, ICCR, INFACT, IOCU (International Organisation of Consumer Unions) OXFAM and War on Want) who criticised them. They had almost a hundred years of experience in dealing with doctors, but they were nonplussed by these groups. How could they manipulate people who were not careerists, were not interested in making money and had nothing to lose themselves in their battle? The outcome of the meeting was the decision to form an International Code of Marketing of Breastmilk Substitutes. Though accepting the idea in principle, industry expressed doubts about an international code, as opposed to local codes, because it might lead to a loss of national sovereignty, a patriotic and philosophical problem which had never worried them when they produced their own ICIFI Code at the time of the Nestlé lawsuit in 1975.[33] Another outcome of the meeting, though it happened outside it, was the evolution of the International Babyfood Action Network (IBFAN) which enabled the various groups struggling to halt the aggressive marketing of baby foods to maintain the links they had forged during this period of hard work.

A set of recommendations came out of the WHO/UNICEF meeting which led to the drafting of a code. At this stage WHO, whose task is to improve world health, and UNICEF, which is concerned with the welfare of children, fell into the role of mediators between the pressure groups and the industry rather than defenders of infant health in their own right. This diversion of their skills gives an insight into the vulnerability of these international agencies. They have to be cautious about taking strong stands on sensitive issues because they are beholden to the world's most powerful groups for their survival. This is not a direct relationship, or at least it was not at the time (in April 1987 the contemporary equivalent of ICIFI, the IFM (International Assembly of Infant Food Manufacturers), achieved the status of a non-governmental organisation within WHO, which changes the relationship), but it is significant that the United States pays 25 per cent of WHO's budget and that the other major industrialised countries make up 70 per cent altogether. Delayed payment can be used as an implicit threat to pressure WHO (and the other UN organisations) if the organisation attempts any action which is perceived to be against the interests of these governments. As the United States government represents the interests and principles of transnational enterprise it is unlikely that it would support moves that restricted the activities of these companies. Nestlé may have been Swiss, it may have been the market leader in baby foods in the Third World, but it was only doing what the US-based companies wanted to do, namely, dominate the market.

THE US REJECTS THE CODE

After a year of revision and consultation between governments, infant feeding experts, the baby food industry and the non-governmental organisations, the WHO/UNICEF International Code of Marketing of Breastmilk Substitutes (the WHO/UNICEF Code) was produced. At the World Health Assembly in May 1981 it was overwhelmingly approved by 118 countries. There were three abstentions and one vote against it. The US delegate, Dr John Bryant, under orders from the US State department, reluctantly voted against the Code. This was where the corporate/political fusion of US politics was brought to light. Other countries with strong industrial interests against the Code, such as New Zealand and the EC countries, may have had more to lose economically than the US, but their decision was made on moral and health grounds. The US government's decision shocked and embarrassed many US citizens. There was extensive newspaper coverage, two leading USAID (United States Agency for International Development) officials resigned in protest, public demonstrations were held and 10,000 letters and telegrams were received by the White House and the State Department. Both the House of Representatives and the Senate approved resolutions expressing dismay at the vote. [34]

The pretext for the US vote was that the Code's provisions would 'cause serious and constitutional problems for the US itself'. The WHO/UNICEF Code of Marketing of Breastmilk Substitutes is a recommendation which means that each country is free to implement it according to their customary methods. Neither WHO nor UNICEF are law-enforcing bodies; no coercion could be brought to bear on any country to implement the Code, so that there were no possible constitutional problems. The Code does not restrict the sale of baby milk and it allows industry sponsorship of conferences on condition no promotion is done. It forbids all advertising but permits the provision of scientific and factual information for health professionals. The US government decision did not represent the will of the US people, who rejected the idea of their companies, as well as Nestlé, being implicated in infant illness and death. But the Reagan administration, under baby food industry pressure, acted to keep the door open for the companies to push their products wherever they could, regardless of their effects. The details of the relationships involved in the collusion of the US government and the baby food industry over the anti-Code vote are more fully detailed in Andrew Chetley's book *The Politics of Baby Foods*.

History has shown repeatedly that the baby food industry has never controlled itself voluntarily and that the medical profession, in spite of its supposed authority, lacked the solidarity, the will or the skill to deal with the marketing practices alone. It took the energy and dedication of a mixed band of people, brought together through their common sense of responsibility, to say, 'This cannot continue,' and to do something. The baby food activists were conspicuously moderate in their protests and there is no illegal or violent action to their record. The WHO/UNICEF Code was produced in an open forum, respected and accepted by governments spanning all shades of political colours. There are international rules for sports, and players agree that following them is the only workable way of running tournaments. When the US government representatives declared the Code to be against the interests of free trade and 'competition' it was only because they knew that an International Code of Practice concerning any product might restrict their own companies, who wanted to be free to change the rules as they went along so that they could always 'win'.

WHAT IS THE CODE? A SUMMARY OF TEN KEY POINTS

Reluctantly, I am going to devote a few pages to the WHO/UNICEF Code of Marketing of Breastmilk Substitutes.[35] Rules, codes and laws rarely make good reading because the need for a definitive clarity stretches them into boredom. They are often misunderstood because few of us have the patience to read them. Lawyers thrive because they have the tenacity to plough through documents which make the ordinary mortal collapse into a coma. The WHO/UNICEF Code of Marketing of Breastmilk Substitutes (the WHO Code) is not too bad, but it is no adventure story and its very moderation crushes any dramatic possibilities. It is important because it is at present the only tool there is for establishing a basis for consistent international practice to protect babies, parents and health workers from commercial pressures. Here is a brief explanation of the Code's main points. The Code's aim is:

> To contribute to the provision of safe and adequate nutrition for infants, by the protection and promotion of breastfeeding and by the proper use of breastmilk substitutes, when these are necessary, on the basis of adequate information and through appropriate marketing and distribution.

Most babies are less likely to die or get ill if they are breastfed, so breastfeeding should be protected and information about it disseminated. The current reality that, for many reasons, some babies have to be fed with a breastmilk substitute means that the carers of these babies must be well informed about the use of artificial milks. The marketing of milks, bottles, drinks or anything used instead of breastfeeding must be appropriate for babies' health and survival and not undermine breastfeeding.

The WHO/UNICEF Code is a minimum requirement; individual governments may make the provisions stronger. As a 'recommendation' each government may bring the Code into effect according to each country's usual way of implementing health measures, so it can be a law or a voluntary Code. The Code includes the following ten main provisions:

(1)   No advertising of breastmilk substitutes.
(2)   No free samples or supplies.
(3)   No promotion of products through health care facilities.

(4)   No contact between company marketing personnel and mothers.
(5)   No gifts or personal samples to health workers.
(6)   No words or pictures idealising artificial feeding, including pictures of infants, on the labels of the product.
(7)   Information to health workers should be scientific and factual only.
(8)   All information on artificial feeding, including labels, should explain the benefits of breastfeeding and the costs and hazards associated with artificial feeding.
(9)   Unsuitable products should not be promoted for babies.
(10)   All products should be of a high quality and take account of the climatic and storage conditions of the country where they are used.

1   No advertising of breastmilk substitutes

Copywriters would not get paid if advertising did not work. Would a company waste money on an ineffective sales tactic? Defenders of advertising argue that it is a source of information, but most baby milk advertisements are singularly uninformative. They rarely give truly relevant facts such as, for example, a baby milk's beef fat content, which is of concern to Hindu or vegetarian families. One brand claimed that 'of all the baby-milks you can buy it's the one that is nutritionally closest to breastmilk'.[36] Since all artificial milk is supposed to conform to standards which attempt this feat, then either this manufacturer is lying or all the others who make similar claims are.

Bottle-feeding parents do not need advertisements but rather impartial information from health professionals, and in Scandinavia they get it. The constant presence of images of artificial feeding in advertisements maintains the 'normality' of it when there is no comparable bombardment of the imagery of normal breastfeeding.

2   No free samples or supplies

Given during the sensitive perinatal period, baby milk samples can encourage the doubt that reduces the possibility of breastfeeding success. Health workers who give them out are demonstrating their own lack of conviction that a mother can breastfeed. If she ends up bottle-feeding, research shows that most women stick to the product they were given in hospital, which is why companies are so keen on this form of promotion which takes away informed choice from parents.[37] The free sample has been implicated in the deaths of thousands of poor babies when its use reduced their mothers' breastmilk and made the purchase of more artificial milk necessary. Too poor to buy sufficient amounts, many mothers have 'stretched' the milk by overdilution so that their babies gradually starved. If a mother is not helped to restimulate her own supply (and it is harder to do this with a sick baby), she is in a desperate situation. She cannot afford the replacement product and she may have lost her own milk. Every health worker handing out a free sample is taking a stand against breastfeeding. Something as important as an artificially fed baby's food needs to be chosen in consultation with an impartial infant feeding expert and not as a result of a good commercial deal between a company rep and a hospital administrator.

One source of samples comes from the free or low cost milk supplies which companies foist on maternity hospitals. In 1986, a World Health Assembly (WHA) Resolution clarified ambiguities in the Code on this issue and called for free supplies to end. The companies ignored this, prompting IBFAN groups to renew boycotts and other action. In 1991 UNICEF tried to persuade the baby food companies to stop free supplies by the end of 1992 and obtained a statement from the International Association of Infant Food Manufacturers (IFM) that they would do so if governments made the practice illegal. To date (February 1993) free supplies persist the world over, particularly in North America where take-home packs are standard practice, but also in many poor countries. Health professionals' collusion in this practice cannot be denied, but ignorance and intimidation exonerate some.

3   No promotion of products through health care facilities
Since the advent of the milk depots (see page 193) clinics and hospitals have been associated with the provision and supply of

milks, bottles and teats in many parts of the world. This practice undermines any affirmation of the value of breastfeeding, as do all other petty forms of promotion. Most health workers have become so used to their clinics being plastered with company posters, notepads, pens and diaries that they do not perceive their function. Each time a health worker scribbles a note or writes a prescription on a paper with a company logo they are endorsing that company's product. Many claim that their use of a notepad does not link them with the company, but how many doctors would be happy to write their prescription on a paper bearing the name of a local bar?

Though direct corruption can exist, most health workers are unwitting participants in this game and receive little personal benefit through acting as unpaid salespeople for the companies. As Dr Natividad Clavano, the Paediatric Chief at Baguio General Hospital in the Philippines, said, 'We allowed the companies to touch the lives of our babies, not because we did not care, but because we did not realise the consequences of granting such a privilege.'[38] When Doctor Clavano decided to do something about breastfeeding, her most difficult task was persuading not the mothers but the hospital staff, who could not believe that you could run a maternity ward without company endorsement. Health worker practices have proved hard to change, because the commercial links have become such an intrinsic part of their work that they fail to notice them. Once a doctor from a tropical country said, 'But I must have samples. I have to have something to give a poor mother to take away.'[39] He perceived the consulting room as the boundary of his responsibilities and thought that to maintain the doctor/patient relationship he must act as a benefactor and hand over an object as a token of his solicitude. In his country he might as well have handed a mother a lump of bad meat for her baby.

The record from the US in the early twentieth century shows how vital it was for companies to establish themselves within the health care system. This is still the case and it is the area where companies struggle most fiercely to resist Code implementation. They know medical endorsement is vital for sales.

4 No contact between company marketing personnel and mothers

Thanks to the pressure of the 1970s, companies have phased out the notorious 'milk nurses' (see page 228) only to replace them with such devices as telephone counselling services, video tapes (with free samples tucked inside) and hijacking of baby care materials. Many governments blithely let companies publish infant feeding brochures thus establishing a channel of contact between mother and company. Some national codes have mistakenly allowed reps to contact mothers (such as through presentations at clinic classes) if a health worker gives permission: this transfers responsibility to the health worker who is usually ill-trained about these ethical issues.

5 No gifts or personal samples to health workers

This is difficult, not just because of personal temptation, but because gifts are often given so subtly. A paediatrician in a private Bangkok hospital describes one of the ways a company managed to get its baby milk used:

> One of my colleagues who wields a lot of influence with the director invited us to a birthday party. Of course we thought he was doing it all, but when we arrived, a representative from a drug company with a formula offering was present. They had financed the celebration. And the next month, that brand was served in the nursery. [40]

Health workers need to get on with their colleagues and it is hard for individuals to go against the workplace norm. If one midwife tries to take a stand by refusing to use notepads or diaries she may be viewed as petty or sanctimonious. Resisting company pressure when your superiors do not is an implied criticism of their principles and in the hierarchy of most health systems this is not going to make working life easier. The Code makes it easier for everyone because it provides a clear, realistic base for practice; everyone can refer to it and can know where they stand.

The issue of receiving small gifts is often viewed as a trivial matter. In a poor country these things might be hard to buy so that their value as a gift is not small. A health worker can feel very obligated to the salesperson who has given much-needed pens, notepads and diaries, and of course this is why it is done. There is no such thing as a free biro; a profit-making company is just that and it is very inefficient and unbusinesslike if it spends money on public relations tactics that do not improve sales.

6   No words or pictures indealising artificial feeding, including picture of infants, on the labels of the products
Parents want their baby to be healthy and the picture of the gorgeous child on the tin of milk conveys the message that theirs will be equally chubby and happy; this is a lie which is why the Code bans the baby pictures. Some companies have removed the baby pictures but replaced them with an equally seductive image. For example Mead Johnson have depicted the well-known character 'Peter Rabbit' with his mother. Doubtless, skilled marketing psychologists advised that this image conveyed trust, security and motherliness. The only example of full Code compliance in this respect is in Iran where the Ministry of Health rules that milks carry a plain, beige label with standardised information and instructions. Company names are printed in small type in case the origin of the milk needs to be traced. Other countries have attempted national milk labels, purchasing the product from companies such as Nestlé or Nutricia, but such is the power of packaging imagery that the public often believes the branded tin is superior even when the milk in the national tin is the same product. All baby milk, and bottle and teat packaging project idealised images of product-consuming glamour. If you lead a hard life this picture can provide a fantasy of health and wealth, but if the product leads your baby to illness and death it can prove a costly one. The allure of packaging is universal, and rich and poor alike select products on this superficial basis, which is why companies invest so much in its design.

7   Information to health workers should be scientific and factual
When companies change their products or bring out a new one, it is important that health professionals know exactly what is in the product, and the companies may announce these facts as fully

as possible in straightforward product information. In Sweden and Norway for instance a company would simply provide a factual leaflet to health workers. In countries where the Code is not in practice, they print misleading advertisements. For example, there was a spate of advertisements which emphasised the addition of taurine to a milk. One company advertisement filled three-quarters of the page with a naked woman cuddling a full-term healthy baby.[41] In fact there is as yet no scientific evidence that additional taurine in artificial milk makes any difference to a bottle-fed full-term baby, whereas taurine is definitely important for premature babies. This advertisement was deliberately trying to make health workers believe that this milk was better for all normal babies, yet if anyone had time to read the scientific references cited in the advertisement, they would discover that there was no evidence for this claim. If taurine is found to be so significant, then it should be made statutory to add it to all brands. An informative advertisement would have dispensed with the mother and baby picture and used the space to present an honest and responsible comparison of data.

8   All information on artificial feeding, including labels, should explain the benefits of breastfeeding and the costs and hazards associated with artificial feeding

Electric plug instructions carry warnings about the risks of improper use. Baby milk can be as risky a product as an electric plug, so the potential hazards of misuse must be clearly explained. Baby milk is an economic hazard as much as a nutritional one where there is poverty.

9   Unsuitable products should not be promoted for babies

Throughout the debate during the 1970s, when the companies claimed to be following their own ethical code, unsuitable products were not only advertised for babies, but instructions for infant feeding were put on the tin. Several companies who argued that their infant milks were necessary because ignorant mothers would use inappropriate foods, were at the same time promoting products such as sweetened condensed milk and custard powder for babies.

Since the Code came into existence, several companies have picked out verbal loopholes in the Code and cynically launched other products, such as sweetened teas and follow-up milks which they claim are not breastmilk substitutes and therefore promote without restriction. Sweetened teas are used extensively in Europe and have damaged babies' teeth. They are merely well packaged equivalents of the sugar water that the companies have criticised poor mothers for using. Any product other than breastmilk (even water) used during infancy is a breastmilk substitute, can interfere with breastfeeding and therefore jeopardise an infant's health.

10 All products should be of a high quality and take account of the climatic and storage conditions of the country where they are used

Most consumers take it for granted, if they buy a tin of baby milk, a bottle or a teat, that the contents are of high quality, but they are overly complacent. Maureen Minchin and FORMULA have documented the worryingly high incidence of inadequate or substandard products. Some were nutrient-deficient and this fact was only discovered after babies became ill. Others are cases of poor quality control or inadequate packaging and storage. Contamination is yet another problem which is possible even with a well-designed breastmilk substitute. The possibility of faulty products being sold in poor countries is far greater, for consumer awareness and pressure may be weak and the expensive infrastructures for challenge have not yet been developed. Transport, climate and storage problems make products more vulnerable. If laws do not exist to demand sell-by dates, companies do not put them on the package. Quality control is difficult to maintain even in ideal conditions. In 1986 in the UK, Farleys eventually had to close down a factory because they could not eliminate persistent salmonella in their powdered baby milk, Ostermilk. Though the product was withdrawn from sale throughout Britain relatively quickly, the logistics of withdrawal from tropical countries, where contamination was potentially more lethal, meant it was inevitably less speedy.[42]

If the Code were adhered to the number of these accidents would be reduced. If it were law, as it is in some countries, the threat of prosecution would make manufacturers take more care. If companies stopped promotion they could spend the money saved on better quality control. Suggest this and marketing managers admit that sales would fall without promotion, which belies their claim that they only sell baby milk to fulfil a need.

COULD THE CODE WORK?

Even before the Code's adoption, one country, Papua New Guinea, had, in 1977, introduced legislation to control the use of feeding bottles and artificial milk and as a result had dramatically reduced malnutrition. In 1976 a third of the children under 2 in the capital, Port Moresby, were being artificially fed and over two-thirds of these were malnourished. In just two years, bottle-feeding had dropped from 35 per cent to 12 per cent and malnutrition had been reduced by a third. It is illegal to sell a bottle without a prescription and a health worker has to prove it is in a baby's interests to be bottle-fed before writing one. There is a high level of awareness among health workers and the policies were able to be implemented fully because the baby milk companies had not yet established themselves. The authorities were resolved to make the policy work so at that time, the companies did not attempt to sabotage it. In 1991 Papua New Guinea, where 85 per cent of the population live in rural areas and only 34 per cent have safe drinking water (Brazil 97 per cent), had an infant mortality rate that at 55 per 1,000 is comparable with those of Brazil and South Africa and lower than that of Turkey, all countries which are considered to be at a more 'advanced' level of development. Papua New Guinea's health policies worked because the government and health workers were united in their efforts to implement them. Unfortunately satellite TV, now (1992) beams advertising into the country and bottle-feeding is increasing. Designed to function internationally, the Code is hard to implement if a neighbour flouts it. Guatemala has a strong Code and has prosecuted individual violators, but cannot stop the US TV stations which broadcast baby food company advertising into their country. The international action of the 1970s and 80s motivated the baby food

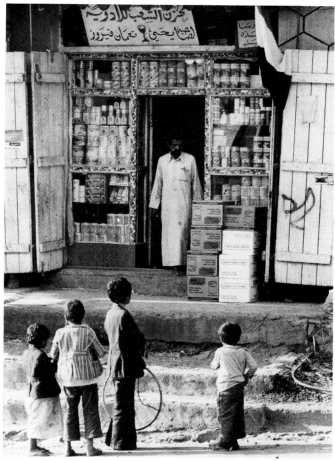

22 Grocer's shop in the Yemen stocked with imported powdered milk products (*Photo:* David Green; courtesy of OXFAM)

companies to form an alliance (ICIFI) which transmutated into the International Association of Infant Feeding Manufacturers (IFM). Not only do they work together to evade and distort the Code's provisions, but IFM enjoys recognition as a non-governmental organisation (NGO) within the World Health Organisation. The UN agencies are not immune to industry influence and Code advocacy has been remarkably absent from their agendas.

THE HEALTH AGENCIES' ROLES

It is a measure of the limitations of the international health agencies' adequacy that, in spite of their skill in drafting the Code in a compromise form to suit everyone, including the baby food industry, they cannot achieve a health advocacy which enables governments to resist the less acceptable influences of business interests. WHO and UNICEF have only moral authority; they cannot prosecute a government or a company which ignores the tenets of the Code. It is the member states who create the consensus for WHO to formulate its policies and what a health minister agrees to at an international forum might prove difficult to implement at home. Some countries, such as New Zealand, Sweden and Norway, have brought in the Code as a voluntary measure and a relatively high level of awareness has kept abuse to a minimum. Other countries, such as the UK, Singapore and Nigeria, invited the baby milk industry to write their codes for them and inevitably these weak industry codes maintained the status quo. Some countries, including Guatemala, Sri Lanka, and Peru, have implemented the Code as a law, but enforcement is often difficult. With an overburdened legislature and political instability, a public prosecutor is unlikely to prosecute a powerful foreign company when other problems are so pressing. Developing countries desperate to keep their fragile economies cobbled together are at the mercy of the transnationals and the international moneylenders. They cannot take truly effective stands against such issues as environmental pollution, let alone something as taken for granted as advertising and promotion. Besides, national governments are mostly dominated by men and any issue which affects the daily lives of women is of secondary importance to the 'serious' concerns of 'defence' and 'trade'.

WHO's constitutional objective is 'the attainment by all

peoples of the highest possible level of health', but as they say themselves, this can 'only be achieved to the extent permitted by the manpower and budgetary resources available'. [44] As shown on page 251, their financial support is weighted and it is difficult for WHO to attempt to implement policies which offend the big paymasters. These are the governments who are beholden to big business for political and financial support. WHO employees spend their lives balancing on a rickety fence. Their task is to battle for health and in the modern world much ill-health comes not only from nature or lack of knowledge, but also through the effects of the international economic system and the might of transnational companies. This can apply to hunger caused by the appropriation of good land for export crops, the Bhopal disaster or the infiltration of a hospital system by a baby milk company. The old definitions of 'left' and 'right' have become obscured as in the Former Soviet Union (FSU), communists are called 'conservatives' and in the UK, conservativism has been dubbed 'radical'. A government's stance is immaterial, for international trade is dominated by those who control the markets and the so-called 'free market' policies of both elected and non-elected governments are under their influence. The developing nations are at the mercy of the controllers of international trade and finance. Any moves to redress the balance of power can ricochet back on the poor. For example, when the oil-exporting nations invested their burgeoning wealth during the 1960s and 1970s, they did so within the international banking system which is dominated by the industrialised nations. The last thing any moneylender wants to do is pay out interest and the financiers quickly solved the problems of high deposits by flinging money in the form of loans into the poorest nations, thus creating the state of devastating indebtedness which now cripples poor nations. The now notorious International Monetary Fund packages, which bail out countries on condition that they cut down on internal investment in health and social welfare, keep millions poor and sick. The World Health Organisation cannot make statements on these issues lest the rich country governments get angry and withhold their subscriptions.

There is some evidence which shows that poor people do better during phases of world economic recession because as the market for cash crops declines they can grow more useful food crops for themselves.[45] In the same way periods of shortage of supplies of baby milk can lead to falls in infant mortality and illness because breastfeeding increases. Destroying the support systems for breastfeeding and replacing it with an industrialised product has the same effect as appropriating food-supplying land for cash crops. It creates dependency and malnutrition.[46] In spite of its own indebtedness, the US still dominates the world economy and its political protection can feel like a stifling embrace when any country attempts to establish policies which put human welfare above profit making. When the US voted against the WHO Code they made a grand gesture, which no other country dared make. They had enough power to put two fingers to WHO, to the medical profession, even to the moderates in industry who were concerned about the unacceptable face of capitalism. The anti-Code vote was a way of saying 'screw you' to the poor countries struggling to protect their children from colonialism's own child, unrestricted marketing.

THE NATURE OF THE BEAST

The transnational enterprises work hard to integrate themselves with governments, because this is the best way of achieving their ends. Conflict with them is counter-productive to business advancement. This is why companies are so chameleon-like. If they can advertise on television in one country they will, if they are not allowed to in another they will not. They will boast of their innovative marketing in the one and of their ethical marketing in the other. Because public relations departments are skilled at projecting a benign image, we tend to forget that companies do not exist to do good or to provide useful products. A director of US Steel (later significantly called US X) remarked that the company's purpose was not to make steel but to make money. He was right and the pursuit of profit and the welfare of the less powerful are often conflicting goals. Enterprises which market less aggressively find themselves pushed out in the market place by their less squeamish competitors, so that it is difficult for companies who want to behave well to do so. History has shown that without legal restraints companies will behave unethically and when this happens others must follow suit or shut up shop. It is up to us to say when to stop and if we really do live in democracies, we must demand that our representatives, governments, establish the checks. If international measures are the only way of doing this, then we must work to secure them. If we find that the channels for protest and challenge are blocked, then democracy does not truly exist.

It is a waste of energy focusing on whether the director of a company is a 'nice person' or not. The participants in the trans-national enterprise game (and most of us who use money are participants) are not evil beings plotting destruction, they are players (some willing and some not) in a system that is out of control. What we must be suspicious of are the protestations of companies that they are principally concerned with human welfare. That is not their role; the 'caring' image is simply part of marketing and has nothing to do with the realities of big business.

THE PHILIPPINE EXPERIENCE

Because of the US vote, any country dependent on their political and economic patronage would be reluctant to implement the Code fully because it had been declared to be against US interests. For example, in the Philippines, an ineffective Industry Code had been drafted. The Marcos government would never have taken action to disturb multinational marketing. When the actress Liv Ullman visited the country in 1983 in her capacity as an ambassador for UNICEF, she was booked to appear on a TV chat show which happened to be sponsored by Nestlé, and she was told not to mention breastfeeding. Liv Ullman was appalled; she declared that she had never been censored in her life and she made sure this story was given to the press. Of course the TV producers were embarrassed and the Marcos government feigned shock and surprise. The Marcoses' daughter had just given birth and it was quickly announced that she was now going to breastfeed her baby.

There was however no mention of withdrawing TV sponsorship. Liv Ullman had by chance stumbled across the free market in action and found that it involved some curtailment of other freedoms for it to function.[47]

When the Aquino government was elected, a Philippines Code was made law in 1986. It bans free milk supplies but has the major weakness of allowing advertisements if they are approved by a government committee. In 1987 the US company Wyeth was threatened with legal action by BUNSO (the National Coalition for the Promotion of Breastfeeding and Childcare) for breaking the Code by advertising one of their so-called 'follow-up' milks, to be used in a feeding bottle. Taking on a powerful multinational company is a courageous step for a small third world health group. Wyeth was one of the companies that lobbied the US government to vote against the WHO Code. The US government has often criticised the human rights records of other countries, yet it is a US-based company which seems willing to violate the human right of Filipino babies to be breastfed.

If the US had taken a moral stand (something they repeatedly claim to be doing when they charge into the conflicts of other nation states) on this issue, it could have led the world in implementing the changes. Of course the companies would have had to reduce their markets, but tax incentives could have been devised to help companies to 'demarket' milks and to diversify into other products. The so-called 'free' market system is manipulated through fiscal measures by most industrialised country governments, and many products are supported by both open and hidden subsidies. The US was one of the first governments to support 'demarketing' when they paid farmers not to produce certain food crops because this was judged to be for the common good. Surely this was a far more draconian infringement of free market principles than setting guidelines for the marketing of a product whose improper use could kill children?

Every baby in the world is an individual and has a right to the life and liberty that the US has claimed to be defending in many a military conflict, yet when it came to the commercial exploitation of babies, these rights were set aside. Now aid agencies, many of them partly staffed and financed by US workers and money, urge women to breastfeed as though mothers themselves had established the sales and promotion of the artificial products and the damaging medical customs. The head of UNICEF is a US citizen, yet he is restricted by an unwritten code of practice from publicly criticising his government for their stance on this issue. It would be more than his job was worth to do so. Where is this freedom that the US proudly claims to fight for worldwide? The US corporations have benefited from being treated like individuals under the 'due process' clause of the Fourteenth Amendment and yet are not accountable as individuals for any damage that they cause worldwide.

I may have been unfair in focusing on the US companies when others are no better in their marketing behaviour. Some are worse than others; the Japanese baby food industry is now particularly zealous, but it is not worth comparing the marginally better behaviour of one with another because this could change by the time these words are in print. The companies are both dynamic and transnational. The UK-based company Cow & Gate is now owned by the Dutch firm Nutricia and the US company Carnation by the Swiss Nestlé.[48] The balance of share ownership can shift from day to day. The dynamism is such that companies are constantly changing identity and ownership in order to maximise their profits. A new director, a shift of targets, and stock market movements are all cogs in the ever-mobile company machine.

THE BOYCOTT CONTINUES

After the 1981 adoption of the WHO/UNICEF Code, each company wrote its own weakened version, of the original. Nestlé still took little action to change their marketing practices, so the boycott continued and strengthened. By this time Nestlé had invested in a new public relations system, whose director persuaded the diehards within Nestlé that it might even be commercially expedient to make concessions. The company issued a statement saying that they would keep to the

WHO/UNICEF Code, but their practices showed scant improvement. The boycott continued and under this pressure Nestlé eventually brought out guidelines for their employees. Nestlé made an agreement with the International Nestlé Boycott Committee (INBC) in which it gave an undertaking to abide by the WHO/UNICEF Code and to concede to WHO's final decision in any dispute about the details of implementation. As a result, the boycott was suspended in early 1984 at the INBC conference in Mexico City, and after a six-month test period when evidence in eight regions indicated that reforms were taking place, the boycott was ended.

Not everyone was happy about this move, especially those from the developing countries. With their limited purchasing power, a boycott could not function effectively in a poor country, so it citizens were dependent on the activists in the industrialised countries to make their protest felt. Many health workers from developing countries were worried that the ending of the boycott would mean that the issue would fade and they would be at the mercy of industry once again. Another matter concerned both the Third World and the European delegates at the Mexico City conference. In the horse trading that happens in every conciliation meeting, Nestlé had resisted on one count. It refused to keep to the WHO/UNICEF Code in Europe until the other companies agreed to.

By 1986 the European Parliament had debated the issue and voted for the Code to be made law in the EC in three separate sessions. Each time the European Commission (the EC Civil Service) drafted a Code which echoed almost to the letter the weak industry Codes, EC commissioners deny company influence

23 (*opposite page*) Mother of twins. The child with the bottle is a girl – she died the next day. Her twin brother was breastfed. This woman's mother-in-law told her she didn't have enough milk for both children, so she breastfed the boy. She certainly could have fed both, because suckling induces milk production. Even if she could not produce sufficient milk – unlikely as that would be – a better alternative would have been a wet-nurse. Ironically, this could have been the grandmother, a common practice before the advent of bottle-feeding. (UNICEF 1992: *Photo* by Mushtaq Khan)

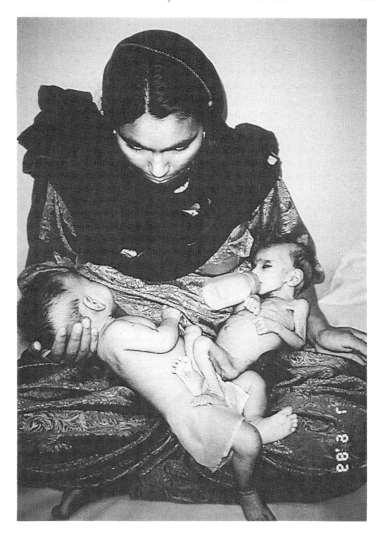

and from one aspect it is hardly necessary. Both the Scientific Committee for Food which advises the EC Commission and The Codex Alimentarius Committee which lays down food compositional standards, are comprised mainly of individuals with food industry connections. The Commission's Code drafting-group included representatives from each EC member state, few of whom knew about breastfeeding, the original Code or marketing. One who did was a UK representative, a civil servant who just happened to be the father of a breastfed child, with a personal interest in the subject. Such is the chance nature of politics. When the 'European Commission Directive on Infant Formulae and Follow-on Milks' was finally adopted in 1991, it did not directly contradict the WHO/UNICEF Code, for the Commission had heard the concerns of many hundreds of groups and individuals. However the final document omitted and weakened many key points. Meanwhile Nestlé led the way in intensifying promotion in Europe revealing the mendacity of their statements to the INBC. A group of sincere activists had been duped by the sweet talk of a cynical public relations exercise.

THE 1990S: HOPE OR DESPAIR?

In 1990, a British TV team visited Pakistan and were shocked by what they found. Five million babies are born each year of whom half a million die. Almost half die from diarrhoea; most of these would live if fully breastfed. Only a quarter of babies under three months are exclusively breastfed. With contraceptive use at only 12 per cent and with such disrupted breastfeeding, birth rates and short birth intervals are unacceptably high, jeopardising the health and survival of Pakistani women as well as their babies. Just half the population have access to safe water and less than a quarter to sanitation. Female illiteracy is 80 per cent, 30 per cent of people live below the absolute poverty level* and a tin of baby milk costs the average daily wage of about US$3.

* Absolute poverty level is defined as being unable to afford a nutritionally adequate diet.

These conditions have not inhibited the companies. Abbott-Ross, American Home Products (Wyeth), Boots (Farleys), Mead Johnson, Meiji (the market leader), Morinaga, Nestlé, Nutricia and its subsidiary Cow & Gate and Snow Brand together enjoyed a doubling of sales during the 1980s. In 1987 an estimated 9 to 18 million dollars' worth of baby milk was sold and 4.5 million feeding bottles imported. The film team met company reps in hospitals who almost innocently stated: 'My job is to promote my product,' as they produced samples. A doctor responsible for a large newborn unit enthused about follow-on milks as the rep showed her a glossy promotional brochure. There were company posters in the wards, and in the streets billboards advertising follow-on milks and bottles.

The film team followed babies dying of diarrhoea into the emergency rooms and discovered a complicating factor. Many had been given immodium (Ioperamide), an anti-diarrhoeal drug made by Janssen (a subsidiary of Johnson & Johnson) sold over the counter in the form of paediatric drops unavailable in Europe or North America. Immodium immobilises the gut, making death more likely for children (see page 91). It was as though the jackals had followed the vultures for any leftovers. But within days of the film's transmission Johnson and Johnson announced the withdrawal of its paediatric formulation.

The milk and bottle companies whose products triggered the initial diarrhoea did not follow Johnson and Johnson's example. In 1991, the US company, Abbot-Ross was promoting Similac as 'comparable to the nutritional characteristics of breastmilk fat'. The Japanese firm Meiji advertised its follow-on milk 'Meiji Fu' on TV as 'the secret of health'. Cannon, a British bottle and teat manufacturer claimed on billboards that they had had 'mothers' confidence for 50 years'. Free supplies from eight main companies were found in Pakistani maternity hospitals in 1991. [49]

These marketing tactics are not unique to Pakistan, nor is government inertia. In the United States where 200,000 babies a year are hospitalised for diarrhoea, promotion has intensified. In the absence of a Code, the American Academy of Pediatrics (AAP) and the companies had a gentlemen's agreement to forego public advertising. Nestlé scuppered this when they bought

Carnation and started TV advertising and Bristol Myers/Mead Johnson and Gerber followed suit. Formula sales rose and within 5 years there was a 24 per cent decline in infants being breastfed at 6 months. The gentlemen in the AAP are impotent.[50]

And what about Nestlé, who boast of keeping to 'every dot and comma' of the Code? In 1991, IBFAN monitoring discovered more Code violations by Nestlé than any other company, partly because it is the most ubiquitous. They gave free supplies in 55 countries. Nestlé knew the results of these 'donations', for having ignored the experts' consensus at the 1986 World Health Assembly, in 1988 they embarked on their own research.

During the first boycott, Nestlé had set up the 'independent' Nestlé Infant Formula Auditing Committee (NIFAC) in Washington D.C., chaired by a venerable US Senator called Edward Muskie. Several years of inaction became untenable so they hired a team of reputable researchers to investigate infant feeding practices in Mexico. The study results were damning. Most mothers went into hospital planning to breastfeed. Almost all had their babies snatched away to suffer the barbaric and useless medical ritual of gastric lavage, put into nurseries and routinely bottle-fed with free supplies provided for the most part by Nestlé, but also by the Mexican state food company, Conasupo. Many mothers went home with free tins of baby milk. By 3 months, 45 per cent of mothers were bottle-feeding and 55 per cent mixed feeding. Only one mother exclusively breastfed! Mothers who had received free samples were significantly more likely to be giving formula by 2 weeks. Nestlé closed NIFAC down before the study was published. When asked why, a Nestlé UK Executive, Ron Hendey said; 'Well, they were all getting on a bit.'[51]

But some powerful people do seem to care. In 1990, 32 Governments and 10 UN Agencies developed and signed the 'Innocenti Declaration' which called for a radical approach to national and social policies in order to create a breastfeeding culture. If your government participated in this hold them to their words. The declaration is a magnificent statement (see Appendix 3). This paved the way for breastfeeding rights to be included in the under-implemented 'Convention on the Rights of the Child' adopted in 1990.[52]

In 1991 most of the organisations involved in breastfeeding met and formed the 'World Alliance for Breastfeeding Action' (WABA) to co-ordinate their efforts. Soon after, UNICEF launched its 'Baby Friendly Hospital Initiative' (BFHI) in an effort to motivate all maternity facilities to implement 'The Ten Steps to Successful Breastfeeding' (See Appendix 4). UNICEF also extracted a promise from the IFM that all free and low cost supplies would be stopped by the end of 1992. However, the promise was only for developing countries and then only on condition individual governments passed laws banning free supplies. Twelve 'lead' countries which included Pakistan and Mexico were named. There has been no revolution but some important improvements. UNICEF hopes that hospital practices will be transformed in all countries by 1995. When in early 1992, the director of UNICEF was asked why companies were starting to co-operate with plans for change he answered 'because of the boycott'. This renewed action against Nestlé has been led from Europe (49 per cent of world sales of all products) and by 1992 was in 14 countries across the world. In the UK, by 1992, Nescafé (a targetted boycott product) sales were falling. There were some 'Baby Friendly Hospitals', but overall free supplies and many other promotional tactics were still much in evidence. [53]

Although the Code deems that 'independently of any other measures', the companies should conform to its provisos, they refuse to restrain themselves unless the governments bring in laws. But what happens when countries do make laws? In 1986, the Philippines Code outlawed free supplies; the companies merely invoiced the hospitals and never collected payment. Then a bill was drafted to make rooming-in mandatory. The companies sent a critique of the bill to the Health Ministry claiming that rooming-in was dangerous and increased infection. A perturbed doctor in the Philippines Senate sent copies to the Institute of Child Health in London and Baby Milk Action (UK IBFAN). Industry's claims contradicted medical evidence (a baby is exposed to more infection in a nursery than in her mother's arms), yet lack of access to good data made this doctor feel unable to prove the case.

Despite the obduracy of the companies and the timidity of

governments, there has been some progress. About 75 countries have taken some action to implement all or part of the Code but only nine countries have legislated the Code in full. Brazil, Guatemala and Kenya shine out for having achieved reversals in breastfeeding decline. A key to success in those countries is that aware and talented individuals have educated the powerful. [54] But there are other constraints. In Canada, the federal government threatens to cut funds from hospitals who do not take the industry bribes. The Women's College Hospital in Toronto is under pressure to sign a deal with Mead Johnson for $1 million in return for taking free supplies and take-home packs for mothers. The staff are being asked to break their code of professional ethics and risk their patients' health and some are angry. What can they do when their own government colludes with Code violation? [55]

In Brazil there is concern that low-income mothers stop breastfeeding before 6 months because: '. . legislation supporting working women in Brazil by giving them time off to nurse and by providing nurseries for child care is not complied with by most companies in Sao Paulo.' [56] Brazil, a highly indebted country, had a huge export drive in the 1980s which led to impressive growth. Much of the profits go into debt-servicing. As Brazil developed into one of the world's largest food exporters, child malnutrition rose alarmingly mostly among the quarter of Brazilians who live below the absolute poverty level. The mothers in Sao Paulo, whose employers refuse them time to breastfeed, contribute to Brazil's astounding economic performance through their work, yet to achieve this output they must sacrifice the health and often the lives of their children. In Sao Paulo babies who are not breastfed are fourteen times more likely to die of diarrhoea.

Finally, a tale from Europe: in 1990, a relief agency requested EC Aid for medical kits to distribute in Romania. EC Aid agreed to provide the kits on condition the agency also distributed milk powder, including branded baby milks. There was disagreement within the agency but finally the urgent need for medical kits made them submit to the EC Aid conditions. The health worker put in charge of the milk distribution was horrified by the Romanian situation; breastfeeding rates are low and the infant death rate is the highest in Europe. She considered the milk distribution harmful but felt powerless to defy her superiors. If manufacturers can manipulate a European Community body to break the Code and market their products for them, no wonder more vulnerable regions succumb to company pressure.[57]

THE ENDURING ATTRACTION

Why do the medical bodies allow this state of affairs to continue? Once again we return to the old love affair. An important proportion of medical and nutritional research is financed by the baby milk companies. The professional health bodies (whom the Code asks to report violations) frequently receive funding for salaries, grants and conferences from manufacturers. Research is prestigious, but it is costly and researchers' careers depend on the generosity of their funders. Both companies and researchers earnestly claim that there are no strings attached to the funding, but coincidentally the same recipients of company money are often those most reluctant to speak out in support of the Code. But, I hear many researchers cry, they never influenced my research. Here is money, say the companies, and do what you like, we are only too happy to support open research. Good, if this is true let it be publicised. I have yet to meet a researcher with baby milk industry funding who is actively criticising their unethical practices and there is as yet no company that is blameless.

Often company influence is so subtle it is almost subconscious. Once IBFAN offered their materials for a resource centre. The doctor who ran the centre said, 'Oh I can't take that because we're supported with Nestlé money.' There had been no conditions with Nestlé's donation; if asked they would probably have denied any wish to control or censor this doctor's selection of materials. The doctor changed his mind and used the IBFAN materials, because he was so startled by his own spontaneous complicity with the company, but it is a natural human reaction to feel bounden by someone's generosity. No one wants to bite the hand that feeds them. Scientists pride themselves on objectivity, doctors dedicate themselves to the prevention and cure of disease, but both set boundaries to their thinking. Like all of us, they have their price, they are dedicated to their work and the threat of having it taken away is powerful. They think they are free pipers, but out of an innate sense of tact they avoid playing a tune that he who pays does not like, for in their hearts they realise that if they play something discordant to the paymaster's ears, their pipe is taken away and given to another player.

After research showed a link between cows' milk protein in baby milks and insulin dependent diabetes, Dr John VanderMeulen, a paediatric endocrinologist at McMaster University, Ontario, was asked by the *Hamilton Spectator* if there was cause to make recommendations regarding infant feeding. He replied, 'It would be irresponsible to avoid cows' milk protein . . . It would be unfair to the dairy industry . . . to the infant formula industry.'
Reported in INFACT Canada Newsletter, Summer 1992

· 9 ·

Money, Work and the Politics of Waste

THE ECONOMIC VALUE OF BREASTMILK

In 1973, in his book *The Nutrition Factor*, Alan Berg calculated the market value of breastmilk for several different countries. He valued breastmilk by determining the costs of securing an equivalent amount of nutrients through commercial milks. For example, in the Philippines 31 per cent fewer mothers breastfed in 1968 than a decade earlier and this was equivalent to a loss of US$33 million that year. Since then other health economists have estimated the value of existing or lost breastmilk. The Jelliffes estimated in 1973 that it would take a herd of 114 million lactating cows to replace the milk of the women of India.[1] In 1982, John Eliot Rohde published a detailed analysis of breastmilk in relation to the Indonesian economy. He found that mothers produced over 1· billion litres annually with a conservatively estimated market value of over US$400 million. Additional monetary savings in health and fertility reduction added a further $120 million to the economy. 'Mother milk', as he called it, was one of Indonesia's most precious natural resources, exceeding tin and coffee in gross monetary value and approaching that of rubber.

> Its value exceeds twice the national budget for health and roughly equals the cost of imported rice, for which Indonesia has become, unenviably, the world's largest buyer. This great source is not only renewable, but also equitably distributed, benefits consumer and producer alike and gives far ranging non-monetary benefits to society.[2]

Other researchers calculated the values for Ghana, Ivory Coast, Tanzania and parts of the Caribbean, and each time the magnitude or this resource was illustrated. It seemed that at last women's unique contribution to their countries' economies was getting some acknowledgment. Some women reacted against this. Fran P. Hosken in *The Women's International Network News* referred to Alan Berg's calculations and comparisons and stated 'The obvious obscenity of such an equation points out dramatically the basis of the reasoning that was pursued by all the groups who, by all means, promoted breastfeeding.' (Actually she is wrong, for in her own country the most active group, INFACT, was never a breastfeeding promotion group and was only concerned with ethical marketing behaviour.)[3]

ATTITUDES TO WEALTH AND PAYMENT

This ambivalence towards the monetary evaluation of breastmilk matches other areas of women's production, In most cultures wealth brings social prestige, but how it has been acquired affects the measure of respect the wealthy earn. Sometimes money brings power but not status. There are numerous nineteenth-century European novels with the theme of moneymakers from peasant or worker backgrounds having to marry into ancient noble families in order to consolidate their social position. Today, in western society, though there are vestiges of the honouring of certain non-wealthy groups such as clergymen and intellectuals, increasingly wealth is the chief badge of social prestige. In the United States, the clergy, artists and left-wing intellectuals may be rich without shame. Psychotherapists and other nurturers who replace the shamans of pre-industrial societies charge high sums for their services without losing honour. Even the 'doula'* or mother/nurturers who have supported the new mother to breastfeed in both traditional and modern societies may now be

---

* I thank Monique Frangouli of La Leche League Greece for informing me that the word 'doula' means slave. Understandably Greek breastfeeding supporters dislike the term and I will not use it again.

the lactation consultant who charges fees for her services. The other side of this fusion of honour and wealth is that unpaid work is disregarded and despised. Anyone who works in the voluntary sector and whose work becomes salaried knows that suddenly society regards what they have always done as 'a real job'.

If wealth ownership is no disgrace what is wrong with the idea of putting an economic value on breastmilk and breastfeeding? Since the establishment of a dominating monetary economic system everything, including time, labour and services, is costed. Lawyers, doctors and other 'consultants' raise their fees with their reputation, yet many of the female-dominated jobs are not only low-paid but viewed as necessarily low-paid in order to preserve their spiritual value. Nursing is an example; in Britain, the Florence Nightingale ethos decrees that its 'vocational' nature is such that high pay might attract 'the wrong sort', those who are 'only in it for the money'. At the same time other servers of public welfare such as judges and admirals get pay rises because 'we must have good salaries to attract the right calibre of man'. It is not a coincidence that nursing is a predominantly female profession and judging a male one.

A parent couple who mutually agree for the father to support the mother of their children have made an informal contract whereby she relinquishes economic power and is dependant on his goodwill. When a whole society endorses this arrangement by restricting the economic advancement of women there is a significant loss of power. This marginalisation of mothers developed with industrialised capitalism and yet is falsely depicted as 'traditional'. A highly sentimentalised and unrealistic ideology of motherhood was needed to justify cutting women off from such a fundamental human right as inclusion in economic production. The gathering, peasant and trading women of pre-industrial societies have usually had more economic autonomy than the average western mother. In West Africa, women such as the Yoruba have been the principal traders for years and they have integrated breastfeeding and childrearing into their lives without loss of prestige or economic advancement. [4]

When men are so advantaged in the market place, it makes sense at family level for them to be the breadwinners, if parents want to care for their child in a way they think is good, and the market place makes no provision for this nurture. The resentment that many western women feel against their children is often the expression of bitterness at their own exclusion from the outside world, and this discrimination continues long past the phase when it is justified for child survival. It also affects childless women who lose out because of a hypothetical potential for childbearing. There is no reason why a mother could not give birth and breastfeed, but a male partner could perform all the attendant work and be the main childcarer for the rest of the children's growing life. One of the main reasons that this does not happen is because none of these activities is rewarded with money.

THE MARGINALISATION OF CHILDCARE

In most societies, a mother who is not economically productive, either as a peasant producer, trader or through some form of paid employment is rare. The existence of the dependent and allegedly unproductive woman in the West is a hiccough in history that has been given a disproportionate amount of attention in influencing attitudes to women's lives. The export of these attitudes has triggered such long-term disasters as the expanding food crisis in Africa because the denial of the reality of women's production has led to the diversion of resources and support. It suited the owners of capital to have their workers' physical needs attended to by an invisible, unpaid workforce and women's traditional skills were utilised to achieve this. It also suited them to expand the ideology of the home as a unit of consumption so as to consolidate markets for their goods. The woman who buys artificial milk and bottles and props her baby in a cot with a bottle while she cooks her husband's meal or washes his socks is serving both these ends.

Childcare has been marginalised because it happened to remain in the 'domestic' sphere, which was once the unit of economic production. Thus the most important task of all, sustaining new and vulnerable humans through the most crucial and influential phase of their lives, has become a low-prestige job, underpaid or unpaid and disregarded. Even 'professional' nursery workers are low-paid in most societies. Many mothers who can survive economically, may seek out work in the market place that is far less vital for the greater social good than infant nurture simply to gain self-esteem and escape their marginalisation. The very fact that men avoid childcare is a measure of its low prestige in the minds of both sexes. The assumption that all childcare must take place in the home has led to the exploitation of women in a new way that reverses the effects of factory organisation, without regaining the flexibility and communality of traditional household production. Transnational companies are turning increasingly to home-based labour because in doing so they can reduce the costs and the responsibilities of worker welfare. Swasti Mitter's book *Common Fate, Common Bond*[5] describes these changes and shows how they have increased the exploitation of women in the global economy. Women work at home for shockingly low rates of pay, often without insurance or even the most basic health and safety provision. They use dangerous machines and chemicals in conditions which escape the inspection of any official eye, whether government or trade union. This change is spreading almost unnoticed because it is affecting women more than men and both management and unions have disregarded part-time or home-based women's work. This happens in both industrialised and developing countries. The nineteenth-century myth of the 'hearth and home' puts women and their children at risk.

> *A mother who worked at home putting catalogues into envelopes told an inquest in Southwark, south London, yesterday that she would always feel guilty about the death of her 2-year-old son who was crushed to death under a pile of mail order catalogues.* (Guardian, 5 December 1987)

Young children are a 'nuisance' because they distract from economic production. The mother who worked at home with the mail order catalogues feels guilty, but she had little choice in her means of survival. Her society does not provide her with an adequate income to care for her child. At the same time it excludes mothers from the centres of group production and condemns this woman, while it boasts of economic advance if the catalogue company increases its profits. Do the shareholders feel guilty?

A MODEL SOON TO BE LOST: THE BAKA

There are still human societies where there are few rigid divisions between men and women, and children are cherished. The Baka, the small people of the Cameroon Rain Forest, treat children with a wisdom and sensitivity that makes any psychology book redundant. A film made in 1987 showed a father being utterly involved in preparing his son for and supporting him through the experience of the arrival of a new sibling. His mother was as completely involved in the communal hunting procedures as her husband was with his child's physical and psychological welfare. Naturally children are breastfed for a very long time in this society, but women are not confined nor denied involvement in the process of production. Sadly, the Baka way of life is threatened by the forces of 'development'. [6]

ECOLOGICAL POWER

The irony of industrialised society is that women are still oppressed by the concept of their biological destiny, yet they have less involvement with their own biological powers than their 'primitive' sisters. Women still take responsibility for a whole range of tasks that were supposed to lead 'naturally' on from lactation. Women of all classes continue to prepare meals for adult men or supervise other women to do so, yet increasing numbers have lost the ability to feed their own children and are deterred from doing so.

So why should women not be rewarded for producing breastmilk and for breastfeeding? Human milk is a commodity which is ignored in national inventories and disregarded in food consumption surveys, yet it does actually save a country millions of dollars in imports and health costs. The Mozambican Ministry of Health calculated in 1982 that if there were a mere 20 per cent rise in bottle-feeding, in just two years this would cost the country US$10 million,and this did not include fuel, distribution or health costs. They also calculated that the fuel required for boiling the water would use up the entire resources from one of the major forestry projects. Inventors of fuel-saving cars are rewarded, why not energy-sparing women? For every 3 million bottle-fed babies, 450 million tins of formula are used. The resulting 70,000 tons of metal in the form of discarded tins is not recycled in the developed countries.[7]

Even in industrialised countries milk is not cheap. Its relatively low market price has only been achieved through massive subsidies to dairy farmers, and milk powder is stored at vast public expense. In the Europe Community it costs every household almost £16 per week to pay for the Common Agricultural Policy.[8] The human breast makes milk in exact quantities to order and there are no storage problems or costs. If the free market were truly allowed to function, cows' milk would not be the low-priced commodity we all know and are persuaded to love. The costs of every facet of production from cow to baby are astronomical, but the current world economic system is based on the profligate usage of resources without the real costs ever being put on the balance sheets. It has been estimated that it will cost £200 million to clean up the nitrate-polluted waters of just one agricultural region of Britain. Nitrate fertilisers are used to grow feed for dairy cows. Are the dairy farmers, the baby milk companies or the milk consumer going to pay for this salvage?

Breastfeeding puts far more into the renewable resource issue than taking bottles to the glass recycler. The women who complained of Alan Berg's calculations are presumably not ashamed when they, their partners or friends get a pay rise for whatever their work is. Do they consider all workers who produce primary food products as engaged in 'obscene' acts? Comparing the value of women's milk production with that of any other mammal is not 'obscene' but comparing women's breasts with prosthetic objects of plastic and rubber is.

Many trades and professions include the skilled and patient delivery of a service, together with a product, often to an individual. Why should a lawyer earn high fees for giving his or her time and skill to a client yet the same patience and time to a child must not be evaluated in these terms? Every baby needs continuous physical and emotional contact with one or two people who become sensitive to its needs. When people say bottle-feeding is convenient, they forget that someone has to prepare the food and give it to the baby. If the baby is left with a propped bottle, there is risk to both physical and emotional health.

CHILDCARE IS NOT HOUSEWORK

Regrettably, in women's struggle for justice, a lot of economic and personal exploitation of women by other women takes place, most often in the field of childcare and what is now seen as exclusively domestic labour. The linking of the two tasks of domestic labour and childcare has marginalised them both. Why is housework linked with childcare when being a business executive is not linked with office cleaning? Often a woman who relinquishes a paid job to 'stay at home' with her baby, finds herself engaging in an increased proportion of domestic tasks which have nothing to do with the baby. Vacuuming the carpet or preparing adults' food does nothing for the baby, but it is assumed to be a mother's task.

However committed to 'free market' capitalism, all the industrialised countries subsidise commercial food producers either directly or indirectly. If they get rich it is seen as fair reward. Subsidies are criticised, but in the discussion of alternatives, food security is seen as a priority. Why is this policy not applied to breastfeeding mothers who produce the highest quality, most efficiently produced, food in the world.

I for one am not happy with the monetary evaluation of every part of our lives, but I also object to the penalisation of women who are so often deprived of economic independence if they want to care for their children in this way and are impeded by the discrimination against mothers in the sites of economic activity.

Since the start of human life women have breastfed and have been engaged in economic production. Millions of women still take this integration for granted, but social endorsement of the system is essential for this to work. Research has shown that work itself does not stop women breastfeeding. In Norway women who went back to work within the first twelve months after childbirth breastfed more than those who stayed at home. Women who want to breastfeed use a lot of ingenuity in their arrangements so as to continue breastfeeding, but they are working against a system that perceives it as an enemy of productivity when this process is the most efficient and multi-faceted production system ever. Maternity leave is usually viewed as the only answer to this issue and haggling over how much they can get takes place. However, in one US hospital workers returned to their jobs before the end of their maternity leave when they were offered the facilities for them to continue breastfeeding. [9]

The private arrangement that some women are able and willing to make with the baby's father makes them dependent on a man's economic survival in the market place and also his personal grace and favour. Thousands of mothers find themselves poor and destitute simply because their children's fathers abandon economic responsibility for their children. Every health and development report bemoans the problem of the number of households headed by women, as though the very femaleness of the main breadwinner were the cause of the problem. The problem is that all economic production, employment and reward is weighted against women. In many traditional societies, women were and are the main food producers and their children would not have starved if good land had not been appropriated for cash crops which in the majority of cases are in the hands of men. Modern production methods do not take a baby into account. Breastfeeding does not work like a machine, like 'clockwork', and the attempt to reduce it to this has helped to damage the breastfeeding process. This has not only affected the health of infants but has also had a devastating effect on women's fertility. It has disrupted not only individual lives but also, through too-rapid population expansion, the welfare of entire societies.

EXTRACTED VALUE

When a mother uses a breastmilk substitute, money goes from a mother's pocket into that of the manufacturer. Even the baby milk industry acknowledges the superiority of breastmilk and its method of delivery, so why are the producers of this product not better off than the manufacturers of the inferior product? Carolyn Campbell summarises the denial of the economic value of breastmilk aptly:

> The discussion of whether or not breastmilk is the ideal infant food is like asking whether or not the kidneys are the ideal means to eliminate wastes from the body and suggesting that dialysis machines ought to replace human kidneys. Human breastmilk is controversial because it is a highly valued product produced by the family for family consumption, and at least up to now has been totally removed from capitalist market control. Subsistence production is contrary to the needs of capital which, to be effective, must incorporate into the market as many goods necessary for or 'desired' by humans. Without commodity production and distribution via the market, there is no surplus value extraction, i.e. no profit.[10]

There is a consensus that poverty is a great enemy of child health. On every level from governments to the household, from bank accounts to the meal table, women are worse off than men. Women who care for children are usually poorer than women who do not. If every mother were entitled to proper economic reward, this would facilitate a redistribution of resources that could only benefit any society on every level. Women could feed their children better, they could pay for their own education as well as their children's and they could benefit their country's economy at the same time. Child health would improve if breastfeeding rates were improved and fertility would be lowered, reducing population pressure and dependency on expensive and fallible family planning programmes and services. Without denying the efforts made by a significant minority of fathers, the reality is that worldwide women have the main responsibility for childcare. There is no evidence why men could not carry out every aspect of childcare except birth and breastfeeding.

The first obstacle, usually from economists working within the system, is the cry of 'We can't afford it'. Society has always found the resources to do what is believed by the powerful to be important. The development of armaments, of extravagant prestige projects such as the Concorde aeroplane, of nuclear power stations and dozens of other government-subsidised schemes have soaked up millions with little benefit to most people and often creating horrific problems for them. Westinghouse nuclear reactors in Brazil and the Philippines (constructed on a site vulnerable to earthquakes) are being paid for in billions of dollars' worth of debt repayments and they have never given a kilowatt of power. Presidential security and royal families use up millions of pounds worth of undebated expenditure. Global military expenditure exceeds US$1000 billion a year, about US$166 for every human being on the planet, which is more than the annual income of millions. That does not include the peripheral services, administration and research which cushions the arms industry. Despite dominant free market ideology, tax payers foot this giant bill for killing.[11]

The justification for profit seeking is that 'growth' leads to prosperity and improved human welfare. This is obviously untrue, though it keeps the lives of a powerful minority comfortable. The redistribution to mothers of money diverted from baby food manufacturers would change the direction of the economy, not depress it. Women could spend money on food, housing, clothing and all the other commodities which really do improve health and the quality of life. Worldwide women energetically work for their families' welfare; giving them adequate means to do this can dramatically change a society. An example of this is the effect of national policies during the Second World War in Britain. The country's resources were severely limited, yet health and nutrition improved and infant mortality fell because resources were fairly distributed. Child welfare was given priority and women were involved in decision making and national economic production. (Interestingly, public breastfeeding, which had virtually disappeared during the

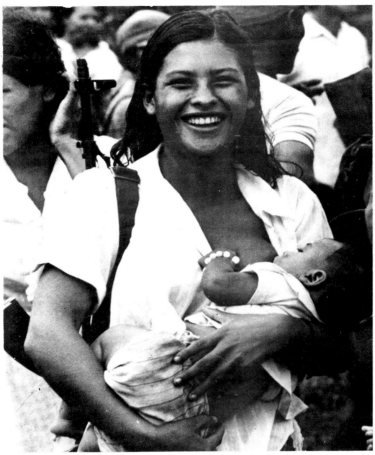

24 Member of the Nicaraguan popular militia feeding her baby (*Photo:* courtesy of AMLAE)

twentieth century, became socially acceptable during the Second World War. [12]) Sadly I suspect that health also improved because so many men were away and not competing with women and children for limited household resources.

The term 'children' in any fund raising appeal has an immediate emotive effect and people give generously when confronted with the images and idea of suffering children, yet the question that must be asked is what sort of world is it that allows there to be 'children in need'? Why don't we have fund raising appeals for weapon development or royal family weddings, presidential expenses and nuclear reactors?

In a world where obsession with 'wealth' creation motivates the pillage of the earth's resources to such an extent that we are organising the destruction of the source of all our wealth, we can turn to our most neglected and abundant resource, people. The level of communication, knowledge and organisational skills that we have attained through the experience of industrial development can be diverted and utilised to build a truly productive society where waste is not the God but the Devil. Women on the whole do not benefit from wealth; it trickles past them rather than to them. Women use up fewer resources than men; we are biologically more energy-sparing and yet most women are penalised economically simply for being female.

IS THE LEFT ANY BETTER?

In Herbert Biberman's 1954 film *The Salt of the Earth*, an account of a zinc mine workers' strike in New Mexico, there is a scene when the strikers' wives, who are imprisoned for their part in the action, demand 'formula' for one of their babies. My heart sank when I saw this film, for it has become a classic in political film making for its sensitive examination of the relationships between employers and workers and men and women. However it displays an obliviousness to one aspect of women's power. The main character has a baby and though there is a scene of her breastfeeding, the shot conveys that this act is one of poverty and pathos. In the prison scene, the baby is being bottle-fed with 'milk that makes him sick'. The women know that 'formula' is the answer, set up a shout of 'We want formula' and finally the warder gives in and gets it, presumably from the company store. It is a scene of triumph. The real strikers and their wives were involved in the film making, so I presume the story is true and it illustrates how widespread was the belief in the superiority of a commercial product over a natural one, even among radicals who were aware of the exploitative nature of commerce. The women (and presumably the film makers) were unaware of their power to keep the baby alive, even if they had no access to manufactured products. Ignorance is so powerful it can restructure political demands; consider the other prison situation, the Japanese Internment camp where all the British women fed their babies. They did not have to demand baby milk because they had Cicely Williams's knowledge that lactation was possible in the worst of circumstances (see page 209).

It has been one of the tenets of socialism that people are more important than profits, yet there is no evidence that women achieved real equality with men in any socialist country, though in some ways, particularly in regard to education and employment, they were better off than many in the capitalist countries. The record of the socialist countries in protecting breastfeeding is better than those of the 'free' market economies principally because maternity provision was a right and there was no aggressive promotion of baby foods. Political upheaval is undermining these benefits. The Former Soviet Union (FSU)'s legislation forbade employment discrimination against a pregnant or breastfeeding woman. The statutory 112 days' maternity leave was fully paid and could extend to a year with partial payment. Breastfeeding breaks were a right. Most socialist bloc countries had similar provision and are trying to maintain this support. However, the destructive ignorance of western medicine has crossed all political boundaries and legislative support is useless if breastfeeding is sabotaged by other means. In the FSU and surrounding regions babies are separated at birth and tightly swaddled, making suckling difficult. Free or cheap baby milk was also provided by the state and health workers handed out milk as a panacea for breastfeeding problems.

In China maternity leave ranges from 6 months to one or two years according to region and a proportion of salary is paid, but urban breastfeeding rates have plummeted in recent decades. This is partly due to bad hospital practices, but also to the milk companies, mainly Nestlé, who have created a lucrative market. In the Scandinavian countries, Sweden has the best legislation, but although good by European standards, breastfeeding rates are lower then in neighbouring Norway where women have less maternity leave. [13]

That beacon of capitalism, the United States, shines out with its conspicuous absence of maternity provision. As a cartoon depicts: 'Like many American companies we treat giving birth to a human being just as we would if you skipped town for a bowling convention.' [14] Paid breastfeeding breaks are unheard of. Increasingly in many countries, what ever the ideology, a proportion of women cannot claim their rights and most find the logistics of work and mothering difficult. It would therefore seem obvious that radical groups, trade unions and political activists would be fighting for the fundamental right of women to feed their babies and not be economically penalised or forced to stay at home if continuation of their trade or profession is vital to them. I have yet to come across a trade union or labour organisation that has fought hard to implement the basic ILO Convention No. 103 (see page 78) adopted in 1919, that women should be entitled to nursing breaks without loss of pay. When I discussed this issue with a trade unionist, she said that the struggle for equality with men was so hard that they were reluctant to demand any right that highlighted their femaleness. When the few women who can, claim their meagre maternity rights they frequently meet hostility and discrimination on a more subtle level, often from other women. Equivalent social commitments such as jury or military service cost far more money and decrease a worker's productivity more drastically than breastfeeding a baby, yet they are not used as reasons for discrimination. Many academics have the right to take sabbatical years in order to focus on one important research project which then adds to their prestige.

BREASTFEEDING AS 'ALLIED CRAP'

Breastfeeding has provoked scorn and been trivialised by some sectors of the political left. In 1986, a British magazine, *New Socialist*, published two articles about breastfeeding which were followed by a spate of letters, many expressing interest in the authors' experiences. However, some readers expressed outrage that such a subject should be discussed in a serious political journal: 'It is unbelievable and tragic that in this time of terrible want and social breakdown, so-called socialists preoccupy themselves with image, fashion, high-brow art forms, and concerns like food additives, the "politics" of breastfeeding and other allied crap.' The writer then declares, 'Northern (meaning from the north of England) mothers queue for free milk and vitamins for their babies, many of whose own milk may be of poor quality as a result of inadequate diet.'[15] As a man he is ignorant of the fact that women's bodies always produce good quality milk and as a socialist he is oblivious of the commercial manipulation of this part of the National Health Service which undermines British women's attempts to breastfeed. He equates breastfeeding with 'image' as though it is immaterial that millions of babies have died because of bottle-feeding. His ignorance blinds him to the fact that breastfeeding represents a defiance against a dependency upon the owners of capital.

Another correspondent wrote that she only wanted to read about breastfeeding in baby books, not political journals and breastfed at home while her husband went to the political meeting, presumably because she believed that political participation was out of bounds while she was lactating. Hence she theoretically excluded most women from the poorest countries, almost a fifth of all adult women, from any political involvement. Another letter writer was so eager in his quest for equal parenthood that he 'imposed a bottle' on his daughter, ensuring that 'the mother was not around' in order to do this. He found his 'success' 'emotionally very rewarding'. But the gem of the correspondence lay in the information that there had been a report in *Tribune* (another socialist magazine) of a plot to remove Glynis Thornton from the chair of the Greater London Labour

Party because 'the fact that she's a woman, and sometimes brings her baby to meetings, and even occasionally feeds it in public hasn't helped'. The writer of this letter commented that these attitudes survived because 'class politics' meant 'male politics'. [16]

I do not believe that even those who criticise the power of industrialised capitalism have sorted out their feelings about women's fertility and parenthood. The eastern bloc countries stated the rights and established laws, but talk to any woman from that region and though she might be shocked to discover the lack of unconditional maternity rights in capitalist society she will still say, 'Of course I suffer discrimination, of course my male colleagues grumble when I take time off to care for my sick child. Of course my husband refuses to do this and he never washed or changed the nappies.'

Oppression comes right from the heart of the family. How can men who are oblivious at home push forward sensitive rules and legislation in the seats of power?

THE BRAVE NEW WORLD

When, in 1970, Shulamith Firestone expressed a demand on behalf of women that technology should take over all reproductive functions she opened a Pandora's box. [17] More than two decades later, biotechnological science is hurtling towards this end and women have woken up to the fact that something that was theirs is being taken away from them. The motive for much of the research into embryo survival outside the uterus, is not the relief of suffering but the quest for money and power. Already companies are arguing for the right to patent such methods so that royalties could be charged and shares from the profits launched on the stock market. [18] The 'Brave New World' that the novelist Aldous Huxley depicted in 1932 is becoming a possibility. [19] What has been seen by so many for so long as the burden of women is now perceived as a power and a right that may soon be lost. So far women are still giving birth themselves, but technology is rapidly taking over this function. There has been no dramatic decline in maternal or infant mortality since these changes have been implemented and in fact increased risk of post-natal infection has been shown to be linked to some interventions.[20] The safety of mother and baby during childbirth has far more to do with high levels of health, hygiene and midwifery skills and low levels of poverty and stress than with the provision of sophisticated technology. This can be appropriate, but in a world where full-term newborns still die unnecessarily of tetanus (see page 71) the introduction of technology whose value is still unproven seems crazy. In one developing country, I saw a full-term normal baby in a special care ward because he had been pierced through the chest by the amniocentesis procedure, used, it was claimed, to judge whether he was overdue for delivery. Not only are there better methods of judging lateness (which is only rarely dangerous), but in this particular country induced abortion was illegal. Why was amniocentesis being introduced? Where was the equipment manufactured and who was making a profit from the sale?

In the western nations where infant mortality statistics have changed little in the last decade and have worsened in the United States, more women are asking why they must be wired up to instruments if neither they nor the baby in their uterus is actually in danger.[21] As more machines are used, the old skills die out; foetal heart monitors are useless during an electricity cut, yet modern midwives and obstetricians may have had little chance to become experienced listeners with an ordinary foetal stethoscope. Sometimes sacrosanct medical practices which humiliate women are found to do more harm than good. Shaving pubic hair was done in the name of hygiene, much to women's discomfort, until someone actually counted the bacteria and discovered that the procedure increased the risk of infection. Another misused practice is episiotomy: cutting the vagina during labour. A 1991 Swedish survey revealed that complications and pain were worse for women who had undergone episiotomy than for those with a spontaneous tear and their pelvic floor muscle strength was weaker. The procedure did not protect against perineal trauma nor urinary incontinence. Episiotomy actually does harm yet it has become routine worldwide. Giving birth on your back makes tearing more likely and with skilled assistance most women could deliver without damage. The Swedish mothers who suffered episiotomy were less likely to be breastfeeding at 3 months and the researcher speculated that the extra pain might affect their early breastfeeding experience. My own feeling is that if you are told that your vagina is so ill-designed that it must be cut open to perform a normal function, you are less likely to believe that your breasts can work well. [22]

The story of infant feeding has followed the same sad pattern. The zeal to solve the problems of nature actually created more problems and women lost a power that their ancestors took for granted. The errors and the sabotage created the acceptance of the normality of a prosthetic instrument, the bottle, and of a second-class substitute for an amazing fluid that our own bodies miraculously produce. It is as if crutches intended for those with damaged legs were issued to everyone, in case their legs ached a bit after a long walk. When muscle wasting follows everyone actually does need crutches and normal walking becomes impossible. People who dare to run freely are viewed with dismay or ridicule by those who are afraid to try, and especially by the crutch makers whose livelihoods depend on their use.

A WORLD FIT FOR WHOM?

In the industrialised world our capacity to feed our children was almost destroyed by the interaction of medical ignorance and authoritarianism with commercial interests. Some of our grandmothers' generation might have considered a world without childbirth and childrearing a paradise. But now the reverse is happening; women want to have children, but those who have gained the few hard-won economic and educational gains do not want to lose these rights. The divide between privileged and poor women is widening all over the world and this will suit the men in charge. Because the modern ruling structures originated from a male-dominated world there is resistance to the acknowledgment of intimate childcare as a human right and need. In saying this I realise that there are many women, both rich and poor, who are having to make enormous compromises, because society still wants to slough off childcare into a shadow world of lesser status. It is they who suffer the private conflict and guilt when it is society's responsibility.

A common argument for the exclusion of children and babies from everyday economic activity is that it is too brutal, too rough for a tender child. If the world is too brutal for a child then it is too brutal for all of us. A world fit for children is a world fit to live in. We must question why all the frenzied wealth creation and reorganisation of human life is taking place when it does little to improve the lot of human beings, creates divisions that lead to more conflict and wars, to famines, displacement and the destruction of the planet.

'May I also take this opportunity to draw your attention to the fact that your wish to breastfeed your baby is causing considerable alarm amongst the staff at the Nursery.' (Letter to Alicia Salazar Dawes from the spokesman of the Nursery Management Committee of a leading Scottish university, May 1986.)

Alicia begged to be allowed to breastfeed her seven-month-old son during the lunch break and was told by the Matron, 'If that is what you wanted you should stay at home with your children.'

(The UK Department of Health recommends that children should be breastfed until they are a year old.)

There is no niche for men and women who want to integrate their childcare and their means of earning a living, though this was normal for most of human existence. There is an enforced separation of reproductive and economic functions; the new moves towards 'homework' do not allow for childcare, for invariably it is isolated women who perform this function, yet the compromises necessary for the integration of parenthood and production depend on willing co-operation and social cohesiveness. The style of nurseries and day care centres do not allow for the needs of the breastfeeding couple and can never ensure the continued physical and emotional intimacy which many believe all babies need. Some crèches and nurseries actually forbid breastfeeding mothers to visit their infants.

To any mother who is able and willing to stay at home with her child there is the eternal question, 'Do you work?' The 'working woman' is the woman who earns money. The 'non-working' woman may in fact work harder than the woman in waged employment, often because she is poorer and poor people work harder. Most people who are not in the formal labour market work extremely hard. They have many skills – the skills of surviving on minimum income, bearing with irrational bureaucracy, wasting hours of time with the agents of welfare if they exist, finding ways of supplementing income without being punished, foraging for cheaper goods in the marginal economy of charity, discarded goods and food, and learning to tolerate hunger, cold, scorn and boredom. Mothers who do not delegate their childcare and do not have paid employment are officially unemployed, but they can avoid the miseries if they arrange one vital factor. They must somehow manage to get someone to support themselves and their child or children. The common idea in the modern world is that the father of the child should do this. Many do not and even within the conventional father-supported family, women and children are often deprived because resources are withheld by the man.[22] Only the women who happen to live in societies and within the class where fathers are able and prepared to do this do not suffer. Many have a pleasant experience during the time when they can intimately care for their children. However, the woman who leaves paid employment because she, and maybe her partner, have certain ideals about 'good' childcare still lacks status and she risks losing her place on the ladder of prestige and economic security. She is a dependant; economically she changes from an adult into a child and often her self-esteem and her partner's attitude to her changes. A woman has to be supremely self-confident to survive this backward step in social status, which will affect her standing for ever. Her period of childcare will never contribute to the value of her *curriculum vitae* or gain her increments in her salary. No wonder that some women reject this humiliating episode and delegate their childcare in order to stay in the swim. For poor women there is not even the choice. In Central and South America, in some areas as many as 75 per cent of households are headed by women; this is a euphemism for saying that the father of her children has run away from the responsibilities of a family.

While health agencies urge breastfeeding they do little to dismantle the system which makes it so difficult. In the industrialised countries many scoff at the practice of purdah, the system in many Islamic countries whereby women must hide their faces from the eyes of strangers. It is seen as restrictive and oppressive. We do exactly the same to mothers and especially to breastfeeding mothers. When I was in Mozambique, babes-in-arms were accepted as normal in cinemas, theatres, restaurants and at parties. Because they were breastfed whenever they cried, there was no disturbance, and friends were astonished to learn that in my country I was forbidden to take my baby to places of entertainment.

In Britain and in many other 'advanced' countries there is an apartheid of those who care for their young children and those who do not. Many women who have control over their fertility still want to bear children and this is increasingly becoming a momentous decision. The prestigious worlds of business, academia and politics have grudgingly let women put one foot in the door only on the condition that they behave like men. They must hide their reproductive functions. Sylvia Rumball, a biochemist from New Zealand, noted that women scientists in California were facing agonising choices about whether they could risk having a child. The competition in academic life was so stiff that they knew that any sign of weakness, any time off, any diminution in the number of papers published would mean they would be pushed down a rung of the ladder of prestige and promotion. Sylvia Rumball has four children, all breastfed. When she decided to have children she said to her professor: 'I am going to have children and I want to reduce and change my timetable to suit my changed situation. I also want to keep my tenure and to get my deserved promotion; this is perfectly reasonable; I have two jobs to do and there will be no reduction in the quality of my work, you could equally arrange this contract to someone who wanted to run a farm as well as be an academic.' Sylvia got exactly what she wanted because she is a highly respected scientist and has the self-esteem to demand justice, but what she was demanding should be the right of all women. It is up to women with some measure of power to push for these rights. [24]

Every mother who is breastfeeding is caring for a child in the best possible way. She is nurturing and forming a future member of society. She is saving finite resources which is beyond valuation and billions of dollars' worth of health care costs. But the way our society is organised means that those who control and use up the earth's resources are the richest and the most revered. Waste is favoured because it produces what is defined to be wealth. The production of the perfect food delivered in the ideal way actually benefits a child and his mother, but this production and service does not make money for any company; in the economic terms of our world, it does not 'create wealth'.

There is nothing intrinsically wrong with production. It is the way we produce and the scale of production that cause the problems. It is the fact that we are eating up at an exponential rate all the non-renewable resources, producing goods which are sometimes useless and often harmful. The injustice is that the really useful products never reach a large proportion of humanity. To keep this system going we destroy intrinsically useful products and processes.

During this century a vast array of means have been used to interfere with the process of breastfeeding. Women have been separated from their babies for many reasons: for custom, for labour, for sexual and other services to men and because people got in the habit of doing this and forgot why it was done. The production and aggressive promotion of commercial artificial milks took power away from women and gave it to industry. Industry got richer and women got poorer. There is enough human milk in the world for the few infants who cannot get their mother's milk. The majority of women can easily produce enough milk for two babies, so milk donorship could suffice for orphans, the abandoned and for the minority of women who cannot breastfeed such as those with AIDS. Where there is political will and social consensus, the blood donor system works well, especially when it is not commercialised and people feel proud to donate blood to save lives. So it is with breastmilk and wherever breastmilk banks are established, women are more than willing to donate milk and the necessary HIV testing has not deterred them. [25] In Scandanavia where milk donation is part of normal life, special care baby units even create nutrient supplements from human milk for the tiny babies who need them. This is not done on a worldwide basis because the 'profit motive' is absent from this process. No company will get rich from women's generosity so it is discouraged, yet it could save millions of lives and health costs.

THE GROWTH FACTOR

The hardest thing about writing this book has been coping with my own despair as I confront the facts of human 'progress'. It is not simply breastfeeding that is destroyed before it has even begun to flow, but oxygen-giving, climate-maintaining forests, the food abundant sea and the fertile earth. All the wealth, beauty and resilience that nature has provided for so long is being damaged irretrievably. As I check one fact with a biologist he casually uses the throwaway line 'with this endgame' as he refers to the state of affairs in the contemporary world. I admire him for being able to work so well while his consciousness of reality is so brutal. His words paralyse me for days. Another biologist offers me the image of a wave breaking to illustrate the crisis that is upon us and she convinces me that there is no hope. I cannot turn away from their considered judgments, but my only response is a denial of passivity. If the solidarity of Hadza women can keep the violence of their menfolk at bay, why cannot the solidarity of women worldwide keep the violence of the economic system from causing so much human suffering and from destroying life itself?

I started out with the idea that breastmilk and breastfeeding was of such economic value that it should be recognised and valued in these terms. I find myself in a dichotomy, for I now realise that 'economics' has become a religion which is deliberately kept obscure so that the ordinary person does not rumble the truth. In medieval Europe the Christian church controlled the masses through a set of ideas which few dared to doubt or challenge. The threat of excommunication kept thousands subdued, although they could not understand the language, Latin, in which the threat was made. The concept of condemning their immortal souls to hell kept millions subject to a social order that benefited the powerful. In the modern world millions of the poor are kept down by the religion of economics whose priests use an equally obscure language and who threaten whole communities with excommunication if they do not obey their commandments. Like the medieval priests, many modern economists may sincerely believe in their own religious edicts and accept the suffering of the poor as part of the overall plan. Perhaps even I could accept it if I thought there was some long-term good, but I see none. The word growth is apt to describe the aims of modern economists because it is also used for a tumour that eats away at the body. The principle of economic growth is like a tumour. The sources of thousands of beneficial products, the forests, are obliterated to provide a few hamburgers served in a carton that destroys the ozone layer which protects all life on earth. The producers say it is 'uneconomic' to stop this production. The sea and land are poisoned with radioactive waste and chemicals that are designed specifically to resist the healing cycle of nature and contaminate all living tissue. Women are led to believe that breastfeeding is not possible, or that it demeans them or that it is a trivial function, yet cows must consume poor people's food crops to produce expensive milk so that more women can participate in this relentless growth. More nuclear power stations are built so 'production' and growth will expand even faster. The tumour must be fed.

But, say the economists, we need this wealth to invest for our future. Where is this investment? I do not see the wealthy investing in good. I see enormous sums spent on drugs, alcohol, tranquillisers, tobacco, cocaine and heroin, because people desperately need to escape from themselves, their pain and reality. I see salaries paid to bureaucrats, to police and military forces who are needed as agents of control as 'development' accelerates social breakdown. Contrasts of poverty and wealth, more horrifying then any of those which precipitated the French Revolution, widen across the world. Technology means that the poor can watch the rich at play (the soap opera *Dynasty* was shown on public TV screens in impoverished areas of Bangladesh), while the rich can watch the poor starve. Rich, powerful men spend millions on entertainment, on the sexual exploitation of those who have only their bodies left to sell. Money goes to the purveyors of pornography, of videos, magazines and live shows so that a man's flagging virility can be stimulated for long enough for him to have sex with a stranger so that he can feel alive for ten seconds. Money is 'invested' in conspicuous consumption, that makes up in opulence and extravagance for the empty soul of the owner. There have always been greedy people and who can prove what causes the emptiness in someone's heart that compels them to seek out more than they need for life and harmony? It is only with this flowering of industrialised capitalism that it has become a duty to maintain a system which depends on the greed and infinite consumption of the few and the stoicism and infinite degradation of the many. Greed has always been with us, but it has never had such ideological support. When Ghengis Khan brutally conquered half the world few of the crushed peasants actually cheered. Now the transnational companies who are laying waste the world and enslaving the people boast about their conquests in TV commercials, and worldwide people innocently display their badges.

A detective novel by Michael Gilbert, *Fear to Tread* (1953), describes a company that sells a charlatan cure for skin trouble. The 'cure' uses two products. The first is applied to the diseased skin, whereupon it 'draws out the toxins', and the second is the balm that soothes the inflammation. The first product is merely itching powder that causes irritation. Industrialised capitalism works on the same principle; many of its products are designed to sooth the itching it has itself caused.

There are other ways to solve problems. For example, cassava, a vital food crop in Africa, was being ravaged by a mealy bug, but the same blight was not happening in South America where cassava had originated. An entymologist researched for two years and discovered a predator wasp. This was introduced to Africa, colonised and kept the cassava pest under control. [26] But who will get rich from a solution that distributes itself and only benefits the poor household consumer? Where is the extracted value? Who has the incentive to pay for more research of this beneficial nature? It is the same problem with breastfeeding; breastfeeding would save millions of lives and drugs and drips, but how would the baby milk manufacturers survive if it were truly endorsed by the social and economic system? With the free market there must be the 'incentive', which is not the drive to make the world a pleasant harmonious place for everyone, only using technology when it is appropriate and beneficial. Rather the motivation must be the desire to do better than your fellows at all costs – competition to destruction. A 12-year-old boy I knew said, 'I don't understand socialism because surely the whole point of working is to get richer and have more than your mates, to have a bigger car, better clothes and more toys.' The world is managed by little boys who still think like this, only they are twice the size of the 12-year-old and their toys include real guns and nuclear weapons and factories that make as many poisons as useful products.

The baby milk companies and many misguided individuals spent a century telling women that their own milk was not there or was not good enough. Now many women have lost faith in their own bodies, the milk has gone and they believe they 'need' these products to keep their children alive. Nestlé are among the transnational companies who are now exploiting and destroying the tropical rain forests. [27] Doubtless they will be among the first to find some way of marketing oxygen if there is any left to sell. Other companies are no different. They started by destroying our milk and making us believe their cocktail of coconut and cow juice was better. They will end by destroying our planet and making us believe their wasteland is what we want.

Artificial Feeding Mishaps

A PRELIMINARY LIST

Before the 1960s babies who were were not breastfed were fed on varieties of dried, evaporated, condensed, and whole milk modified according to various methods; with cod liver oil, juices, and other supplements given to make up for the deficiencies of cows' milk. Brand name products such as SMA, Similac, Lactogen and others existed but were nothing like the complicated mixtures they are now and were used by a minority only. These inadequate feedings resulted in morbidity and mortality from infection, malnutrition, brain damage, anaemia, and much else. Problems included:

low levels of folic acid and lack of vitamin C caused megaloblastic anaemia;

pyridoxine deficiency caused fits, cerebral palsy and retardation;

excessive protein loads caused dehydration, uremia and brain damage;

protein imbalance in some formulas caused brain damage;

vitamin E deficiency caused haemolytic anaemia;

insufficient iron caused anaemia and increased infections;

excessive iron caused gut bleeding, anaemia and immunological disorder;

excessive vitamin D caused convulsions and kidney damage due to hypercalcaemia; this had long-term mental consequences;

excessive phosphorus caused convulsions due to hypocalcaemia;

vitamin C deficiency caused scurvy;

zinc deficiency caused retardation, failure to thrive, and distressing skin disorders (acrodermatitis enteropathica);

essential fatty acid deficiency caused skin, gut and eye disorders, and failure to thrive;

vitamin A deficiency caused diarrhoea, facial palsy, and symptoms in liver, spleen, breasts and elsewhere.

These problems were physiological in origin and were recognised more quickly than more subtle ones. Companies modified their products at different rates, and some problems continued into the next decade. No regulations existed to monitor defective formulas nor legal impediments to continued sale on domestic or foreign markets.

Problems included:

Lactobezoars (tough indigestible curds) caused bowel obstruction requiring surgery most commonly in premature infants on the early high-calorie prem. formulas;

neonatal hypocalcaemic fits occurred at one week in about 1 per cent of bottle-fed babies, but not in breastfed babies. These fits are still being reported in 1985. Late hypocalcaemia also developed in some;

hypomagnesaemic fits only in bottle-fed infants;

lead and other heavy metal contamination (which is cumulative and can result in brain damage) was realised to be a matter for concern;

neonatal metabolic alkalosis with failure to thrive in the second and third weeks of life occurred in infants fed the early 1970s formulation of Nutramigen, despite the fact that this formula met 1974 guidelines for composition;

goitre occurred because of improperly heated soy formulas and/or lack of iodine;

prolonged prothrombin time due to vitamin K deficiency led to acute epidermal and retinal bleeding in some infants;

bacterial contamination of some American and Australian formulas caused salmonellosis, vomiting and diarrhoea;

necrotising enterocolitis reported in infants fed formula with very high osmolarity. The mortality rate is high, and there is a strong association with artificial feeding, although it can happen rarely in breastfed infants;

high solute loads in formulas led to hypernatraemic dehydration; consequences included 'permanent brain damage, gangrene and disseminated intravascular coagulation'.

Particular products involved since 1978 include:

1978—Enfamil with iron contaminated with bacteria (E. coli);

1979—SMA recalled because improper homogenisation led to gastro-intestinal upsets;

—Neo-Mull-Soy and Cho-free were deficient in chloride, causing metabolic alkalosis. Other formulas were checked and some were too low in (but not totally lacking) chloride;

1980—Soy-a-lac and I-Soy-a-lac contained excess vitamin D;

1980—Enfamil with iron recalled because some had curdled and was green, sour and contaminated;

1981—Enfamil with iron (ready to use) recalled because of contamination with solvents from excessive can-lining material.

1982—Wyeth

More than 3 million cans of SMA and Nursoy were recalled because they lacked vitamin B6;

SMA Concentrate (Maine) contained black foreign matter;

SMA Concentrate (Maine) had a bad odour and the fat had separated.

1983—Loma Linda

Soy-a-lac recalled because of problem with vitamin A stabilisation.

Filmore Foods

Naturlac recalled because lacking in thiamine, copper and B6.

Abbott-Ross

Similac and Isomil found to contain carcinogens, trichloroethylene (TCE) and perchlorethylene (PCE) due to contaminated well water. The US Food and Drug Administration considers these 'weak' carcinogens and did not order a recall.

1984—Neo-Ag-U

A Taiwanese formula, deficient in calcium, causes tetany.

De-lact Infant

Contains calcium caseinate, dangerous for infants. Difficulty in tracing cans.

Bristol Myers

Sealed bottle of Enfamil found to contain Enterobacter cloacae.

Powdered formulas

The Food and Drug Administration discovers loophole in the US Infant Formula Act: 'The manufacturer can (and routinely does) refuse to allow FDA access to records not directly related to nutritional quality.'

1985—**Scott Treadway** (Kama Nutritional)

Kama-Mil Powder recalled by Wishing Well Distributing Co. and Threshold Enterprises because the product is deficient in folacin (folic acid), zinc and vitamin D. Product never registered with the Food and Drug Administration, which someone notified anonymously.

Nutra-Milk Powder recalled. Nutrient deficiencies and lack of registration. Manufactured from 1980–1985 without the knowledge of the Food and Drug Administration, which had difficulty in locating this manufacturer.

Gerber Foods

Gerber Meat Base Formula (MBF) recalled because some lots contained excess vitamin A. Vitamin pre-mix had been purchased from Watson Food Co.

Ross-Abbott

Three reformulations made without notifying the Food and Drug Administration.

Edensoy Drink

Pamphlets suggesting suitability as infant food withdrawn after case of severe malnutrition in infant fed solely on this product.

Carnation (Australia)

Evaporated milk mislabelled Prosobee, potential risk to cows' milk-intolerant baby.

1986 **Loma Linda**

Soyalac Powder (physicians' samples) recalled because of progressive vitamin A degradation.

Watson Foods Co.

The US Department of Justice filed a motion for a preliminary injunction because 'as a result of inadequate control, numerous Watson vitamin and mineral mixes (used in infant formulas) have been misbranded and adulterated'.

Source: Maureen Minchin, *Breastfeeding Matters*, Alma Publications, Alfredton, Australia, 1985, and 'FORMULA', PO Box 39051, Washington DC 20016, USA, 1986.

1986 Over 50 per cent of commonly used baby milk brands purchased
to   in 37 different countries contain **dangerous levels of Entero-**
1989   **bacteriacae** (which can cause diarrhoea) in the tin. (Muytjens
       et al., J. Clin. Microbiol., 1988)

Babies choke (but survive) on Pur brand **silicone teats and
dummies** (pacifiers). Well known brands of rubber teats
including Cannon Babysafe, Chavalin, Cuddles, Maws,
Pigeon, Playtex and Twinkle Tots were found to contain **high
levels of nitrosamines** (which can be carcinogenic). There are
no international standards for the quality control of bottles,
teats and dummies. (Choice 1986, Baby Milk Action 1986)

Aluminium levels in cows' milk-based baby milks are 10–20 fold
greater than in breastmilk and 100 times greater in soy-based
milks and may be in water used to mix feeds. Aluminium has
caused brain and kidney damage. Nutritionists recommend that
soy-based baby milks be on prescription only and that
aluminium contents should be labelled. To date (1993) soy-
based baby milks are on the open market and aluminium content
is not on the labels. (Bishop, McGraw, Ward, Lancet 1989)

Aggressive promotion has expanded the market for **sweetened
drinks and infant herbal 'teas'** (1992) 17 per cent growth in the
UK) which damage children's teeth. In Europe there have been
thousands of law suits and compensatory settlements out of
court. Brands include Cow and Gate, Farleys, Milupa and
Ribena. A breastfed baby needs no other fluid and extra drinks
reduce breastmilk intake. An artificially fed baby may need
plain boiled water but sweetened drinks not only damage teeth
and current nutrient balance, they also establish a long term
'sweet tooth'. In the UK, in one year, 25,000 children under four
years have needed multiple extractions under anaesthetic
because of dental caries. (AIS 1992)

The US 'Nelson: Textbook of Pediatrics' recommends formula be
made up with water low in **fluoride**. Some commercial milk
labels recommend using bottled deionised water to make up
feeds. The UK Department of Health considers that there is no
risk to mixing powdered milk with water in fluoridated areas
(UK DOH 1988). The main concern is fluorosis (mottling of
the teeth), but long term effects are unknown. (Ekstrand J.
Nutr. 1989)

'Nelson' state that **iodine** 'should be lowered by dairies'. Iodine levels in artificial baby milk may be 10 times higher than in breastmilk and this may adversely affect thyroid function. (Fisher D.J. Nutr. 1989)

High **differences in mineral contents** (deviating from label contents) were found in 'a common formula for pre-term infants' after babies showed high renal acid excretion. (Tolle et al., J. of'Trace Elements, and Electrolytes in Hlth and Dis., 1991)

A study found a high correlation between use of **high-iron formula** and salmonellosis (gastroenteritis caused by the bacteria, salmonella). (Haddock, RL et al., Am. J. of Public Health, 1991)

The risks of iron-fortified formula were noted in 1972 and restated in 1985. One scientist notes that the wealth of literature showing the ill effects of iron 'has aroused surprisingly little concern in the medical and nutritional communities,' (Dallman, J. Nutr. 1989)

Two babies had severe reactions to **peanut oil** in formula and it is recommended that this should not be used. (Moneret-Vautrin, D et al., The Lancet, 1991)

Chloride deficient formula still shows its effects 9 years later. Children show a range of learning difficulties. (Silver et al., J. Pediatr. 1989)

Excess vitamin D raises calcium levels in the blood (hypercalcaemia) which can lead to brain damage and death. Seven of 19 samples of baby milk contained more than 200 per cent of label claims of Vitamin D contents; one had 419 per cent of label claim. (Holick et al., New Eng J. Med, 1992)

Early fits (neonatal tetany) still occur in artificially fed babies born full term and healthy. (Fabris et al., Acta. Paed. Scand. 1988)

Hydrolysate baby milks are still promoted for allergic babies when experts state that they should not be used for these infants and could even be life-threatening. In materials given to German health professionals, Nestlé claimed that their 'hypoallergenic' formula Beba HA would prevent allergy in at-risk newborns (Nestlé Nutrition Workshop 1988). Their US product Carnation Goodstart caused several cases of severe anaphylaxis (allergic attack). The US FDA has requested all manufacturers to submit evidence to substantiate their claims of 'hypoallergenicity'. Meanwhile Mead Johnson promote Nutramigen for cows' milk allergy claiming 'there's no substitute for clinical proof' in medical journal ads. One allergic child showed greater skin test reaction to these products (the two above plus Ross Alimentum) than to cows' milk. (Saylor and Bahna, J. of Pediatr., 1991)

Over-concentrated feeds causing hypernatraemia (excess sodium in the blood) led to kidney failure, gangrene and amputation, coma and death in the 1970s, yet the risk remains with labelling errors on tins of Ross Similac in 1989 and yet again in 1993. Errors in making up artificial milk feeds are common, with scoop measurements ranging twofold between users. One study found doctors were particularly inept at knowing how to make up a feed correctly. (Jeffs, J. Royal Coll. Gen. Practs., 1991; Oates and Lilburne Aust. Paediatr. J., 1987; INFACT Canada 1993)

Sources: Cunningham, Jelliffe and Jelliffe's Annotated Bibliography (see notes), IBFAN, Marsha Walker's compilation of Hazards of Infant Formula for ILCA and my own searches.

The Economics of Bottle-Feeding

The milk industry in the Philippines has two major characteristics:

1. It is foreign-dominated. Transnational companies such as Bristol Myers (Mead Johnson), American Home Products (Wyeth-Suaco), and Nestlé (Filipro) control the infant formula in the Philippines; 60 per cent of total sales is controlled by Nestlé.
2. The milk industry is only an importing, compounding and packaging industry. The country imports 100 per cent of the raw materials. The milk industry in the Philippines covers only:

   (a) importation of finished goods and raw materials in bulk;
   (b) processing of raw materials into powder using local manufacturing facilities;
   (c) packaging of finished products using either local or imported containers and printing equipment;
   (d) brand management and distribution to drug stores, physicians, hospitals and other outlets.

In 1975–76, the Philippines imported 79,500 tons of milk in powder and granules at a cost of US$89.7 million.

In 1979 combined sales of Wyeth-Suaco, Filipro and Mead Johnson amounted to US$200 million. Its market has been growing by 15 to 25 per cent yearly.

Specific marketing strategies applied are:

Advertisements in media, and distribution of baby booklets with misleading claims.

Aggressive hospital promotions.

The milk companies employ a substantial number of medical representatives: in 1982 Nestlé had sixty while Mead and Johnson and

Wyeth-Suaco had about thirty to forty medical representatives each. A medical representative's job is to influence hospital policies and the medical professionals' prescription for infant feeding practice.

One company training manual for sales personnel reports:

> Hospitals represent one of the most critical markets . . . for infant formula. When one considers that for every 100 infants discharged from the hospital on a particular formula brand, approximately 93 infants remain on that brand, the importance of hospital selling becomes obvious.

Milk companies sponsor medical conventions including travel expenses and accommodation.

In 1980–81 Nestlé sponsored the Continuing Regional Seminar of the Integrated Midwives' Association of the Philippines knowing that in the Philippines' health structure midwives have the best access to rural mothers.

Researchers exemplifying artificial infant feeding are funded by milk companies. These researchers supplant the gaps in the medical curriculum which are deficient in breastfeeding technicalities.

Fellowships abroad for medical practitioners are granted by milk companies in return for favouring its product prescription.

Hospital architectural designs and nursery equipments are fully donated.

> That's why some hospitals are called 'Nestlé hopsital' or 'Mead Johnson hospital' –'because of the benefactor. Thus, all babies born are captive consumers of certain brands. This explains the so-called 'flavour' of the month, or 'house formula'.

Doctors are given one year's supply for their own babies. Mothers, through doctors or nurses, are given starter formula samples.

Country's loss due to importation

The estimated sales volume and market value of different types of milk food in the Philippines for 1975–76 have reached immense proportions. Milk companies assiduously court hospital administrators and staff in order to promote their product regardless of cost to infant lives.

7,000 tons of infant formula costing US$22.2 million;
4,500 tons of milk-based products at US$11.2 million;
6,800 tons of condensed or evaporated milk at US$56.3 million.

(1976 dollar rate, 8 pesos to US$1)

Source: World Health Organisation Collaborative Study on Breast-feeding.
Dr Virginia de Guzman, University of the Philippines Institute of Public Health

Philippine import commodity classification milk powder/granules*

1981	Quantity kilograms	Free on Board $	Cost Insurance Freight $
(a) *Bulk*	10,405,458	15,445,529	16,669,713
(b) *Consumers*	15,318,551	36,600,447	39,591,377
Total for (a) and (b)		52,045,976	56,261,090
1982			
(a) *Bulk*	11,895,506	18,142,184	19,557,345
(b) *Consumers*	19,193,426	48,777,021	52,412,249
Total for (a) and (b)		66,919,205	71,969,594
1983 January-September			
(a) *Bulk*	11,142,470	13,271,209	14,411,880
(b) *Consumers*	11,611,908	27,800,820	29,816,077
Total for (a) and (b)		41,072,029	44,227,957

*Does not include skimmed milk
Source: Foreign Trade Statistics of the Philippines 1981, 1982
Foreign Trade Statistics of the Philippines

In 1983, the equivalent cost of 106.7 metric tons of milk importation was US$145 million.
(1983 dollar rate, 17 pesos to US$1)
Source: 'Milk imports cut sharply', *Bulletin Today*, 27 January 1985

Individual's loss

Family expense for one month of low-income group (net income P900) for a two-month-old baby bottle-feeding on infant formula:

Alacta 400 g. (January 1985 price) at P27.90	
×8 cans per month	P223.20
Water consumption	20.00
Kerosene fuel	24.00
Detergent soap	8.50
Cost of bottles, nipples, cap, brush for washing	P15.00
(only a portion derived from total costs,	
usage extends to a few months)	
Doctor's fee	30.00
Medicines (when the baby gets sick)	90.00
Transportation	20.00
Total	**P430.70**

Source: This data was gathered from a community meeting with low-income mothers in Parang, Marikina, the Philippines, in January 1985.

Family expense for one month of a middle-income group (net income P3,000) for a two-month-old baby bottle-feeding on infant formula:

S-26 400 g. (January 1985 price) at	
P43.50×8 cans per month	P348.00
Water consumption	20.00
Electric fuel	40.00
Detergent soap	8.50
Cost of bottles, nipples, cap, brush for washing	15.00
(only a portion of total cost, usage extends to a few months)	
Doctor's fee	60.00
Medicines (when the baby gets sick)	90.00
Transportation	20.00
Total	**P601.50**

Source: Data gathered from Mothers' Meeting of residents (office employees) of Bliss Sikatuna, Quezon City, the Philippines, in January 1985, and BUNSO (Balikatan at Ugnayang Naglalayong Sumagip sa Sanggol/National Coalition for the Promotion of Breastfeeding and Childcare).

UPDATE 1993

Since 1986 per capita income has declined and even more Filipinos (58 per cent) live below the absolute poverty level. There are now 25 pesos to US$1 so people must work more to pay for the import of the raw materials to make the milk which damages and kills their babies. In 1992 a month's supply of Nestlé Nan costs P 1,124 (US$45) and a minimum wage earner get P 3,323 (US$133), so it uses up more than a third of family income instead of a quarter as in 1985.

(Sources: Lim Fides in Aldana-Benez (ed.) 'Unmasking a Giant' IBON Philippines 1992 and UNICEF 1993)

Artificial feeding as an economic drain is not unique to the South. Baby milk can cost $500 to $1000 a year in the USA, $150 a month in Canada. The US government (i.e. the US taxpayer) spends $500 million a year providing baby milk for low income mothers in the Women, Infants and Children (WIC) programme which accounts for about 40 per cent of the US market, the biggest single baby milk market in the world. If all mothers in the WIC programme could be helped to breastfeed for just one month US$29 million could be saved annually. The savings on medical costs have not been estimated, but it is known that dental damage (caries leading to malocclusion) occurs in 50 per cent of Native American children and can cost up to US$1000 per child.

(Source: Batten J. Pediatr. 117 (2) 1990 and Prevention Reports of the US Public health Service 1990)

THE INNOCENTI DECLARATION ON THE PROTECTION, PROMOTION AND SUPPORT OF BREASTFEEDING

Recognising that

Breastfeeding is a unique process that:

- provides ideal nutrition for infants and contributes to their healthy growth and development;
- reduces incidence and severity of infectious diseases, thereby lowering infant morbidity and mortality;
- contributes to women's health by reducing the risk of breast and ovarian cancer, and by increasing the spacing between pregnancies;
- provides social and economic benefits to the family and the nation;
- provides most women with a sense of satisfaction when successfully carried out; and that

Recent research has found that:

- these benefits increase with increased exclusiveness[1] of breastfeeding during the first six months of life, and thereafter with increased duration of breastfeeding with complementary foods, and
- programme interventions can result in positive changes in breastfeeding behaviour;

---

[1] Exclusive breastfeeding means that no other drink or food is given to the infant; the infant should feed frequently and for unrestricted periods.

> *The Innocenti Declaration was produced and adopted by participants at the WHO/UNICEF policymakers' meeting on "Breastfeeding in the 1990s: A Global Initiative", co-sponsored by the United States Agency for International Development (A.I.D.) and the Swedish International Development Authority (SIDA), held at the Spedale degli Innocenti, Florence, Italy, on 30 July – 1 August 1990. The Declaration reflects the content of the original background document for the meeting and the views expressed in group and plenary sessions.*

We Therefore Declare that

As a global goal for optimal maternal and child health and nutrition, all women should be enabled to practise exclusive breastfeeding and all infants should be fed exclusively on breastmilk from birth to 4–6 months of age. Thereafter, children should continue to be breastfed, while receiving appropriate and adequate complementary foods, for up to two years of age or beyond. This child-feeding ideal is to be achieved by creating an appropriate environment of awareness and support so that women can breastfeed in this manner.

Attainment of the goal requires, in many countries, the reinforcement of a 'breastfeeding culture' and its vigorous defence against incursions of a 'bottle-feeding culture'. This requires commitment and advocacy for social mobilization, utilizing to the full the prestige and authority of acknowledged leaders of society in all walks of life.

Efforts should be made to increase women's confidence in their ability to breastfeed. Such empowerment involves the removal of constraints and influences that manipulate perceptions and behaviour towards breastfeeding, often by subtle and indirect means. This requires sensitivity, continued vigilance, and a responsive and comprehensive communications strategy involving all media and addressed to all levels of society. Furthermore, obstacles to breastfeeding within the health system, the workplace and the community must be eliminated.

Measures should be taken to ensure that women are adequately nourished for their optimal health and that of their families. Furthermore, ensuring that all women also have access to family planning information and services allows them to sustain breastfeeding and avoid shortened birth intervals that may compromise their health and nutritional status, and that of their children.

All governments should develop national breastfeeding policies and set appropriate national targets for the 1990s. They should establish a national system for monitoring the attainment of their targets, and they should develop indicators such as the prevalence of exclusively breastfed infants at discharge from maternity services, and the prevalence of exclusively breastfed infants at four months of age.

National authorities are further urged to integrate their breastfeeding policies into their overall health and development policies. In so doing they should reinforce all actions that protect, promote and support breastfeeding within complementary programmes such as prenatal and perinatal care, nutrition, family planning services, and prevention and treatment of common maternal and childhood diseases. All healthcare staff should be trained in the skills necessary to implement these breastfeeding policies.

Operational Targets:
All governments by the year 1995 should have:

- appointed a national breastfeeding coordinator of appropriate authority, and established a multisectoral national breastfeeding committee composed of representatives from relevant government departments, non-governmental organizations, and health professional associations;
- ensured that every facility providing maternity services fully practises all ten of the *Ten Steps to Successful Breastfeeding* set out in the joint WHO/UNICEF statement[2] 'Protecting, promoting and supporting breastfeeding: the special role of maternity services';
- taken action to give effect to the principles and aim of all Articles of the International Code of Marketing of Breastmilk Substitutes and subsequent relevant World Health Assembly resolutions in their entirety; and
- enabled imaginative legislation protecting the breastfeeding rights of working women and established means for its enforcement.

We also call upon international organizations to:

- draw up action strategies for protecting, promoting and supporting breastfeeding, including global monitoring and evaluation of their strategies;

[2] World Health Organisation, Geneva, 1989.

- support national situation analyses and surveys and the development of national goals and targets for action; and
- encourage and support national authorities in planning, implementing, monitoring and evaluating their breastfeeding policies.

UNICEF AND WHO
TEN STEPS TO SUCCESSFUL BREASTFEEDING

Every facility providing maternity services and care for newborn infants should:

1. Have a written breastfeeding policy that is routinely communicated to all health care staff.

2. Train all health care staff in skills necessary to implement this policy.

3. Inform all pregnant women about the benefits and management of breastfeeding.

4. Help mothers initiate breastfeeding within a half-hour of birth.

5. Show mothers how to breastfeed, and how to maintain lactation even if they should be separated from their infants.

6. Give newborn infants no food or drink other than breastmilk, unless *medically* indicated.

7. Practise rooming-in – allow mothers and infants to remain together – 24 hours a day.

8. Encourage breastfeeding on demand.

9. Give no artificial teats or pacifiers (also called dummies or soothers) to breastfeeding infants.

10. Foster the establishment of breastfeeding support groups and refer mothers to them on discharge from the hospital or clinic.

Notes

CHAPTER 1   WHY BREASTFEEDING IS POLITICAL

1 *Watchdog,* BBC1, 6 March 1987.
2 This figure was calculated by Andrew Chetley, American Home Products 1991 sales figures for infant formula were US$686 million (SCRIP, no. 1718, 15 May 1992) on the premise that they have 10 per cent of the global market, the US$38 billion figure has been calculated by Dr Idrian Resnick of Action for Corporate Accountability.
3 'Confronting the US infant formula giants', *The Corporate Examiner,* vol. 2, no. 7–8, July–August 1982.
4 Steinem, Gloria, 'If men could menstruate', in *Outrageous Acts and Everyday Rebellions,* London, Fontana, 1984, p. 336. Steinem speculates that if 'suddenly, magically men could menstruate it would become an enviable, boast-worthy, masculine event'.
5 Chase, Marilyn, 'GenPharm to Use Bull to Enter Market for Infant Formula', *The Wall Street Journal,* 13 January 1993.

CHAPTER 2   THE RIGHT TO CALL OURSELVES MAMMALS: THE IMPORTANCE OF BIOLOGY

1 Jelliffe, D.B. and Patrice Jelliffe, E.F., *Human Milk in the Modern World: Psychological, Nutritional and Economic Significance,* Oxford, Oxford University Press, 1978, p. 4.
2 Elia, I., *The Female Animal,* Oxford University Press, 1985. In the US an estimated 4 million women are beaten by their husbands or boyfriends each year, more than are hurt in motor accidents, rapes or muggings. See 'Home is where the hurt is', *Time Magazine,* 21 December 1987.
3 Prentice, A.M. and Whitehead, R.G., 'The energetics of human reproduction', in Lowden, A.S.I. and Racey, P.A. (eds), *Reproductive Energetics in Mammals* (Symposium of the Zoological Society of London), Oxford, Clarendon Press, 1987.

CHAPTER 3 EVERYTHING YOU WANTED TO KNOW ABOUT BREASTFEEDING BUT FORGOT TO ASK

1 There is also evidence that men can and have lactated and suckled babies. See Marieskind, Helen, 'Abnormal Lactation', *Journal of Tropical Pediatrics and Environmental Child Health,* vol. 19, 1973, pp. 123–8.

2 Cadogan, W., *An Essay Upon Nursing and the Management of Children,* 1772 (first edition 1769).

3 Rendle-Short, Morwenna, *Father of Childcare,* Bristol, Wright, 1966.

4 Latham, Michael, statement made at workshop on 'Ethics and ideology in the battle against malnutrition', Fifth International Congress of Nutrition, Brighton, 18–23 August 1985.

5 Fildes, Valerie A., 'Neonatal feeding practices and infant mortality during the 18th century', *Journal of Biosocial Science,* vol. 12, 1980, pp. 313, 324. In 1991 UNICEF and WHO launched the 'Baby Friendly Hospital Initiative' and implementation of the '10 Steps' (see Appendix 3) is a first goal of the campaign.

6 Lunn, P.G., 'Maternal nutrition and lactational infertility: the baby in the driving seat', in Dobbing, J. (ed.), *Maternal Nutrition and Lactational Infertility,* Vevey, Nestlé Nutrition, New York, Raven Press, 1985.

7 Short, Roger V., 'Breastfeeding', *Scientific American,* vol. 250, no. 4, April 1984, pp. 23–9.

8 White, A., Freeth, S. and O'Brien, M., *Infant Feeding 1990*, Office of Population Censuses and Surveys, Social Surveys Division, London HMSO, 1992.

9 Romito, Patrizia, 'The mother's experience of breastfeeding', paper presented at Society for Reproductive and Infant Psychology's Sixth Annual Conference, Pollock Halls, Edinburgh, 26th August 1987.

10 Marchione, Thomas J. and Helsing, Elisabet (eds), 'Project report, results and policy: implications of the cross-national investigation: rethinking infant nutrition policies under changing socio-economic conditions', *Acta Paediatrica Scandinavica,* Supp. 314, 1984; Jelliffe, D. B. and Jelliffe, E. F. P., *Human Milk in the Modern World,* Oxford, Oxford University Press, 1978, pp. 364–5.

11 Ibid., p. 88.

12 Masters, William H. and Johnson, Virginia E., *Human Sexual Response,* Boston, Little, Brown, 1966.

13 Koplick, H., *The Diseases of Infancy and Childhood,* London,

Henry Kimpton, 1903, pp. 52–3.

14 Meier, P. and Cranston Anderson, G., 'Responses of small preterm infants to bottle and breastfeeding', *Maternal and Child Nursing,* New York, vol. 12, March/April 1987.

15 *The Baby Book,* presented free by hospitals and clinics to expectant mothers, ed. Prof. Norman Morris (Professor of Obstetrics and Gynaecology, Charing Cross Hospital). The new booklets have improved information, though they still contain baby milk advertisements. Many hospitals and clinics continue to give out outdated literature until stocks have run out.

16 *Present Day Practice in Infant Feeding: Third Report,* Report of a Working Party of the Panel of Child Nutrition, Committee on Medical Aspects of Food Policy, DHSS Report on Health and Social Subjects no. 32, London, HMSO, 1988.

17 Prentice, A.M., Paul, A.A., Prentice, A., Black, A., Cole, T. and Whitehead, R., 'Cross-cultural differences in lactational performance', in Hamosh, M. and Goldman, A. (eds), *Human Lactation 2. Maternal and Environmental Factors,* London, Plenum Press, 1986.

18 Uddoh, C., *Nutrition,* London, Macmillan (Macmillan International College Editions), 1980, p. 114.

19 Conton, L., 'Social, economic and ecological parameters of infant feeding in Usino, Papua New Guinea', *Ecology of Food and Nutrition,* vol. 16, 1985, pp. 39–54.

20 Specker, B.L. *et al.,* 'Sunshine exposure and serum 25-hydroxy-vitamin D concentrations in exclusively breastfed infants', *Journal of Pediatrics,* vol. 107, 1985, pp. 372–6.

21a Kiles, R.V. *et al.,* 'Vitamin K content of maternal milk: influence of the stage of lactation, lipid composition and Vitamin K supplements given to the mother', *Pediatric Research,* vol. 22, no. 5, 1987, pp. 513–7; *Present Day Practice in Infant Feeding,* op. cit. note 16. I am indebted to Michael Crawford of the British Zoological Society for illuminating my tentative ideas about vitamin K contamination during childbirth.

21b Source of information about fats and oils in artificial milks are Betty Sterken of INFACT Canada and nutritionists at Farleys (Boots), Wyeth (AHP), Cow and Gate (Nutricia).

22 Task Force on the Assessment of Scientific Evidence Relating to Infant Feeding Practices and Infant Health, *Pediatrics,* vol. 74, no. 4, 1984 (Supplement); Prentice, A. *et al.,* 'The nutritional role of breastmilk IgA and Lactoferrin', *Acta Paediatrica Scandinavica,* vol.

76, 1987; Minchin, M., 1987, 'Infant Formula: A Mass Uncontrolled Trial in Perinatal Care', *Birth* 14: pp. 97–100; Karjalainen, J., et al, *New England Journal of Medicine*, 1992, 336, pp. 269–71; NB There are numerous studies describing the essentiality of certain fatty acids for brain development eg Hoffman, D.R. and Uduz, R., 1992, 'Essentially of dietary w3 fatty acids for premature infants', *Lipids* 1992 27 (11) pp. 886–95.

23 Jelliffe, op. cit. (note 10), p. 10; Hamosh, M. and Goldman, A.S. (eds), *Human Lactation 2. Maternal and Environmental Factors,* London, Plenum Press, 1986; Davis, Margaret K., et al. 'Infant Feeding and Childhood Cancer', *Lancet*, 13, Aug. 1988, pp. 365–8; Hahn-Zoric, M. et al 1990 Antibody responses to parenteral and oral vaccines are impaired by conventional and low protein formulas as compared to breastfeeding. Acta Paediatr. Scand. 79: pp.1137–42; Savage, F., 'Breastfeeding and SIDS', *MIDIRS Midwifery Digest*, 2, 1 March 1992; See also Cunningham, A.S., Jelliffe, D.B., Jelliffe, E.F., Patrice, *Breastfeeding, Growth and Illness: an Annotated Bibliography,* 1992, UNICEF New York for a range of references giving evidence for protective effects of breastfeeding.

24 Bitman, J. *et al.,* 'Lipid composition of prepartum, preterm and term milk', in Hamoth, M. and Goldman, A.S. (eds), op. cit., pp. 131–41.

25 Whitehead, R.G. and Paul, A.A., 'Growth charts and the assessment of infant feeding practices in the western world and in developing countries', *Early Human Development,* vol. 9, 1984, pp. 187–207.

26 Lucas, A., and Cole, T.J., 'Breastmilk and necrotising enterocolitis', *Lancet* 1990; 336; pp. 1519–23; Lucas, A. 'Summary and future directions' (Symposium on assessment of bone mineralisation in infants), *J. Pediatr,* 1988; 113:248. Also Lucas, A. Pers. Comm. Jan. 1993; Whitelaw, A. and Sleath, K., 'Myth of the marsupial mother: homecare of very low birth weight babies in Bogota, Columbia', *Lancet*, vol. 1, 1985, pp. 1206–8.

27 Rattigan, S., Ghisalberti, A.V. and Hartmann, P.E., 'Breastmilk production in Australian women', *British Journal of Nutrition,* vol. 45, 1981, pp. 243–9; Goodall, J., Hans Gadow Lecture, 26 November 1987, Cambridge University. (See also *In the Shadow of Man* by Jane van Lawick Goodall, London, Collins, 1971.); Victora, C.G., et al, 'Infant Feeding and deaths due to diarrhoea', *Am. J. Epidemiol.* 1989; 129: 1032–41; Oski, F.A. and Landow, S.A. 'Inhibition of iron absorption from human milk by baby food', *Am. J. Dis. Child,* 134, 459–60, 1980; Oski, F.A., 'Is bovine milk a health hazard?' *Pediatrics,* 75(2) 182–6 (1985).

28   Fytianos, K. *et al.,* 'Preliminary study of organochlorine compounds in milk products, human milk and vegetables', *Bull. Environ. Contam. Toxicol.,* vol. 34, 1985, pp. 504–8; Lukens, J.N., 'The legacy of well-water methaemoglobinaemia', *Journal of the American Medical Association,* vol. 257, 1987, pp. 2793–5; Pearce, Fred, 'The hills are alive with nitrates', *New Scientist,* 10 February 1987; Personal communication from present and former staff of Thames Water Authority and Cambridge Water Company; Link, Ann, 'Chlorine, Pollution and the Parents of Tomorrow', *The Women's Environmental Network,* London 1991; Rogan, W.J., 'Cancer from PCBs in breastmilk? A risk benefit analysis', *Pediatr. Res.* 1989; 25: 105A: Van Tram, D. et al. 'Survey on Immunisation, diarrhoeal disease and mortality in Quang Ninh Province, Vietnam', *Journal of Tropical Paediatrics,* vol. 37, December 1991, pp. 280–5; Shanon, M. and Graef, J., Hazard of lead in infant formula (letter), *New England Journal of Medicine,* 326 (2): 137, 1992; *Good Housekeeping* (US edition), August 1992; BBC World Service 'Science in Action', 'Aluminium in Baby Feeds'. Interview with Dr Neil Ward of the University of Surrey, 27 Nov. 1988. Also personal Communication with Dr N. Bishop, Dunn Nutrition Unit, Cambridge, UK; Brown, Paul, 'Trans-sexual trout swallow the pill from sewage outfall', the *Guardian,* 11 Feb. 1993. See also: Radford, Andrew; 'The Ecological Impact of Bottle-Feeding,' *Baby Milk Action,* Cambridge, 1991.

29   Di Lallo, D. *et al.,* 'Radioactivity in breastmilk in Central Italy in the aftermath of Chernobyl', *Acta Paediatrica Scandinavica,* vol. 76, 1987, pp. 530–1; Haschke, F., *et al.,* 'Radioactivity in Austrian milk after the Chernobyl accident' (letter), *New England Journal of Medicine,* vol. 316, no. 7, pp. 409–10; Swedish National Institute of Radiation Protection, Box 60204, S–10401 Stockholm, Sweden (May 1987); Baby Milk Action Coalition, 1987/8.

30   Zeigler, J.B. *et al.,* 'Postnatal transmission of AIDS-associated retrovirus from mother to infant', *Lancet,* i, 1985, pp. 896–7; Van de Perre, Philippe et al, 'Postnatal Transmission of HIV Type 1 from Mother to Infant'. *New Eng. J. of Med. 325,* 9, August 29, 1991; Newell, M.L. et al., 'Risk Factors for Mother-to-Child transmission of HIV-1, The European Collaborative Study', Paper presented to WHO/UNICEF Consultation Meeting, 30 April 1992; Newburg, David S. et al., 'A human milk factor inhibits binding to the CD4 Receptor', *Ped. Research, 31,* 1, pp. 22–8, 1992; Consensus Statement from the WHO/UNICEF Consultation on HIV

transmission and Breastfeeding, Geneva, 30 April – 1 May 1992.

31 Film 'Breastfeeding: The Baby's Choice' 1991. Available from the Department of International Health Care Research, Karolinska Institute, Box 60400, S–104 01 Stockholm, Sweden.

32 Klaus, M.H. and Kennell, J.H., *Maternal Infant Bonding,* St. Louis, Missouri, Mosby, 1976.

33 Lucas, A. et al, 'Breastmilk and Subsequent Intelligence Quotient in Children Born Preterm', *Lancet,* vol. 339, 1. Feb. 1991; Task Force on the Assessment of Scientific Evidence Relating to Infant Feeding Practices and Infant Health, op. cit.

34 Advertisement for Mead Johnson's Enfamil showing a man bottle-feeding in *Journal of Pediatric Gastroenterology and Nutrition*, vol. 4, no. 2, 1985.

35 Still, G.F., *The History of Paediatrics,* London, Oxford University Press, 1931, p. 305.

36 The World Bank, World Development Report 1991, *The Challenge of Development*, Oxford University Press, p. 156.

37 Ibid.

38 Gilman, R.H. and Skillicorn, P., 'Boiling of drinking water: can a fuel-scarce community afford it?', *Bulletin of WHO* (1985), vol. 63, no. 1, pp. 157–63 (En) (*Trop. Dis. Bull.,* vol. 83, no. 3, 1986); The World Bank, op. cit.

39 'The cost of powdered infant formula', *IBFAN Africa News,* Dec. 1989. Cutting, W., 'Breastfeeding and HIV: Advice depends on circumstances', *British Medical Journal,* 305, 3 Oct, 1992. UNICEF 1993 'The State of the World's Children'. Oxford University Press.

40 UNICEF, op. cit.

41 Habicht, J.P. *et al.,* 'Does breastfeeding really save lives or are apparent benefits due to biases?', *American Journal of Epidemiology,* vol. 123, no. 2, pp. 279–90.

42 Carpenter, R.G. *et al.,* 'Prevention of unexpected infant death: evaluation of the first seven years of the Sheffield Intervention Programme', *Lancet,* 2 April 1983, pp. 723–7.

43 Minchin, Maureen, *Breastfeeding Matters: What We Need to Know About Infant Feeding,* Alfredton, Australia, Alma Publications, p. 250.

44a Howie, Peter, W. et al., 'Protective effect of breastfeeding against infection'. *British Medical Journal,* 1990; 300; 11–16.

44b Barker, D.J.P., 'Childhood causes of adult diseases', *Arch. Dis. Child.* 1988; 63:867–9; Davies, D., Changing patterns of growth in children. Presentation at Scientific Meeting 'Recent Advances in

Mother and Child Health in Developing Countries'. Institute of Child Health, London, 26, 10, 1992; Karjalainen, J. et al., *New England Journal of Medicine,* 1992, 327, 302–7.

45   Birch-Johnsen, K. *et al.,* 'Relation between breastfeeding and incidence rates of insulin-dependent diabetes melitis', *Lancet,* vol. 2, 1984, pp. 1083–6.

46   Kois, William E., 'Influence of breastfeeding on subsequent reactivity to a related renal allograft', *Journal of Surgical Research,* vol. 37, 1984, pp. 89–93. (I thank Penny Stanway for bringing this fact to my attention.)

47a Hull, David and Johnston, Derek, *Essential Paediatrics,* Edinburgh, Churchill Livingstone, 1986.

47b Personal communication Chris Carson Infant Feeding Tutor, Birmingham Maternity Hospital.

48   Petterson, B. *et al.,* 'Menstruation span: a time-limited risk factor for endometrial carcinoma', *Acta Obst. Gynecol. Scand.,* vol. 65, 1986, pp. 247–55.

49   Aloia, J.F., 'Risk factors for postmenopausal osteoporosis', *American Journal of Medicine,* vol. 78, 1985, pp. 95–100; 'Nutrition Reviews: Parathyroid hormone, 1-25-Dihydroxy-vitamin D3 and calcitonin in women breastfeeding twins', *Nature,* vol. 43, no. 10, 1985; Hreschyshyn, M.M., et al., 'Association of parity, breastfeeding and birth control pills with lumbar spine and femoral neck bone densities', *Am. T. Obstet. Gynecol.* 1988; 159; 318–22; 'More people are fracturing more bones more often', *Nutrition Reviews,* vol. 49, 1, 1991 (Jan.) p. 24; Huang C.Y., Georgia G., Dai X.Z., et al, Incidence in hip fracture in Chengdu China. Abstract of Fourth Sichuan Nutrition Conference, 1991, cited in 'Diet and Bone Density among elderly Chinese', *Nutrition Reviews,* vol. 50, 12, 1992 (Dec.) pp. 395–7.

50   Ing, Roy, Ho, J.H.C. and Petrakis, Nicholas L., 'Unilateral breastfeeding and cancer', *Lancet,* 16 July 1977, pp. 124–7; Byers, T. *et al.,* 'Lactation and breast cancer: evidence for negative association in premenopausal women', *American Journal of Epidemiology,* vol. 121, no. 5, 1985, pp. 664–73; Kuen-Young, Yoo et al., 'Independent Protective Effect of Lactation against breast Cancer: A case Control Study in Japan.' *American J. of Epidemiology,* 135, 7, 1992, pp. 726–32.; Reiping, Elisabeth, J., 'Breast cancer and early contact with bovine milk'. Paper presented at meeting of European Society of Gynaecological Oncology, 1987.

51 For an analysis of mother/baby nutrition arguments in emergency situations see: Armstrong, Helen, 'Milk for hungry children: some questions', a discussion paper for IBFAN – Africa Newsletter, February 1985. (Available from IBFAN.) See also: Kelly, Marion, 'Infant Feeding in Emergencies.' Disasters 17 (2) June 1993. De Waal, Alexander, 'Famine that Kills.', *Oxford Studies in African Affairs.* Clarendon Press, Oxford, 1989.

CHAPTER 4 POPULATION, FERTILITY AND SEX

1 Shelter, The National Campaign for Homeless People, 5th Floor, 88 Old Street, London EC1V 9HU.
2 *New Internationalist*, no. 176, October 1987, p. 9.
3 *Man-Made Famine,* Channel 4, May 1985.
4 Tanner, J.M., *Foetus into Man: Physical Growth from Conception to Maturity*, London, Open Books, 1985 (first published 1978).
5a Bongaarts, J., and Greenhalgh, S., 'An alternative to the one child policy in China', *Pop. and Dev. Review,* vol. 11, no. 4, December 1985.
5b McKenna, J., 'An Anthropologicla Perspective on Sudden Infant Death (SIDS) the role of parental breathing cues and speech breathing adaptations'. *Med. Anthr.,* Special Issue 10 (1) 92pps (1986).
6 McNeilly, A.S., Howie, P.W. and Glasier, A., 'Lactation and the return of ovulation', in Potts, M. and Diggory, P. (eds), *Natural Human Fertility – Social and Biological Mechanisms,* in press.
7 Dewart, P., MRC Reproductive Biology Unit, Edinburgh, 'Contraception and breastfeeding', paper presented at the Sixth Annual Conference of the Society for Reproductive and Infant Psychology, Edinburgh, 26–28 August 1987.
8 *Guinness Book of Records*, 1984, p. 17.
9 Prentice, A.M. *et al.,* 'Dietary supplementation of Gambian nursing mothers and lactational performance', *Lancet*, ii, 1980, pp. 886–8; Lunn, P.G., 'Maternal nutrition and lactational infertility: the baby in the driving seat', in Dobbing, J. (ed.), *Maternal Nutrition and Lactational Infertility,* Vevey, Nestlé Nutrition, New York, Raven Press, 1985; Howie, P.W. *et al.,* 'Effect of supplementary food on suckling patterns and ovarian activity during lactation', *British Medical Journal,* vol. 283, 1980, pp. 757–9; Pérez, A., Labbock, M.H. and Queenan, J.T., 'Clinical study of the lactational amenorrhoea method for family planning', *Lancet*, vol. 339, 18 April 1992.

10 Dix, Carol, *The New Mother Syndrome,* London, Allen & Unwin, 1986.

11 Jack, Malcolm and Jack, Marjorie. I am indebted to Malcolm and Marjorie Jack for this and many other descriptive accounts of parent/child relations in Nepal.

12 Hardyment, Christina, *Dream Babies: Child Care from Locke to Spock,* Oxford, Oxford University Press, 1984, p. 181.

13 Van Estrick, Penny, *Infant Feeding Options for Bangkok Professional Women,* Ithaca, New York, Cornell University Press (Cornell Int. Nut. Mon. series no. 10), 1982, p. 61.

14 Short, R.V., 'The biological basis for the contraceptive effects of breastfeeding', in *Advances in International Maternal and Child Health,* vol. 3, pp. 27–39; Morley, David, *Paediatric Priorities in the Developing World,* London, Butterworths, 1978, p. 103.

15 Masters, William H. and Johnson, Virginia E., *Human Sexual Response,* Boston, Little, Brown, 1966.

16 Alder, E.M. *et al.,* 'Hormones, mood, and sexuality in lactating women', *British Journal of Psychiatry,* vol. 148, 1986, pp. 74–9.

17 *Living* magazine, February 1986.

18 Silkin, Trish, 'Marriage and social change in the "liberated zones" of Eritrea controlled by the Eritrean People's Liberation Front', paper presented at the conference of the Review of African Political Economy at the University of Liverpool, 26–28 September 1986.

19 Personal communication with Maureen Minchin, 1987.

CHAPTER 5   FROM THE STONE AGE TO STEAM ENGINES: A GALLOP THROUGH HISTORY

1 Mead, Margaret, *Male and Female,* Harmondsworth, Penguin Books, 1950.

2 Truswell, A.S., 'Diet and nutrition of hunter-gatherers', in *Health and Disease in Tribal Societies,* Ciba Foundation Symposium no. 49 (new series) Amsterdam, Elsevier-Excerpta Medica North-Holland, 1977.

3 Sahlins, Marshall David, *Stone Age Economics,* London, Tavistock, 1974.

4 Pharaoh, P.O.D. (Liverpool School of Tropical Medicine), film of toddlers catching insects, shown at London School of Hygiene and Tropical Medicine, 1985.

5 Woodburn, James Campbell, 'Sex roles and the division of labour in hunter-gatherer societies', unpublished paper presented at the

First International Conference on Hunter-Gatherer Societies, Paris, June 1978 and personal communication.

6 Jelliffe, D.B. *et al.,* 'The children of the Hadza hunters', *Journal of Pediatrics,* vol. 60, no. 6, 1962.

7a World Commission on Environment and Development, *Our Common Future,* Oxford, Oxford University Press, 1987, p. 12.

7b Sadly the !Kung way of life is virtually non-existent now. These self-sufficient people have been 'settled' and these beneficial feeding patterns are threatened by the influences of 'development'.

8 Farb, Peter and Armelagos, George, 'The food connection: new crops and increased production allow populations to soar', *Natural History,* September 1980, pp. 26–30.

9 Conton, Leslie, 'Social, economic and ecological parameters of infant feeding in Usino, Papua New Guinea', *Ecology of Food and Nutrition,* vol. 16, 1985, pp. 39–54.

10 Worsley, Peter, *The Three Worlds,* London, Weidenfeld & Nicolson, 1984.

11 King, J. and Ashworth, A., 'Changes in infant feeding practices in the Caribbean', Dept. of Human Nutrition, London School of Hygiene and Tropical Medicine, Occasional Paper no. 8, 1987, p. 7.

12 Mitter Swasti, *Common Fate, Common Bond: Women in the Global Economy,* London, Pluto Press, pp. 53–4.

13 King and Ashworth, op. cit. (note 11), p. 7.

14 Ibid., p. 9.

15 'Romanian women subjected to "pregnancy tests" at work', *Guardian,* 21 June 1986; Tindall, Gillian, 'In pursuit of liberté, egalité, natalité', *The Times,* 7 December 1985; Jacobson, Philip, 'Lee's tight little island', *The Sunday Times,* 24 November 1984.

16 Bryan, B., Dadzie, S. and Scafe, S., *The Heart of the Race: Black Women's Lives in Britain,* London, Virago, 1985, p. 18; Ashworth and King, op. cit. (note 11), p. 10; Laslett, Peter, *The World We Have Lost – Further Explored,* London, Methuen, 1983, p. 112.

17 Maurer, Harold M., 'The Growing Neglect of American Children', *AJD,* 145, May 1991. The US IMR for 1989 was 9.7 per 1000, but 19.4 for black American babies who have less chance of survival than a Jamaican baby. A Jamaican baby is far more likely to be breastfed than a US baby.

18 Still, G.F., *The History of Paediatrics,* London, Oxford University Press, 1931, p. 141.

19 Faludi, Susan, *Backlash,* Chatto and Windus, 1992.

20. McLaren, D., 'Nature's contraceptive: wet nursing and prolonged

lactation: the case of Chesham, Buckinghamshire 1578–1601', *Medical History,* vol. 23, pp. 426–41.

21 Fildes, Valerie A., *Breasts, Bottles, and Babies: A History of Infant Feeding,* Edinburgh, Edinburgh University Press, 1986, p. 104; Pollock, Linda A., *Forgotten Children: Parent–Child Relationships from 1500 to 1900,* Cambridge, Cambridge University Press, 1983, p. 215.

22 Fildes, op. cit. (note 21), p. 105.

23 Laslett, op. cit. (note 16).

24 Smith, Poppy, 'A place of safety', *New Society,* 21 August 1987; in 1987 in the UK, 79,000 children were in 'care', *New Society* Database, 13 February 1987; Hector Bebenco's 1981 film *Pixote* is based on a real street boy's life in Sao Paulo, Brazil. He and his friends routinely experience incarceration, rape and police brutality. The degradation of their lives easily equals any historical horror stories.

25 Pollock, op. cit. (note 21).

26 Fildes, op. cit. (note 21), p. 160.

27 Ibid., p. 161.

28 Fildes, Valerie, *A History of Wet Nursing from Earliest Times to the Present,* Oxford, Basil Blackwell, 1988.

29 Smith, F.B., *The People's Health 1830–1916,* London, Croom Helm, 1979, p. 83.

30 Jenkins, Liz, 'Mix-up babies back with right parents', *Daily Telegraph,* September 1986.

31 Smith, op. cit. (note 29), pp. 71 and 73.

32 Fildes, Valerie, 'Syphilis as an occupational disease of wet nurses: an international review 1490s to 1980s', paper presented to the Society for the Social History of Medicine, London, 5 February 1988.

33 Khodel, John and Van de Walle, Etienne, 'Breastfeeding, fertility, and infant mortality: an analysis of some early German data', *Population Studies,* vol. 21, 1967, pp. 109–31.

34 'Infantile mortality', *British Medical Journal,* 23 November 1889, p. 1198.

35 Scrimshaw, N.S., Taylor, C.E. and Gordon, J.E., *Interaction of Nutrition and Infection,* WHO Monograph no. 29, Geneva, 1968.

36 Broström, Göram *et al.,* 'The impact of breastfeeding patterns on infant mortality in a 19th century Swedish parish', Newsletter no. 1, ed. Egil Johannson, Demographic Data Base, Umea University, Sweden.

37 Fildes, op. cit. (note 21), p. 330.
38 Broström, op. cit. (note 36).

CHAPTER 6 THE INDUSTRIAL REVOLUTION IN BRITAIN: THE ERA OF PROGRESS?

1 Laslett, Peter, *The World We Have Lost – Further Explored,* London, Methuen, 1983; Thompson, Barbara, 'Infant mortality in 19th century Bradford', in Woods, Robert and Woodward, John (eds), *Urban Disease and Mortality in 19th Century England,* London, Batsford, 1984; Oakley, Ann, *The Captured Womb: A History of the Medical Care of Pregnant Women,* Oxford, Basil Blackwell, 1984.

2 Lewis, Jane, *Women in England 1870–1950,* Sussex, Wheatsheaf Books, 1984, pp. x and 146.

3 Reid, George, 'Infant mortality and the employment of married women in factories', *British Medical Journal,* 17 August 1901, pp. 410–12.

4 'Infantile mortality and the occupation of married women', *British Medical Journal,* 7 September 1901, p. 634.

5 Reid, op. cit. (note 3).

6 Ashby, Hugh T., *Infant Mortality,* London, Cambridge University Press, 1915, p. 45.

7 Thompson, Flora, *Lark Rise to Candleford,* London, Oxford University Press, 1968, p. 139 (first published 1939).

8 Reid, op. cit. (note 3).

9 Rivers, John, *The Health of the Nations,* Milton Keynes, Open University Press, 1985, p. 127.

10 'US Supreme Court agrees to rule on whether pregnant women are entitled to special *disability* [emphasis added] benefits which other workers do not receive; unusual coalition of Reagan admin., business lobbies and women's groups oppose such benefits', *Los Angeles Times,* 21 August 1986.

11 Llewellyn Davies, Margaret (ed.), *Maternity: Letters from Working Women,* collected by the Women's Cooperative Guild, London, Virago, 1978 (first published in 1915 by G. Bell & Sons Ltd).

12 Coutts, F.J.M., 'Inquiry into condensed milks with special reference to their use as infants' foods', *Local Government Board Reports, Food Report no. 15,* London, HMSO, 1911; 'On the use of proprietary foods for infant feeding and analysis and composition of some proprietary foods for infant feeding', *Food Report no. 20,* London, HMSO, 1914.

13   Buffle, Jean Claude, *N comme Nestlé: Multinational et Infanticide, le Lait, les Bébés, et le Mort,* Paris, Alain Moreau, 1986.

14   Drummond, Jack Cecil, *The Englishman's Food,* London, Jonathan Cape, 1958, p. 375.

15   Buffle, op. cit. (note 13); Beaver, M.W., 'Infant mortality and milk', *Population Studies,* vol. 27, 1973, pp. 243–54.

16   Oakley, op. cit. (note 1), p. 60.

17   Enock, A.G., *This Milk Business: A Study from 1895–1943,* London, 1943; Lewis, Jane, *The Politics of Motherhood,* London, Croom Helm, 1980, p. 65.

18   Chamberlain, Mary, *Fenwoman: A Portrait of Women in an English Village,* London, Routledge & Kegan Paul, 1983, pp. 74–5 (first published in 1975 by Virago).

19   *Nursing Times,* vol. 12, no. 59, 16 June 1906.

20   Lee, Laurie, *Cider With Rosie,* Harmondsworth, Penguin Books, 1986, p. 123 (first published in 1959).

21   *The Infant's Magazine,* Annual for 1913, London, S.W. Partridge & Co. Ltd.

22   *Maternity and Child Welfare,* no. 1, January 1917.

23   Davin, Anna, *Imperialism and Motherhood,* History Workshop, no. 5, 1978, pp. 9–65.

CHAPTER 7   MARKETS ARE NOT CREATED BY GOD

1   Conyngton, Mary, *Report on Condition of Woman and Child Wage-earners in the US:* vol. 18, *Employment of Women and Children in Selected Industries,* Washington, Government Printing Office, 1913; vol. 13, *Infant Mortality and its Relation to the Employment of Mothers* 1912 (Fall River Study).

2   Carter, Jenny and Duriez, Thérèse, *With Child: Birth Through the Ages,* Edinburgh, Mainstream Publishing, 1986.

3   Ehrenreich, Barbara and English, Deirdre, *Complaints and Disorders: The Sexual Politics of Sickness,* New York, The Feminist Press, 1973.

4   Apple, Rima D., *Mothers and Medicine: A History of Infant Feeding from 1850–1950,* Madison, University of Wisconsin Press, 1987, p. 21.

5   Rotch, Thomas Morgan, 'A discussion on the modification of milk in the feeding of infants', *British Medical Journal,* 6 September 1902, p. 653.

6   Hardyment, Christina, *Dream Babies: Child Care from Locke to Spock,* Oxford, Oxford University Press, 1984, p. 127.

7   Apple, Rima D., ' "To be used only under the direction of a physician" – commercial infant feeding and medical practice, 1870–1940', *Bull. Hist. Med.,* vol. 54, no. 3, 1980, pp. 402, 417. This and the subsequent ten quotations are taken from Rima Apple's article; see also ' "Advertised by our loving friends": the infant formula industry and the creation of new pharmaceutical markets, 1870–1910', *Journal of History of Medicine and Allied Sciences,* vol. 41, no. 1, January 1986.

8–16   Ibid.

17   Davis, W.H., 'Statistical comparison of the mortality of breastfed and bottle-fed infants', *American Journal of Diseases of Childhood,* vol. 5, pp. 234–47, 1913, ref. 3 in Cunningham, A.S., 'Bottle-feeding and morbidity in industrialised countries: an update 1981', in Jelliffe, D.B. and Jelliffe, E.F. (eds), *Advances in International Maternal and Child Health,* vol. 1, Oxford, Oxford University Press, 1981, p. 129; Woodbury, R.M., 'The relation between breast and artificial feeding and infant mortality', *American Journal of Hygiene,* vol. 2, 1922, pp. 668–87, ref. 4 in Cunningham, op. cit.

18   Victora, Cesar G. *et al.,* 'Evidence for protection by breastfeeding against infant deaths from infectious diseases in Brazil', *Lancet,* 8 August, 1987, pp. 319–22.

19   Grulee, Clifford G. *et al.,* 'Breast and artificial feeding', *Journal of the American Medical Association,* vol. 103, no. 16, 8 September 1934, pp. 735–9. See also *Journal of the American Medical Association,* vol. 104, no. 22, 1 June 1935, pp. 1988–90.

20   Relucio–Clavano, Natividad, 'The results of a change in hospital practices – a paediatrician's campaign for breastfeeding in the Philippines', in *Assignment Children: Breastfeeding and Health,* Geneva, UNICEF, 1981, pp. 139–65.

21   Cunningham, Alan S., Letter to Jane McNeil, Acting Director of Supplemental Food Programs Division, Food and Nutrition Service, US Dept of Agriculture, Washington DC, 1979; Palmer, G., 'Who helps health professionals with breastfeeding?' *Midwives Chronicle.* In Press. To be published May 1993.

22   Deeny, James, report of his article, 'Epidemiology of infantile enteritis', *Lancet,* vol. 253, 23 August 1942, pp. 284–5. Article published in *Journal of the Medical Association of Eire,* vol. 19, 1946, p. 146.

23   Meredith, David, 'The Empire Marketing Board 1926–32', *History Today,* January 1987, pp. 30–6.

24   Note: rubber teats were first patented in the US in 1845, though actual

animal teats and leather ones were still used long after this date.

25 Consumer's Association of Penang, Malaysia, *The Other Baby Killer,* CAP, 1981.

26 King, Jean and Ashworth, Ann, *Changes in Infant Feeding Practices in Malaysia,* Dept of Human Nutrition, London School of Hygiene and Tropical Medicine Occasional Paper no. 7, 1987.

27 Ibid.

28 Manderson, Lenore, 'Bottle-feeding and ideology in colonial Malaya: the production of change', *International Journal of Health Services,* vol. 12, no. 4, 1982, pp. 597–616.

29 Consumers' Association of Penang, op. cit.

30 Williams, Cicely, 'Milk and Murder', Address to the Singapore Rotary Club, 1939, ed. Allain, Annelies, 1986, International Organisation of Consumers Unions, P.O. Box 1045, 10830 Penang, Malaysia.

31 Letter from G.A. Raffé, Nestlé (UK) General Manager to Miss J. Thompson, Public Relations Officer of the Health Visitors' Association, 9 February 1983.

32 Wong Hock Boon, 'Planning for your child', *Child International,* vol. 1, no. 1, pp. 10, 13.

33 Jelliffe, D.B. and Patrice Jelliffe, E.F., *Human Milk in the Modern World,* Oxford, Oxford University Press, 1978, p. 189; Jeanine Klaus of ILCA (see addresses) has suggested that the lactation suppressant bromocriptine could trigger ill-treatment of infants because it stops production of prolactin which is linked with mothering behaviour.

34 Nestlé, Thailand '71, Bulletin Nestlé, no. 3, 1971, cited in Van Esterick, P., *Infant Feeding Options for Bangkok Women,* Ithaca, New York, Cornell University Press (Cornell International Nutrition Monograph Series no. 10), 1982.

35 McLaren, D.S., 'The great protein fiasco', *Lancet,* vol. 2, 1974, pp. 93–6.

36 Rush, D. *et al.,* 'A randomized controlled trial of prenatal nutritional supplementation in New York City', *Pediatrics,* vol. 65, 1980, p. 683.

37 Davidson, S. *et al., Human Nutrition and Dietetics,* Edinburgh, Churchill Livingstone, 7th edn, 1979, p. 196.

38 Trinidad Nutrition Commission, 1938, cited in King, J. and Ashworth, A., *Changes in Infant Feeding Practices in the Caribbean: an historical review,* Dept of Human Nutrition, London School of Hygiene and Tropical Medicine Occasional Paper no. 8, 1987.

39 King, Jean and Ashworth, Ann, *Changes in Infant Feeding Practices in Nigeria: an historical review,* Dept of Human Nutrition, London School of Hygiene and Tropical Medicine Occasional Paper no. 9, 1987.

40 King, Jean and Ashworth, Ann, *Changes in Infant Feeding Practices in the Caribbean: an historical review,* op. cit. (note 24).

41 Ibid.

42 King, Jean and Ashworth, Ann, *Changes in Infant Feeding Practices in Malaysia: an historical review,* Dept of Human Nutrition, London School of Hygiene and Tropical Medicine Occasional Paper no. 7, 1987.

43 UNICEF, *The State of the World's Children,* Oxford, Oxford University Press, 1987.

44 EC Dairy Facts and Figures 1992. Also Personal Communication Declan Ennis, UK Milk Marketing Board.

CHAPTER 8 THE LURE OF THE GLOBAL MARKET

1 Williams, Cicely, Interview in the *Lansing Star,* 18 October 1978.

2 Orwell, S. and Murray, J., 'Infant feeding and health in Ibadan', *Journal of Tropical Paediatrics and Environment and Child Health,* vol. 20, pp. 205–19, 1974.

3 Chetley, Andy, *The Baby Killer Scandal: A War on Want Investigation into the Promotion and Sale of Powdered Baby Milks in the Third World,* London, War on Want, 1979, pp. 58–60.

4 Ibid.

5 Willat, Norris, 'How Nestlé adapts products to its markets', *Business Abroad,* June 1970, pp. 31–3.

6 George, Susan, *How the Other Half Dies: The Real Reasons for World Hunger,* Harmondsworth, Penguin, 1979, p. 180.

7 Ann Ashworth, personal communication.

8 Jelliffe, D.B., 'Commerciogenic malnutrition?', *Food Technology,* vol. 25, no. 55, 1971; Wennen-van der May, C.A.M., 'The decline of breastfeeding in Nigeria', *Tropical and Geographical Medicine,* vol. 21, 1960, p. 93.

9 Chetley, Andrew, *The Politics of Baby Foods: Successful Challenges to an International Marketing Strategy,* London, Frances Pinter, 1986; *WHO Collaborative Study on Breastfeeding,* Geneva, 1979.

10 *New Internationalist,* 'Action now on baby foods', 10 August 1973; Muller, Mike, *The Baby Killer,* London, War on Want, 1973.

11 Chetley, op. cit. (note 9), p. 43.

12 INFACT, *Nestlé in the USA: Giant in Disguise,* INFACT, 1978.

13 Chetley, op. cit. (note 9), p. 45.

14 Ibid.

15 Personal communication: Rev. W. Beaver.

16 Bader, Michael, 'Breastfeeding: the role of multinational corporations in Latin America', *International Journal of the Health Service,* vol. 6, no. 4, 1976, pp. 609–26; Greiner, Ted, The Promotion of Bottle-Feeding by Multinational Corporations: how advertising and the health professions have contributed, Ithaca, New York, Cornell University Press (Cornell International Nutritional Monograph Series no. 2), 1975.

17 Chetley, op. cit. (note 9), pp. 50–2.

18 Krieg, Peter, *Bottle Babies,* film, filmed in Kenya, 16 mm, 30 mins, available to hire from Workers' Film Association, 9 Lucy Street, Manchester 15, tel. 061–848 9782.

19 Buffle, Jean-Claude, *N comme Nestlé,* Paris, Alain Moreau, 1986.

20 Laskin, Carol R. and Pilot, Lynn J., 'Defective infant formula: the Neo-Mul-Soy/Cho-Free incident', in Moss, H.A., Hess, R. and Swift, C. (eds), *Early Intervention Programs for Infants,* vol. 1, no. 4, *Prevention in Human Services,* New York, Haworth Press, 1982, pp. 97–106; Minchin, Maureen, *Breastfeeding Matters: What We Need to Know About Infant Feeding,* Alfredton, Australia, Alma Publications, 1985.

21 Ibid., p. 221.

22 International Baby Food Action Network, Asia, *Babies, Breastfeeding and the Code.* Report of the IBFAN Asia Conference at Sam Phran, Thailand, 5–12 October 1986, p. 22.

23 Willoughby, Anne *et al.,* 'Developmental outcome in children exposed to chloride deficient formula', *Pediatrics,* vol. 79, no. 6, 1987, pp. 851–7; Malloy, M.H. *et al.,* 'Hypochloremic metabolic alkalosis from ingestion of a chloride-deficient infant formula: outcome 9 and 10 years later', *Pediatrics,* 87 (6); 811–22, 1991 Jun; Federal Administration Washington HQ/Division of Regulatory Guidance: telex refusing permission for Syntax request to donate for export recalled formula, 28 September 1979.

24 Makil, Lorna P. and Simpson, Mayerling, *Seven Infant Deaths,* an IPC Working Paper, Institute of Philippine Culture, Ateneo de Manila University, Querzon City, Philippines, November 1984; See also BUNSO ('National Coalition for the Promotion of Breastfeeding and Childcare') information pack, available from

66 J.P. Rizal St., Project 4, Querzon City, Tel. 921 8022.

25 Vaughan, V.C., McKay, R.J., Behrman, R.E. and Nelson, W.E. (eds), *Nelson Textbook of Pediatrics*, Philadelphia, W.B. Saunders, 1979, p. 203.

26 Patrice Jelliffe, E.F. 'Breastfeeding and the working woman: bending the rules', in *Lactation, Fertility and the Working Woman,* Proceedings of the Joint International Union of Nutritional Science/ International Planned Parenthood Federation Conference, Bellagio, Italy, 1977, p. 51; 'Split House panel approves bill requiring employers of 15 or more to provide family and medical leave', *Los Angeles Times,* 14 May 1987.

27 Lichano, Alejandro, 'Disturbing proposals in an incoherent paper', Philippine *Panorama* magazine, 26 August 1984, cited in Center for Women's Resources (2nd Floor, Mar Santos Bldg, 43 Roces Ave, Querzon City, Philippines. Tel. 99 27 55), *How Do We Liberate Ourselves? (Understanding Our Oppression, Working for Emancipation),* 1987; UNICEF, *State of the World's Children,* 1992; Lim, Fides, 'The Silent Slaughter' in Aldana-Benitez, Cornelia H. (ed), *Unmasking a Giant*, 1992 IBON Philippines Databank and Research Centre.

28 *Fortune*, 13 February 1978, p. 81; Buffle op. cit. (note 19), p. 13.

29 Chetley, op. cit. (note 9), pp. 52–4.

30 McComas, M. *et al., The Dilemma of Third World Nutrition. Nestlé and the Role of Infant Formula,* Nestlé, USA, 1985, p. 12.

31 Angst, C.L., 'The social responsibility of the food industry', *Consumer Affairs,* September/October 1985, p. 51.

32 Hunt, E.K., *Property and Prophets: The Evolution of Economic Institutions and Ideologies,* New York, Harper & Row, 5th edn, 1986, p. 99.

33 Note: Individuals in industry often protest about 'the Code' but in fact it was the International Council of Infant Food Industries (ICIFI) who proposed the idea. Also, according to the Nestlé account, it was the head of ICIFI (Ian Butler of Cow & Gate) who suggested to Edward Kennedy that the World Health Organisation should be the forum for formulating an international marketing code. Industry was involved and consulted throughout the whole drafting process.

34 Chetley, op. cit. (note 9), pp. 95–6.

35 WHO/UNICEF, *International Code of Marketing of Breastmilk Substitutes,* Geneva, World Health Organisation, 1981.

36 Note: Wyeth SMA used this claim and it was so successful that many

health workers believe to this day that this brand *is* closer to breastmilk. Chloë Fisher says that when Cow & Gate baby milk was the brand used for bottle-feeding in the John Radcliffe Hospital, Oxford, midwives still used to suggest to mothers who had wanted to breastfeed but 'failed' that they should use SMA instead because it was 'nearer to the real thing'. One health worker told me she believed SMA was closer to breastmilk because it contained vegetable oil. Did she believe that human females were more like coconuts than cows?

37 Hamilton, Robert and Whinnett, Dale, 'A comparison of the WHO and the UK Codes of Practice for the marketing of breastmilk substitutes', *Journal of Consumer Policy,* vol. 10, 1987, pp. 167–92.

38 'The results of a change of hospital practices – a paediatrician's campaign for breastfeeding in the Philippines', *Assignment Children, Breastfeeding and Health,* Geneva, UNICEF, 1981, pp. 139–65.

39 Personal communication.

40 IBFAN information; Cow & Gate Careline service was advertised in several journals in 1988, including *Midwife, Health Visitor* and *Community Nurse,* January 1988; IBFAN, *Breaking the Rules,* 1982.

41 *Health Visitor,* November 1987, advertisement for Wyeth SMA.

42 *Guardian:* 'Farley baby firm closes', 22 January 1986, 'Broken image', 23 January 1986, 'Contaminated baby milk', 10 February 1986, 'Boots gets Farley's for cut price £18m', 8 March 1986.

43 Biddulph, John, 'Impact of legislation restricting the availability of feeding bottles in Papua New Guinea', *Nutrition and Development,* vol. 3, no. 2, 1980; UNICEF, *State of the World's Children,* 1992; Minei, Alfred, Evaluation of the Implementation of the International Code of Marketing of Breastmilk Substitutes in Papua New Guinea. Presentation at Training Course on Code Implementation Code Documentation Centre, IBFAN, Penang, Malaysia, April 1992.

44 *Introducing WHO,* Geneva, World Health Organisation, 1976.

45 Madeley, John, 'The crisis has a silver lining', *UNICEF News,* 1984.

46 For further reading on these issues see Sanchez Arnau, J.C., *Debt and Development,* New York, Praeger, 1983, George, Susan, *Ill Fares the Land,* London, Cooperative Society (144 Camden High Street, London NW1), 1985; *A fate worse than debt,* London, Penguin, 1988.

47 Liv Ullmann, Address at the UK Committee for UNICEF press lunch, 16 June 1983.

48 *Who Owns Whom 1987,* London, Dun & Bradstreet International.

49 IBFAN, *Bottle-feeding in Pakistan: The Marketing of Infant Foods and Feeding Bottles,* February 1988; UNICEF, *State of the World's Children,* op. cit. (note 43); Yorkshire TV, 'First Tuesday' Series, 'Vicious Circles' June 1990.

50 'IBFAN, Breaking the Rules 1991' *The New York Times,* Infant Diarrhea Kills Hundreds Yearly in US, 9 Dec. 1988, Report of Study by Dr. Mei-Shang Ho in *J.A.M.A.;* Ryan A.S., Rush, D., Frieger F.W., Lewandowski G.E., Recent declines in breastfeeding in the United States, 1984 through 1989, *Pediatrics,* 88 (4); 719–27, 1990.

51 Margen, Sheldon *et al.,* 'Infant Feeding in Mexico', NIFAC, Washington 1991, Baby Milk Action, Update November 1991.

52 Clark, John, *For Richer for Poorer: An OXFAM Report on Western Connections with World Hunger,* Oxford, OXFAM, 1986, pp. 37, 66; Victora, Cesar G. *et al.,* 'Evidence for protection by breastfeeding against infant deaths from infectious diseases in Brazil', *Lancet,* vol. 2, 1987, pp. 319–22. Innocenti Declaration, Florence, Italy 1990.

53 Baby Milk Action, Update November 1992, 'Take the Baby – Friendly Initiative!' Pamphlet available from UNICEF.

54 Baby Milk Action Correspondence with Dr D. Morley and with Dr M. Dangilen 1989; Allain, Annalies, and de Arango, Ruth, Training Course on Code Implementation in Mothers & Children, *Bulletin on Infant Feeding and Maternal Nutrition,* 11, (3), 1992.

55 INFACT Canada, Sterken, Betty, personal communication.

56 Monteiro, Carlos Augusto *et al.,* 'The recent revival of breastfeeding in the city of Sao Paulo, Brazil', *American Journal of Public Health,* vol. 77, no. 8, 1987.

57 Marlowe, M., personal communication.

CHAPTER 9   MONEY, WORK AND THE POLITICS OF WASTE

1 Berg, A., *The Nutrition Factor,* Washington, DC, Brooking Institute, 1973; Jelliffe, Derek B. and Patrice Jelliffe, E.F., *Human Milk in the Modern World,* Oxford, Oxford University Press, 1978.

2 Rohde, John Eliot, 'Mother milk and the Indonesian Economy: – A Major National resource', *Journal of Tropical Paediatrics,* vol. 28, no. 4, 1982, pp. 166–74.

3 Hosken, Fran P., book review of *Only Mothers Know* by Raphael, D. and Davis, Flora, in *Women's International Network News:*

Women and Health, date unknown (post-1985).

4 Sudarkasa, N., *Where Women Work: A Study of Yoruba Women in the Market Place and the Home,* Ann Arbor, University of Michigan, Anthropological papers no. 53, 1973.

5 Mitter, Swasti, *Common Fate, Common Bond: Women in the Global Economy,* London, Pluto Press, 1986.

6 Agland, Phil, *Baka: People of the Rainforest,* a DJA River Films production for Channel 4, transmitted November 1987 and January 1988. Written information from P.O. Box 4000, London W3 6XJ.

7 Department of Nutrition, Ministry of Health, Maputo, Mozambique, 1982; Jelliffe, D.B. and Patrice Jelliffe, E.F., op. cit. (note 1), p. 270.

8 *Enough is Enough*, Consumers in the European Community Group, 1986; Ann Davison, Consumers in the European Community Group (CECG) personal communication. Also Office for the European Community, London, UK.

9 Helsing, Elisabet, 'Infant feeding practices in Northern Europe', in *Assignment Children 55/56 Breastfeeding and Health,* Geneva, UNICEF, 1981; Katcher, A.L. and Lanese, M.G., 'Breastfeeding by employed mothers: a reasonable accommodation in the work place', *Pediatrics*, vol. 75, 1985.

10 Campbell, Carolyn E., 'Nestlé and breast vs bottle-feeding: mainstream and Marxist perspectives', *International Journal of Health Services,* vol. 14, no. 4, 1984, pp. 547–66.

11 The World Bank, World Development Report 1991, *The Challenge of Development,* Oxford University Press, p. 140.

12 Longmate, Norman, *How We Lived Then: A History of Everyday Life During the Second World War,* London, Arrow Books, 1973, p. 304.

13 Clearinghouse on Infant Feeding and Maternal Nutrition, Government Legislation and Policies to support breastfeeding, improve Maternal and Infant Nutrition and Implement a Code of Marketing of Breastmilk Substitutes, Report No. 5, 1988, American Public Health Association (APHA), Washington DC.

14 Guisewite, Cathy, 'Cathy' cartoon reproduced in Van Esterick, Penny, 'Women, Work and Breastfeeding', York Centre for Health Studies, Institute of Social Research, York University, Ontario, Canada 1990.

15 Kitching, Jonathan, letter to the *New Socialist*, January 1987.

16 Evans, Jan, letter to the *New Socialist*, February 1987.

17 Firestone, Shulamith, *The Dialectic of Sex: The Case for Feminist*

Revolution, New York, William Morrow, 1970.

18 Betty Sterken, personal communication.

19 Huxley, Aldous, *Brave New World,* London, Chatto & Windus, 1977 (first published 1932).

20 National Childbirth Trust, *Survey of postnatal infection,* London, NCT, 1988.

21 'Infant mortality rises in wealthy US', *Guardian*, 11 March 1988; Office of Population Censuses and Surveys Monitor, December 1987.

22 Röckner, Gunny, 'Reconsideration of the use of episiotomy in primiparas: A study in obstetric care', Karolinska Institute 1991.

23 Murcott, Ann (ed.), *The Sociology of Food and Eating,* Aldershot, Gower, (Gower International Library of Research and Practice), 1983.

24 Sylvia Rumball, personal communication.

25 Dr S. Balmer, personal communication.

26 Hansen, Michael, 'The mealybug gets stung', in *Escape from the Pesticide Treadmill: Alternatives to Pesticides in Developing Countries,* Institute for Consumer Policy Research Consumers' Union.

27 'Myth conceptions', *New Internationalist,* October 1987, p. 9.

Further Reading

Boserup, Ester, *Women's Role in Economic Development,* London, Allen & Unwin, 1970. This is an academic book, but it is very readable. Luckily more has been written about this subject since 1970, but Ester Boserup was one of the first to examine this issue and her book provides an excellent starting point.

Buffle, Jean-Claude, *N comme Nestlé: Multinational et Infanticide, le Lait, les Bébés, et le Mort,* Paris, Alain Moreau, 1986. Fascinating, but with one problem, it is in French. Easy to read, though, if you have a basic grasp of the language. It is a lively account of the struggle between the baby food activists and Nestlé, but it differs from Andrew Chetley's in that Buffle discusses all the personalities involved. You learn which activist had rosy cheeks and about the inner complexes of the Nestlé executives.

Chetley, Andrew, *The Politics of Baby Foods: Successful Challenges to Marketing Strategies,* London, Frances Pinter, 1986. This tells the story of the baby milk issue from the 1970s onwards. It recounts the hard fight to change the companies' unethical behaviour, the Nestlé boycott, the struggle to produce the WHO/UNICEF Code and the commitment of the people involved.

Ehrenreich, Barbara and English, Deirdre, *For Her Own Good (50 Years of the Experts' Advice to Women),* London, Pluto Press, 1979. This outlines the arbitrary changes in US dogmas concerning women's roles during our century. It is written with a sense of humour. It is full of nuggets like the fact that in spite of so much focus on housework (which usually took up more of women's time the more that 'labour-saving' devices were invented), no one has ever researched whether its practice actually improves health. Also a sensitive debunking of the supposed pleasures of being a so-called liberated woman.

Elia, Irene, *The Female Animal,* Oxford, Oxford University Press, 1985. If your own education in biology was scant, this book may seem a bit intimidating, but do not worry about the specialist words, they are only used for accuracy and there is a good glossary. At first you might think that it is merely an accumulation of fascinating facts, but Irene Elia is making a major statement about the primacy of the female and showing how significant is the 'mothering' trait to evolution. This book opened my eyes to the biological basis of so much human behaviour and helped me to understand some of the roots of sexism in human society.

Fildes, Valerie A., *Breasts, Bottles, and Babies: A History of Infant Feeding,* Edinburgh, Edinburgh University Press, 1986. A goldmine. A scholarly gathering of all the available data about infant feeding up to 1800. Lots of fascinating illustrations. My only reserve about this sort of history is that it can give an impression that the evidence (documentation, artefacts, etc.) typifies what happened, when it actually tends to reflect elite practices disproportionately. I disagree with Fildes's thesis that today's third world bottles echo eighteenth-century ignorance. The pundits of that era did not have global marketing strategies, nor the mass media, to impose ignorance. The book is too expensive, but insist that your public library gets it. Essential reading for the enthusiast.

George, Susan, *How the Other Half Dies: The Real Reasons for World Hunger,* Harmondsworth, Penguin, 1979. This woke me up in 1979. It presents a thorough examination of the economic and political forces influencing food production and consumption in developing countries. The results are depressing. It is still relevant.

George, Susan, *Ill Fares the Land,* London, Cooperative Society (144 Camden High Street, London NW1), 1984. Really important. Susan George knows so much and thinks so clearly, but unlike many other clever people her aim is not to show off her brains, but to show how appalling is the injustice of the modern world. Consequently she really communicates well. You must read it, it is more academic in style than *How the Other Half Dies,* but shorter.

George, Susan, *A Fate Worse than Debt: A Radical New Analysis of the Third World Debt Crisis,* Harmondsworth, Penguin, 1988. I claimed in Chapter 9 that economists deliberately made things obscure. This book is a beam of light. Susan George not only explains why we have got into the mess we are in, but makes practical suggestions for sorting it out. Do read it.

George, Susan, *The Debt Boomerang: How Third World Debt Harms Us All,* Pluto Press with the Transnational Institute, 1992. As usual such good sense, but not as engagingly written as her previous books, perhaps because the collaboration clouds her style, but the arguments are as sound as ever and it is packed with facts and figures.

Hampton, Christopher, *Savages,* London, Faber & Faber, 1974. A play should be acted or watched rather than read. However I still re-read this and the production I saw years ago is fresh in my mind. This is because the matters addressed are just as relevant as in 1974. Hampton, in a few scenes, deals comprehensively with issues that take up pages and pages for us poor book writers.

Helsing, Elisabet, with Savage King, Felicity, *Breastfeeding in Practice,* Oxford, Oxford University Press, 1982. However accurate the advice, most breastfeeding advice books tend to assume that all breastfeeding women have houses and husbands. This is aimed at health workers in developing countries, but all parents could benefit from it and if any of the terms are too medical they could ask their health worker. A good way of introducing the topics to those poor victims of medical training in the industrialised world.

Hunt, E.K., *Property and Prophets: The Evolution of Economic Institutions and Ideologies,* New York, Harper & Row, 1986. For those who fall asleep every time they get to page 3 of their economics textbooks, try this, It whips through the entire history of human society in a mere 203 pages and gives you the courage to attempt the dryer tomes.

Jelliffe, D.B. and Patrice Jelliffe, E.F., *Human Milk in the Modern World: Psychosocial Nutritional and Economic Significance,* Oxford, Oxford University Press, 1978. The Jelliffes take your breath away. They, more than any other people, have put breastfeeding on the map. This book amasses a vast amount of information, but it manages to avoid being a dry encyclopaedia, possibly because they are not afraid to express opinions. A bit of fresh air after a surfeit of academic articles. It is a little out of date, but nothing yet matches it for breadth and substantiality. Sadly, in 1992, D.B. Jelliffe died suddenly depriving the world of a rare talent and fund of knowledge. Patrice Jelliffe still contributes to the subject.

Laslett, Peter, *The World We Have Lost – Further Explored,* London, Methuen, 1983. The antidote to those dreadful school history books. The purpose of historians' existences seems to be squabbling amongst themselves about what the past was really like. As we will never be able to prove who is right, we might as well enjoy evocative writing and Peter Laslett gives us that. He also mentions breastfeeding so he scores a point with me.

La Leche League, *The Womanly Art of Breastfeeding.* 35th Anniversary

Edition, LLL International, 1991. This is a sensitive revision of what is now a classic. It still seems to assume that most women have husbands, homes and cars and I suppose most readers do, but it is more realistic about wage-earning work than in the first edition. It refers to 'women who have reshaped the workplace to make it more responsive' but neglects to mention that the US government has the worst legislation and attitude in the world (even Saudi Arabia has paid maternity leave and breastfeeding breaks). Nevertheless this is a beautiful book which addresses almost every aspect of the subject, with delightful pictures, good layout and sound advice not just on breastfeeding but on loving and caring for children. It works too. I am always impressed by the skilled parenting and happy, socially aware children I see when I attend LLL conferences.'

Lewis, Jane, *The Politics of Motherhood: Child and Maternal Welfare in England, 1900–1939,* London, Croom Helm, 1982. This conveys so well how the supervisory, patronising, insensitive attitudes to women as mothers evolved in England. By looking at one society you can see how supposedly worthy aims, like the improvement of child health, led to women being picked on and overburdened with unfair and unrewarded responsibilities. This account is important because the same pattern of bossiness, indifference to commercial and social pressures on mothers, and telling them that they ought to breastfeed while undermining traditional support, is echoed across the world today.

Ling, Chee Yoke, *How Big Powers Dominate the Third World: The Use and Abuse of International Law,* Penang, Third World Network (87 Cantonment Road, 10250 Penang, Malaysia), 1987. This short book (70 pages) succinctly explains some of the glaring biases in international structures. It takes this most turgid of subjects and explains clearly how most of the newly 'independent' countries are still bound by the historical world dominance of Europe. There is a good section on 'Training Third World elites to accept the system', which exposes the psychological pressures on individuals passing through the academic *rite de passage.*

Link, Ann, *Chlorine, Pollution and the Parents of Tomorrow,* The Women's Environmental Network, London 1991. This is the first book dealing with this complex environmental issue that I could understand. It will help you to deal with both the sincere scaremongers and the over-complacent. Anyone who wants to be more effective in finding ways to halt the contamination of our babies and our milk will find this helpful.

Minchin, Maureen, *Breastfeeding Matters: What We Need to Know About Infant Feeding,* Alma Publications (Alfredton, Australia) and George Allen and Unwin, 1985. This is a good 'How to do it and why it went wrong before' breastfeeding book, it is packed with information about the risks of industrialised baby foods. Maureen Minchin writes passionately because she is truly angry at the way parents are duped by the companies and some members of the medical profession into complacency about artificial feeding. It does tend to have an Australian bias and assumes (perhaps correctly) that the reader has enough money to make choices.

Mitter, Swasti, *Common Fate, Common Bond: Women in the Global Economy,* London, Pluto Press, 1986. This describes the conditions of the invisible slaves: women. Increasingly, around the world, they are enduring the misery of factory work, but in the isolation of their homes. I like it because it treats the world as one place and shows how the transnational companies are exploiting women wherever they are. A joy to read because Swasti Mitter can explain the wily complexities of transnational operations in everyday terms. It is relevant to all women, showing us how we are the overused, underpaid and unacknowledged tools of the profit makers, but it rightly focuses on the grosser exploitation of black women worldwide.

Mohrbacher, Nancy and Stock, Julie, *The Breastfeeding Answer Book,* La Leche League International, 1992. This may be written in the North American milieu, but it is so good to have all those nagging questions addressed in one handy ring binder. Its sheer bulk might convince a Health Minister that policy implementation needs more than a few posters.

Moore Lappé, Frances and Collins, Joseph, *Food First: Beyond the Myth of Scarcity,* New York, Ballantine Books, 1978. Still relevant. The bigwigs clearly ignore it. Some details have changed, but the system has not. Good reading, written with passion and no intimidating jargon. It should be a school textbook.

Royal College of Midwives, *Successful Breastfeeding,* Churchill Livingstone, 1991. Originally aimed at British midwives (who still thankfully deliver most UK babies), it should be required reading for every doctor in the world. Its strength lies in its respectability; it is all about sensible behaviour in the maternity ward and every argument is diligently backed up with a scientific reference. UNICEF should use it for the BFHI and it should be distributed and translated globally. Breastfeeding advocates should carry one as protection against ignorant health professionals.

Savage King, Felicity, *Helping Mothers to Breastfeed* (Revised edition), African Medical and Research Foundation, 1992. This is a more accessible, less detailed version of *Breastfeeding in Practice* (see above, Helsing). Beautifully clear and simple. Aimed at Africa but needed everywhere.

Van Esterick, Penny, *Motherpower and Infant Feeding,* London, Zed Books, 1989. As an anthropologist who believes in more advocacy within the academic world, her book struggles between meticulous observation and sadness over the difficulties mothers face. The detailed accounts of the daily lives of real women in urban areas of Columbia, Indonesia, Kenya and Thailand teach far more than a million statistics. Very useful for understanding the complexities of life in the South.

Waring, Marilyn, *If Women Counted: A new feminist economics,* London, Macmillan, 1989. Water carried in a pipe counts in the Gross National Economy, but if a woman carries that water on her head it does not. Just one example in Marilyn Waring's challenge of the whole UN system of accounting. I love this book because it is an economics book written with passion and honesty. I learned so much.

World Commission on Environment and Development, *Our Common Future,* Oxford, Oxford University Press, 1987. I have to admit this is a bit boring, but then anything written by a committee is bound to be. However I keep looking up pertinent facts in it and it is very 'official', so get it and quote from it when you argue with the diehards.

Useful Addresses

1. Breastfeeding information and support:
There are breastfeeding mother support groups all over the world but if you cannot find one in your region contact:

La Leche League International INC., 9616 Minneapolis Avenue, Franklin Park, Illinois 6031, USA
or
The World Alliance for Breastfeeding Action (WABA), Secretariat, PO Box 1200, 10850 Penang, Malaysia

(WABA can also put you in touch with a range of organisations and individuals concerned with different perspectives of this issue.)

Nursing Mothers of Australia (NMA), PO Box 231, Nunawading 3131, Victoria, Australia

(NMA has an excellent resource centre)

International Lactation Consultant Association (ILCA), 201 Brown Avenue, Evanston, Illinois 60202-3601, USA

2. Infant Food Industry
The International Association of Infant Food Manufacturers (IFM/ISDI), 194 Rue de Rivoli, 75001 Paris, France.

3. International Agencies
International Labour Office, CH 1211, Geneva, Switzerland.

There may be a regional United National Children's Fund (UNICEF) near you or contact:

UNICEF, Palais des Nations, CH 1211, Geneva 10, Switzerland

or
UNICEF, 3 UN Plaza, New York, NY 10016, USA

World Health Organisation (WHO), 1211 Geneva 27, Switzerland

4. International Baby Food Action Network (IBFAN)
There are IBFAN groups all over the world, but if you cannot find one or want to start one, contact one of the following addresses.

IBFAN Africa, Centrepoint, PO Box 781, Mbabane, Swaziland

IBFAN Asia and the Pacific, Code Documentation Centre, PO Box 19, Penang, Malaysia

IBFAN Europe, GIFA, CP 157, 1211 Geneva, Switzerland

Baby Milk Action, 23 St. Andrew's Street, Cambridge CB2 3AX, United Kingdom

IBFAN Latin America, Casilla de Correo 10993, Surcursal 2, CP 11100 Montevideo, Uruguay

IBFAN North America, ACTION, 129 Church Street, New Haven, Connecticut 06510, USA

5. Other useful organisations
Action and Information on Sugars (AIS)
PO Box 190, Walton-on-Thames, Surrey KT12 2YN, United Kingdom

AIS acts to halt the promotion and misuse of sugar, particularly with regard to babies' and children's food and drinks.

Health Action International (HAI)
Jacob van Lennepkade 334T, 1053NJ Amsterdam, The Netherlands

HAI works to promote the ethical marketing of pharmaceuticals and other rational health policies

Transnational Institute (TNI)
Paulus Potterstraat 20, 1071 DA Amsterdam, The Netherlands

TNI is an independent fellowship of researchers and activists who develop innovative analyses of world affairs.

Women's Environmental Network (WEN)
22 Highbury Grove, London N5 2EA, United Kingdom

WEN educates, informs and empowers women who care about the environment.

The UK NGO AIDS Consortium
Fenner Brockway House, 37/39 Great Guildford Street, London SE1 0ES, United Kingdom

The AIDS Consortium is a gathering of development, aid and support agencies who share information and take action on global issues concerning HIV and AIDS.

Index